# ABC: AI, Blockchain, and Cybersecurity for Healthcare

Join us in the beginning of a conversation and what we hope will be a community dedicated to leveraging some of the latest technologies for a next generation of infrastructure. After decades of building enterprise systems, a fundamental change is occurring because of **AI**, **B**lockchain, and next-generation **C**ybersecurity (**ABC**). This is poised to affect many industries and areas of society, not least of which is healthcare. We are excited to join like-minded colleagues who have agreed to share their expertise and examples in the early days of integrating these technologies into a unified architecture that can meet operational goals. In the case of healthcare, can artificial intelligence, blockchain, and cybersecurity technologies lead to better, faster, and cheaper healthcare and ease the burden on healthcare providers? This may extend to the whole health ecosystem, not just providers and the hospitals and systems, but also to the insurers and payers, and of course the patients or health consumers interested in wellness and well-being. Benefits to healthcare research, drug discovery, and next generation genomic and novel health discoveries could accelerate discovery, trial, and wider knowledge and adoption of novel tools and techniques. In this book, we will explore the potential synergies and benefits of ABC with particular interest in the way that they can make up for weaknesses and be used appropriately and with proper cautions given the potential power of AI. Blockchain for verification, privacy and trust, along with good cybersecurity practices, often called cyber hygiene -- especially with the potential for new and novel attacks far beyond ransomware as the age of quantum computing accelerates. We hope you will enjoy exploring the breadth of knowledge and expertise represented by the many contributors and early insights and case studies.

# ABC: AI, Blockchain, and Cybersecurity for Healthcare

## New Innovations for the Post-Quantum Era

David Metcalf, PhD
Dexter Hadley, MD, PhD
Max Hooper, PhD
Harry Pappas
Vikram Dhillon, MD

Intelligent Health Series

First published 2024
by Routledge
605 Third Avenue, New York, NY 10158

and by Routledge
4 Park Square, Milton Park, Abingdon, Oxon, OX14 4RN

*Routledge is an imprint of the Taylor & Francis Group, an informa business*



*Library of Congress Cataloging-in-Publication Data*
A catalog record for this title has been requested

ISBN: 9781032797281 (hbk)
ISBN: 9781032797274 (pbk)

Typeset in Georgia

# About the Authors

## David Metcalf, PhD

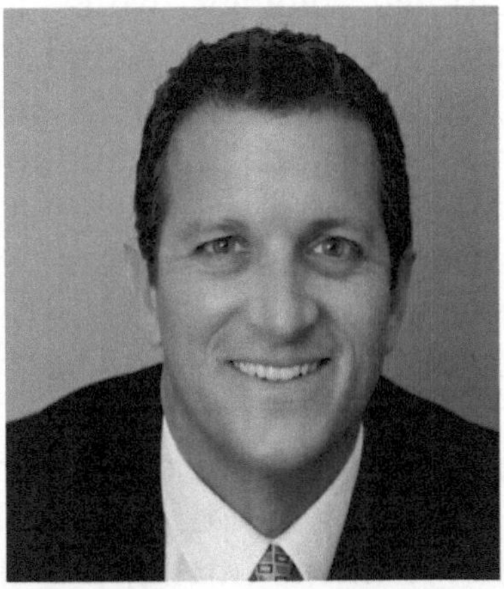

Dr. Metcalf is a General Partner & Managing Director at Global Blockchain Ventures and is a technology specialist. Dr. Metcalf has over 20 years' experience in the design and research of web-based and mobile technologies converging to enable learning and health care. Since 2005, Dr. Metcalf has served as Director of the Mixed Emerging Technology Integration Lab (METIL) at UCF's Institute for Simulation and Training, and formerly held lead research roles for NASA, a consulting executive, and investor. Dr. Metcalf co-authored "Blockchain Enabled Applications" (2017), "Blockchain in Healthcare" (2019), and "Blockchain Enabled Applications" (2021). Dr. Metcalf has worked globally on many projects in and out of the US in enterprise, education, healthcare, and other areas. Dr. Metcalf has a long history working is simulation, AI, mobile, learning, visualization systems, and quantum cybersecurity applications. Dr. Metcalf frequently presents at industry and research events shaping business strategy, discussing the use of technology to improve learning and human performance, and serves on multiple Board of Directors that work to impact global problems.

# Dexter Hadley, MD, PhD

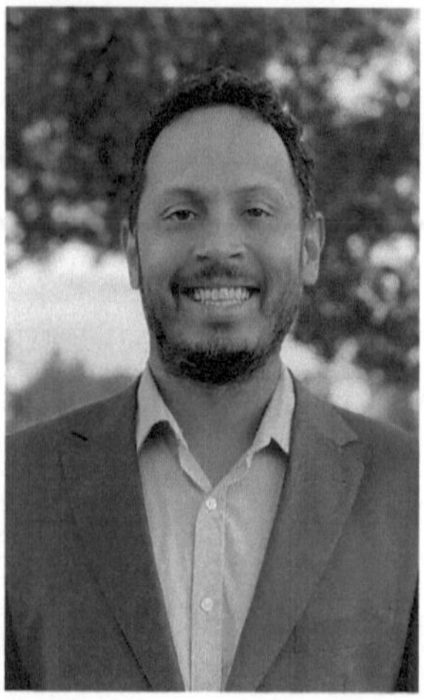

Dexter Hadley, MD/PhD translates big data into precision medicine and digital health. His research generates, annotates, and ultimately reasons over large multi-modal data stores to develop predictive models of clinical intelligence. He earned his PhD in genomics and computational biology while at medical school at University of Pennsylvania, and he trained in clinical pathology while at residency at Stanford. He first became faculty at University of California San Francisco where he won various grant funding for developing deep learning methods in medicine including over $5M from NIH. His contributions have yielded well over 60 peer-reviewed publications in precision medicine to develop novel interventions, identify novel biomarkers and potential therapeutics for disease. He has been giving invited lectures around the globe on leveraging AI/ML in clinical applications. Dr. Hadley is the Founding Chief of Artificial Intelligence at University of Central Florida, College of Medicine where he is building a community of patients, clinicians, and data scientists to turn his vision for Community Driven AI into reality.

# Max Hooper, PhD

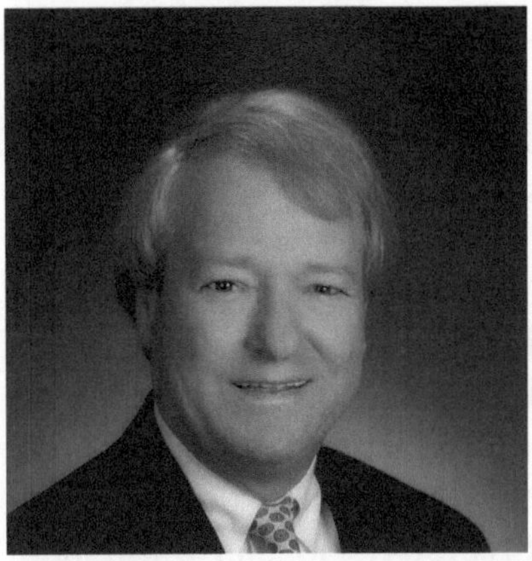

Max W. Hooper, PhD is the chief executive officer of Merging Traffic and co-founder of Global Blockchain Ventures. He is responsible for these company's management and growth strategy, while also serving as the corporate liaison to the financial services industry and various capital formation groups. Prior to starting the company, he was co-founder of Equity Broadcasting Corporation (EBC), a media company that owned and operated more than 100 television stations across the United States. He was responsible for activities in the cable, satellite, investment banking, and technology industries and during his tenure it grew to become one of the top 10 largest broadcasting companies in the country. A lifelong learner, Hooper has earned five doctorate degrees: PhD, DMin, PhD, ThD, and DMin from a variety of institutions. Hooper studied financial technology with cohorts at MIT, and cryptocurrency and business disruption with cohorts at the London School of Economics. Hooper is the co-author of three books about Blockchain Enabled Applications and has taken several companies public on NASDAQ . As an avid runner, he has completed more than 100 marathons and an additional 20 ultra- marathons, which are 50 or 100-mile runs. He has completed the Grand Slam of Ultra Running. Hooper is committed to his family and is a husband, father to five children, and grandfather to seven grandsons. He is active in many organizations and serves on various boards of directors. He works globally with several ministries and nonprofit aid groups, and was honored to speak at the United Nations in New York in 2015.

# Vikram Dhillon, MD

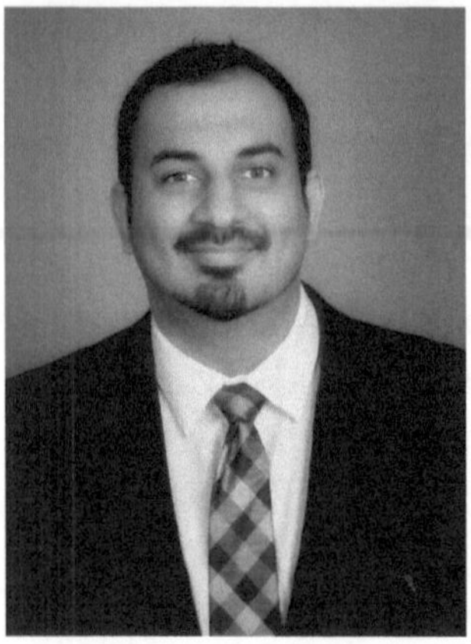

Vikram Dhillon is currently a clinical fellow in hematology/oncology at the Houston Methodist Neal Cancer Center and a research fellow at the Institute of Simulation and Training, University of Central Florida (UCF). He holds a Bachelor of Science degree in molecular biology from the University of Central Florida where his focus was in cancer bioinformatics, a Doctor of Osteopathic Medicine degree, a Master of Business Administration degree and a doctoral degree from Nova Southeastern University. He has published multiple scientific papers and textbooks in the areas of computational genomics, artificial intelligence and blockchain applications. He was previously funded by the National Science Foundation through the Innovation Corps program to study customer discovery and apply it to commercialize high-risk startup ideas. He is a member of the Linux Foundation and has been involved in open-source projects and initiatives for the past several years. He often speaks at local conferences and meetups on artificial intelligence, secure design and blockchain development.

# Harry P. Pappas

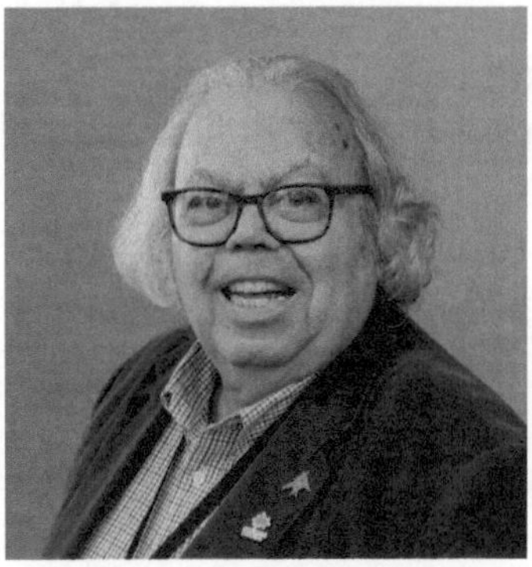

Pappas is a successful, High Tech., Serial entrepreneur in several industries, BUT has a strong focus on the health and wellness technology sector both for consumers and healthcare professionals. He is a strong believer in applying technology to transform the health and wellness community in today's "Continuum of care", and the "WELL CARE" model, from the hospital to the primary care giver, and to the patient's Smart Home. Pappas firmly believes that the world of digital health and wellness needs to be driven by the adoption of technology and personally driven, lifestyle changes, therefore the need for Quality, ON-GOING, education for the consumer and the professionals of the health and wellness community.

Harry is a global, thought leader and has been a tech geek since the age of 12.

He and his team are the producers of the award winning "Intelligent Health Pavilion™" a technology centric, educational platform, A DIGITAL, AI enabled SMART HOSPITAL. You may have visited this pavilion at many trade shows around the world, including at HIMSS over the last TEN years, Canada, Sweden, Saudi Arabia, Dubai, etc.

Pappas is the Founder & CEO of the Intelligent Health Association, a global, educational, Social Purpose entity, that is a technology centric organization dedicated to helping educate members of the Healthcare community on the adoption of new technologies. These technologies can improve patient care, patient outcomes, and patient safety, while driving down the cost of healthcare.

Pappas is the creator of the (i-HOME™), a health and wellness SMART HOME concept that demonstrates, "In Context", a plethora of health and wellness technologies placed in a Digital Smart Home setting for Remote Patient Monitoring (RPM) and Patient Health Management. Harry was developing the concept of the "Smart Home" utilizing Steve Jobs', original Apple "NEWTON" PDA device many, many years ago.

Harry is an internationally recognized thought leader with auto-ID, BLE, NFC, RFID, RTLS, Sensors, Voice, Robotics, Wearables, AI, P 5 G, Biomarkers, and Wireless technologies.

He is clearly an "out of the box thinker" and a long-term strategic player in the world of health technologies for the Digital hospital and for today's Smart Home. He has been presenting educational programs around the world since 2001. Harry is unique in that he has "hands-on" experience with a wide variety of technology and software development projects.

Harry's Goal: To help educate the healthcare community and the consumer on an going bases, so that they may adopt new technologies that can have a dramatic impact on the delivery of improved health, wellness and wellbeing.

Mantra: "Help Others", Do "SOCIAL GOOD" during your lifetime.

# About the Technical Contributors

## *Art Director/ Production Editor:*

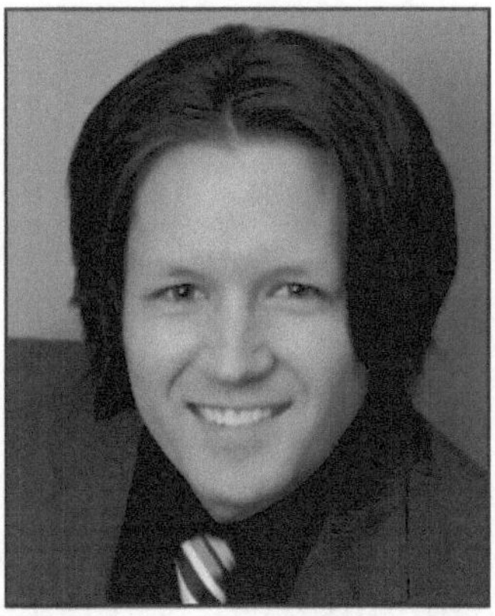

Michael Eakins is the Creative Lead of the Mixed Emerging Technology Integration Lab (METIL) at the Institute for Simulation & Training and has 10+ years of production experience for simulation, training, and gaming. He received his MFA in Digital Media at the University of Central Florida in 2017. Michael has produced a wide variety digital / print publications across multiple industries such as education, industry, and academia.

Cover artwork by Devon Veller

# Acknowledgments

**David Metcalf**
I would like to thank Katy, Adam and Andrew for their patience during the extended hours and effort while putting the book together. and colleagues and students at UCF and through the NSF I-Corps program that identified the power of voice technology years ago and shared their knowledge and future strategies that inspired us to pursue this area of research early. Thank you to my coauthors and our outside collaborators and contributors, and of course to God for the wisdom, ability and grit to bring this effort to life.

**Dexter Hadley**
Many thanks to the UCF College of Medicine as well as the National Institutes of Health for supporting my work and career. I am also thankful to my loving wife and four children to whom I dedicate this work. Finally, many thanks to the amazing community around the Lake Nona Medical City that is building an innovative ecosystem where we can continue to live, learn and discover how this technology can best impact our lives.

**Max Hooper**
Dr. Max Hooper would like to thank his co-authors and colleagues at UCF/METIL Lab, along with a special thanks to Mindy Hooper for her help and support. Additionally, he would like to thank God's inspiration, guidance, direction, and wisdom. He would like to acknowledge His leadership.

**Harry P. Pappas**
I wish to thank my dear wife and girlfriend of many years, Linda who has unstintingly, supported, and encouraged me with my many business interests, many careers, and adventures. I also thank my son, Mark and my daughter, Maria for their patience with me.

**Vikram Dhillon**
Vikram Dhillon would like to dedicate this work to Aaron Hillel Swartz and his legacy.

The authors would also like to thank Stelios Hatzakis, CEO of 1BusinessWorld® for recording, publishing rights, and our ongoing collaboration to advance the state of the art in healthcare and other domains.

# About This Book

Thank you for joining us in the beginning of a conversation and what we hope will be a community dedicated to leveraging some of the latest technologies for a next generation of infrastructure. After decades of building enterprise systems, a fundamental change is occurring because of AI, Blockchain, and next-generation Cybersecurity (ABC). This is poised to affect many industries and areas of society, not least of which is healthcare. We are excited to join like-minded colleagues who have agreed to share their expertise and examples in the early days of integrating these technologies into a unified architecture that can meet operational goals. In the case of healthcare, can artificial intelligence, blockchain, and cybersecurity technologies lead to better, faster, and cheaper healthcare and ease the burden on healthcare providers? This may extend to the whole health ecosystem, not just providers and the hospitals and systems, but also to the insurers and payers, and of course the patients or health consumers interested in wellness and well-being. Benefits to healthcare research, drug discovery, and next generation genomic and novel health discoveries could accelerate discovery, trial, and wider knowledge and adoption of novel tools and techniques. In this book, we will explore the potential synergies and benefits of ABC with particular interest in the way that they can make up for weaknesses and be used appropriately and with proper cautions given the potential power of AI. Blockchain for verification, privacy and trust, along with good cybersecurity practices, often called cyber hygiene -- especially with the potential for new and novel attacks far beyond ransomware as the age of quantum computing accelerates. We look forward to this first foray, which can be seen as a conversation starter to the other books forthcoming in this series and iterative additions given the rapid pace of advances in the emerging areas of ABC.

Thank you,

David Metcalf

# Table of Contents

# Foreword

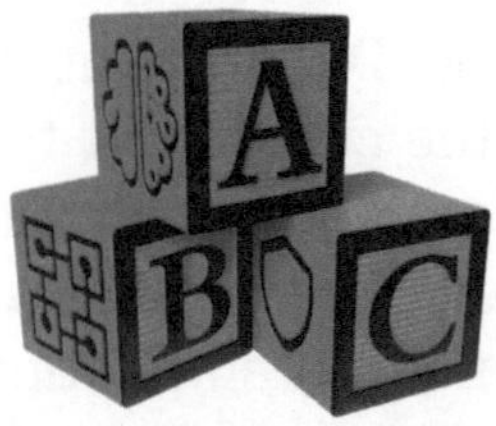


**LTC (Retired) Wilson Ariza**

## *Editor's Note*

Our dear friend and colleague, LTC (Ret) Wilson Ariza was the genesis for a brilliant research direction several years ago that has reshaped our laboratory at UCF and research thesis inside academia and beyond. Without his suggestion of ABC and the unique and powerful integrations that it enables, this book and framework would not have been possible. We thank you Wilson!

- David Metcalf

In the rapidly evolving intersection of healthcare and technology, where efforts to improve physical, mental, and emotional well-being meet innovative applications like AI, Blockchain, and Cybersecurity, we are witnessing a transformative era focused on solving health problems and enhancing life quality.

Amidst a convergence of global events, technological advancements, and the challenges of the COVID pandemic, in 2019, I presented the concept of " Artificial Intelligence, Blockchain, and Cybersecurity (ABC)" at a medical conference. This moment reflected a synergy of world events and innovation, marking a critical juncture where my vision and the needs of a rapidly changing world intersected.

Reflecting on my time at another conference, HIMSS conference, I vividly recall an impromptu meeting with two of the brightest minds in technology, David Metcalf, Ph.D. and Max W. Hooper, Ph.D. What was scheduled as a brief encounter quickly evolved into an hour-long discussion about ABC, sparking a series of meetings that led to numerous business opportunities and a collaborative problem-solving research program that led to better outcomes in the strategy that we were trying to implement in our company. This experience underscored the immense potential of collaborative thinking in driving technological advancements.

My career, deeply rooted in implementing disruptive innovations, began with my pioneering work in the U.S. military, where I introduced for the first time in US history the Electronic Medical Record (EMR) in the battlefield and developed Medical Simulation technologies for the Department of Defense (DoD). These groundbreaking initiatives, like the creation of the first joint program management office for medical simulation, and the collaboration in building the first NATO medical simulation center and being part of the leadership team that established the first medical simulation center in the U.S. Veteran's Affairs, taught me the importance of not only introducing new technologies but also preparing teams and enterprises for the impending disruption. We always need to address the next generation needs of customers.

This experience in the military, and in the battlefields of Bosnia, Iraq & Afghanistan combined with my later private sector work, underscored the need for adaptability and agility in both our innovations and our teams to successfully navigate and leverage the changes brought about by technological advancements. Innovations must be created, developed, demonstrated, evaluated and most importantly put to the test by the user community before a full implementation.

The influence of many General Officers that were my mentors during my military career and Senior Executives in the private sector like Mr. A.J. Ripin in operationalizing and scaling disruptive innovations cannot be understated. Their insights into operational excellence and forward-thinking leadership have been instrumental in guiding my approach to implementing change in Fortune 500 companies and the broader marketplace. I learned that to drive innovation we must incorporate strategies for operations excellence, ensure that your leadership understands that disruption is expensive and that the slogan "Disrupt or be disrupted" can mislead us many times.

As we venture through this book, we will explore various case studies and leading implementations that illustrate the transformative power of AI,

Blockchain, and Cybersecurity in Healthcare. These narratives are not just historical accounts; they are blueprints for future innovation, showcasing how these technologies can revolutionize patient care, data security, and healthcare administration. The time for the ABC revolution in the globe is NOW!

The path ahead in the world of healthcare technology is as thrilling as it is challenging. As leaders and pioneers in this field, we carry the responsibility to not only keep pace with but also anticipate and shape the future of technological evolution. This proactive approach is vital in harnessing the vast potential of innovations in AI, blockchain, and cybersecurity, ensuring they contribute positively to healthcare. Our goal is to create a healthcare ecosystem that is not just technologically advanced, but also more effective, secure, and efficient in delivering patient care. This involves a collaborative effort, where diverse expertise converges to forge a future where technology not only supports but enhances the human aspects of healthcare, thereby making a profound and positive impact on the lives of individuals worldwide.

In conclusion, this book is not just a chronicle of past successes but a guiding light leading us towards a future where the realms of technology and healthcare unite for the collective welfare. It's an invitation to join a journey of continuous learning, adaptation, and innovation. As we step into this bold new era of healthcare technology, let us collaboratively embrace the challenges and opportunities it presents. Our shared goal is to transform healthcare into a space where technological advancements are harmoniously integrated with compassionate care, ultimately enhancing the health and well-being of communities globally.

These three innovations (ABC) and other innovations like Telemedicine are revolutionizing healthcare globally. We need to continue embracing innovations that will transform the healthcare system and will help us to reduce the cost of healthcare, improve access to care, improve outcomes and that will give clinicians more time with the patients.

ABC....Let's identify the next letter and build the future of healthcare together!

# Chapter 1:

# Author Introductions

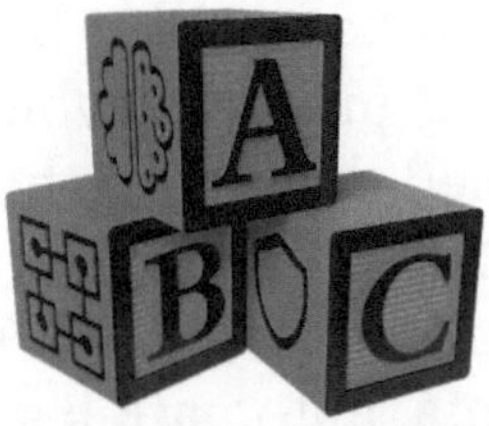



**David Metcalf, PhD**

**Vikram Dhillon, MD**

**Dexter Hadley, MD, PhD**

**Max Hooper, PhD**

**Harry Pappas**

## *Editor's Note*

In our first chapter, each author-editor offers their unique perspective on aspects of ABC from the perspective of researchers, medical doctors, technologists, industry expert, association leaders, and business executives. We hope that this will be thought-provoking and allow our readers from all walks of life and parts of the healthcare ecosystem to understand how AI, blockchain, and cybersecurity may enhance aspects of their role while identifying areas of caution and risks that should be mitigated.

## David Metcalf

Three areas of technology are poised to continue to reshape the landscape of multiple industries, not the least of which is healthcare. A glimpse into the future shows the importance right now in the **ABC**'s of next generation technology – **AI**, **B**lockchain and **C**ybersecurity. Emerging technologies, like these will shape and define the future of our current technology, landscape, and our post quantum future.

There are already substantial strides being made in the use of large language models (LLMs) in AI for novel drug discovery, provider education, and quality of care improvements based on better knowledge and improved patient outcomes. Blockchain technology is not just for cryptocurrency. It is being used to reshape and redefine how trust could be instilled back into our online systems, data, and transactions. Having privacy enabled, immutable records that can have the intelligence applied directly to them through smart contracts and other protocol techniques is fundamental. Blockchain is already having a significant influence in the storage and use of medical records, privacy enable sharing of patient data, automation and verification of billing, and federated learning for healthcare. Cybersecurity is a fundamental building block for medical, health and wellness records, as well as patient privacy. Beyond meeting standards and regulations, the spirit of protecting the rights of patients and providers is fundamental to the oath to do no harm. With the ever increasing waves of ransomware to hospitals, healthcare systems, and insurers the need for protection has never been greater. Cybersecurity in healthcare will continue to be a need with automated phishing techniques, deep fakes, and quantum attacks that can break through all but the most sophisticated encryption. Each of these three areas of technology advancement are moving very rapidly and pose real opportunities and real threats to our organizations and society at large. Protecting health is a fundamental right, and is also a responsibility of sovereign nations that espouse principles of freedom. With the US spending 18% of its GDP (gross domestic product) it is also vital to the stability of the national and international economic landscape. All of these technologies have the potential to enable the quadruple aim of better, faster and cheaper healthcare, that respects and empowers the providers in the process.

Now what happens when you combine these technologies? The ability to supercharge applications that instill privacy, trust, automation, and intelligence could collectively have the type of societal impact we strive to create. Fortunately, many people in organizations are working right at the seams of these fundamental ABC building blocks that will define our future. Best of all, while these technologies may seem far off and complex, they are getting easier to understand and implement every day.

In this book, we will explore the theoretical underpinnings, including a brief history of each of the technologies before diving right into discussions from some of the top authorities in artificial intelligence, blockchain, and cybersecurity and practical, real world examples of where the combination of these technologies form integrated solutions to real world problems in healthcare and deliver real value to society. In the last section of the book, we will explore not only current examples, but look at some of the potential future use cases for integrating technologies that are right around the corner, and further augment the capabilities of our future with ABC Technologies in Healthcare.

## Vikram Dhillon

Artificial Intelligence (AI) has become an integral part of modern technology, enabling machines to perform tasks that would typically require human intelligence. At its core, AI involves developing algorithms that enable systems to learn from data, identify patterns, make decisions, and improve their performance over time through experience. The application of AI spans various domains, including natural language processing, computer vision, robotics, and machine learning. In recent years, there have been growing concerns regarding the ethical implications of using AI, such as issues related to privacy, security, transparency, fairness, and accountability. These concerns necessitate careful consideration when designing, deploying, and managing AI systems.

Blockchain technology is another emerging field that offers significant potential benefits, particularly in areas such as financial transactions, supply chain management, identity verification, and digital voting systems. Blockchain provides a decentralized and distributed ledger system that enables secure and transparent record-keeping without relying on intermediaries or central authorities. By design, blockchains are highly resistant to tampering and fraud due to their consensus mechanisms, which ensure that all nodes maintain consistent copies of the ledger. However, like any other technology, blockchains are not immune to attacks and vulnerabilities, making it essential to implement robust security measures to protect against potential threats.

Cybersecurity refers to the practice of protecting internet-connected devices, networks, and data from unauthorized access, theft, damage, or disruption. Cybersecurity encompasses a wide range of technologies, processes, and practices designed to safeguard sensitive information and prevent malicious actors from exploiting vulnerabilities in software, hardware, and communication protocols. With the increasing reliance on digital platforms for critical infrastructure, finance, healthcare, transportation, and social interactions, the importance of cybersecurity cannot be overstated. Moreover, advances in AI and blockchain technologies introduce new challenges and opportunities for improving cybersecurity defense strategies while also creating novel attack vectors.

The intersection between AI, blockchain, and cybersecurity is becoming increasingly important as these technologies continue to mature and find widespread adoption across industries. For instance, AI can enhance blockchain's functionality by providing intelligent analytics capabilities, automating complex workflows, detecting anomalies, and predicting future trends. On the other hand, blockchain can provide a secure foundation for AI applications by ensuring data integrity, traceability, and provenance. Furthermore, both AI and Blockchain can significantly enhance cybersecurity. AI-powered algorithms can predict and prevent sophisticated cyberattacks, while blockchain can securely manage cryptographic keys and verify digital identities. This synergy promises heightened levels of security for critical infrastructure, financial transactions, and personal data.

However, integrating AI, blockchain, and cybersecurity comes with unique challenges, such as preserving user privacy, maintaining trust, addressing regulatory compliance, and balancing openness with control. As such, further research is needed to explore how best to leverage these technologies' strengths while mitigating their weaknesses. Ultimately, collaboration among experts from diverse fields, including AI, blockchain, cybersecurity, law, ethics, and policy, will be crucial to realizing the full potential of these technologies while minimizing their risks.

Adoption of AI models has gained tremendous momentum in recent years, driven by rapid advancements in computing power, big data availability, and algorithmic innovation. Organizations across various sectors, ranging from healthcare, finance, manufacturing, retail, and marketing, are leveraging AI to streamline operations, optimize resource allocation, reduce costs, and deliver personalized experiences to customers. Some notable examples include chatbots for customer service, automated threat detection systems for cybersecurity, recommendation engines for e-commerce, autonomous vehicles for transportation, and precision medicine tools for healthcare. Despite these successes, several barriers remain to wider AI adoption, such as lack of expertise, high upfront infrastructure investment, limited interpretability, biased decision-making, and ethical concerns. Similarly, blockchain technology has witnessed substantial growth since its introduction more than a decade ago, fueled by its promise of enhanced security, transparency, and efficiency. Various industries, including banking, insurance, logistics, supply chain management, and government services, are exploring use cases for blockchain to address pain points such as fraud prevention, cross-border payments, asset tracking, contract enforcement, and voter registration. Notable examples of successful blockchain adoptions include IBM Food Trust, Maersk TradeLens, Everledger, and Bitfury Group, among others. Nevertheless, blockchain adoption faces several challenges, such as scalability limitations, energy consumption concerns, legal uncertainty, network governance disputes, and integration difficulties with existing IT infrastructures. As a result, organizations seeking to adopt blockchain must weigh its benefits against its drawbacks and consider factors such as cost, complexity, compatibility, and long-term viability.

AI and blockchain technologies offer promising opportunities for businesses and society at large but come with inherent challenges and tradeoffs. To maximize their value, stakeholders must carefully assess their requirements, constraints, and priorities, taking into account factors such as technological maturity, market demand, regulatory landscape, talent pool, and cultural readiness. To unlock the full potential of this technological convergence, fostering collaboration among experts across diverse fields is crucial. AI researchers, blockchain developers, cybersecurity professionals, legal experts, ethicists, and policymakers must come together to address the challenges and maximize the benefits of this transformative fusion.

## Dexter Hadley

The healthcare landscape is undergoing a revolutionary transformation, with artificial intelligence, blockchain, and cybersecurity (*ABCs*) playing central roles in this exciting evolution. These seemingly disparate technologies, when woven together, create a powerful tapestry that promises enhanced patient care, improved data security, and a more robust and reliable healthcare ecosystem. One of the most pressing challenges in healthcare today is the proliferation of misinformation on social media platforms[1]. This misinformation can have detrimental effects on patient health, often leading to delayed diagnoses, incorrect treatment choices, and even vaccine hesitancy. To combat this issue, AI algorithms can be trained to not only identify and flag inaccurate health information online, but to even offer accurate health guidance for most diseases today to both patients and clinicians. However, the success of such AI recommendation systems hinges on access to accurate and reliable patient data.

Health systems and data aggregators are doubtless already training such AI 'copilots' to improve clinical workflows and efficiencies in delivering healthcare and improved outcomes. However, patients are less able to share their valuable patient data with other patients for AI algorithms across health systems due to health information blocking[2] where economic and market conditions create business incentives for some persons and entities to exercise control over electronic health information in ways that unreasonably limit its availability and use. By providing a secure and transparent platform for sharing patient information, adhering to protocols like HL7 and FHIR, blockchain empowers patients to control and share their data seamlessly with authorized healthcare providers and researchers to facilitate Community-driven AI[3]. This data, when anonymized and aggregated, becomes the fuel that propels AI algorithms to new heights of accuracy and effectiveness.

Moreover, patients themselves play a crucial role in this feedback loop as many programs like the Patient-Centered Outcomes Research Institute (PCORI)[4–13] and the National Institutes of Health (NIH)[14] have supported online patient engagement to recruit patients to share data and improve healthcare outcomes. Patients can become more active participants in their own healthcare journey by augmenting these and other programs with AI systems to provide feedback on the possible recommendations and treatment suggestions. This continuous feedback loop must adhere to HIPAA regulations for deidentification of patient data which allows AI systems to learn and adapt, further file-tuning their capabilities and ensuring their alignment with individual patient needs. Blockchain is based a network built of trustless algorithms that provides secure credentials while simultaneously anonymized with secure cryptographic encryption to guarantee fidelity of patients and providers given implicit governance of appropriate and explicit data use in line with existing HIPAA regulations.

However, this interconnectedness of patient data and AI algorithms presents a new frontier for cybersecurity threats and challenges. As AI systems become more sophisticated, they become increasingly susceptible to manipulation by malicious actors[15]. Generative AI algorithms, such as Generative Adversarial Networks (GANs) for images[16] and Generative Pre-Trained Transformers (GPTs) for text[17], can be used to flood AI systems with fake data, leading to inaccurate diagnoses and potentially harmful treatment decisions. Blockchain provides robust security features using distributed ledger technologies to create an immutable record of all transactions, making it nearly impossible to tamper with patient data or inject fake information[18]. Furthermore, the age of quantum computing with massively parallelized computation pipelines allows for implementation of various network algorithms can further bolster security by identifying and neutralizing suspicious nodes or data patterns that might indicate an attempt to manipulate the AI system.

In conclusion, the interplay of AI, blockchain, and cybersecurity (ABCs) in healthcare paints a picture of immense potential. By leveraging the strengths of each technology, we can create a healthcare ecosystem that is not only data-driven and patient-centric but also secure and resilient against emerging threats. In this book, we explore how these technologies holds the key to unlocking a future where patients are empowered, information is trustworthy, and AI serves as a powerful tool for improving health outcomes for all.

## *References*

1. Health Misinformation — Current Priorities of the U.S. Surgeon General. Accessed January 23, 2024. https://www.hhs.gov/surgeongeneral/priorities/health-misinformation/index.html#:~:text=How health misinformation spreads,well as via search engines.

2. (ONC) O of the NC for HIT. Report on Health Information Blocking. Published online 2015:1-39.

3. Hadley D, Kyin C, Sannegowda R, Nedimyer Horner J, Cyrus E, Metcalf D. How COVID-19 Catalyzed Community-Driven AI in the Metaverse of Medical Data. In: Harry P. Pappas PHF, ed. Leveraging Technology as a Response to the COVID Pandemic. 1st ed. Taylor & Francis; 2022:151-180. doi:10.4324/b23264-10

4. Manchikanti L, Falco FJE, Benyamin R, Helm S, Parr AT, Hirsch JA. The impact of comparative effectiveness research on interventional pain management: Evolution from Medicare modernization act to patient protection and affordable care act and the patient-centered outcomes research institute. Pain Physician. 2011;14(3):E249-82. Accessed June 18, 2020. http://www.ncbi.nlm.nih.gov/pubmed/21587337

5. Franck LS, McLemore MR, Williams S, et al. Research priorities of women at risk for preterm birth: Findings and a call to action. BMC Pregnancy Childbirth. 2020;20(1):10. doi:10.1186/s12884-019-2664-1

6. Lo B, Zhang T, Leung K, et al. Identifying best approaches for engaging patients and family members in health informatics initiatives: A case

study of the Group Priority Sort technique. Res Involv Engagem. 2020;6(1):25. doi:10.1186/s40900-020-00203-8

7. Andress L, Hall T, Davis S, Levine J, Cripps K, Guinn D. Addressing power dynamics in community-engaged research partnerships. J Patient-Reported Outcomes. 2020;4(1):24. doi:10.1186/s41687-020-00191-z

8. Esmail L, Moore E, Rein A. Evaluating patient and stakeholder engagement in research: Moving from theory to practice. J Comp Eff Res. 2015;4(2):133-145. doi:10.2217/cer.14.79

9. Forsythe L, Heckert A, Margolis MK, Schrandt S, Frank L. Methods and impact of engagement in research, from theory to practice and back again: early findings from the Patient-Centered Outcomes Research Institute. Qual Life Res. 2018;27(1):17-31. doi:10.1007/s11136-017-1581-x

10. Kraft SA, McMullen C, Lindberg NM, et al. Integrating stakeholder feedback in translational genomics research: an ethnographic analysis of a study protocol's evolution. Genet Med. 2020;22(6):1094-1101. doi:10.1038/s41436-020-0763-z

11. Forsythe LP, Ellis LE, Edmundson L, et al. Patient and Stakeholder Engagement in the PCORI Pilot Projects: Description and Lessons Learned. J Gen Intern Med. 2016;31(1):13-21. doi:10.1007/s11606-015-3450-z

12. Hemphill R, Forsythe LP, Heckert AL, et al. What motivates patients and caregivers to engage in health research and how engagement affects their lives: Qualitative survey findings. Heal Expect. 2020;23(2):328-336. doi:10.1111/hex.12979

13. Forsythe LP, Carman KL, Szydlowski V, et al. Patient engagement in research: Early findings from the patient-centered outcomes research institute. Health Aff. 2019;38(3):359-367. doi:10.1377/hlthaff.2018.05067

14. Murray J. The "All of Us" Research Program. N Engl J Med. 2019;381(19):1884. doi:10.1056/NEJMc1912496

15. Artificial Intelligence (AI) in Cyber Security | FDM Group | UK. Accessed January 23, 2024. https://www.fdmgroup.com/blog/ai-in-cybersecurity/#:~:text=In the context of cybersecurity,information or making incorrect decisions.

16. Goodfellow I, Pouget-Abadie J, Mirza M, et al. Generative Adversarial Nets. Adv Neural Inf Process Syst 27. Published online 2014:2672-2680. http://papers.nips.cc/paper/5423-generative-adversarial-nets.pdf

17. Radford A, Narasimhan K, Salimans T, Sutskever I. Improving language understanding by generative pre-training. Published online 2018. Accessed January 23, 2024. https://www.mikecaptain.com/resources/pdf/GPT-1.pdf

18. Mehta S, Grant K, Ackery A. Future of blockchain in healthcare: potential to improve the accessibility, security and interoperability of electronic health records. BMJ Heal care informatics. 2020;27(3). doi:10.1136/bmjhci-2020-100217

# Max Hooper

The current and future ABC's of technology is developing quickly and will impact the world with changes that are hard to imagine. The "ABC" combination of Artificial Intelligence, Blockchain, and Cyber Security will work together to bring new techniques, innovation, and changes in many areas of life, education, healthcare, commercial industries, government, and in other areas. These next generation technology applications become visible in various use cases and offer the advantages of being trustworthy and secure, bringing about transparency, immutability, and accountability.

As indicated by Sankalp Chenna, "The integration of Artificial Intelligence (AI) and Blockchain technology can enable new use cases and bring about improvements in various industries. These secure applications lead into advanced the cyber security protection. Some of the most promising use cases of AI and Blockchain integration include:

**Finance:** Blockchain-based smart contracts and decentralized autonomous organizations (DAOs) can be used to automate financial transactions and reduce the need for intermediaries. Additionally, AI can be used to analyze financial data in real-time and detect fraudulent activities.

**Supply Chain Management:** Blockchain technology can be used to create an immutable record of the movement of goods, which can help to ensure transparency and accountability. Additionally, AI can be used to optimize logistics and predict demand for goods.

**Healthcare:** Blockchain technology can be used to create a secure and decentralized record of patient data, which can help to ensure data privacy and improve the efficiency of medical research. Additionally, AI can be used to analyze medical images and predict disease outcomes.

**Identity Management:** Blockchain technology can be used to create secure and decentralized digital identities, which can help to prevent identity theft and ensure the privacy of personal data. Additionally, AI can be used to verify the identity of users and detect fraudulent activities.

**Internet of Things (IoT):** Blockchain technology can be used to create a secure and decentralized record of IoT data, which can help to ensure the privacy and security of IoT devices. Additionally, AI can be used to analyze IoT data in real-time and detect suspicious activity.

**Gaming and Virtual Reality:** The integration of AI and blockchain can enable new forms of gaming and virtual reality experiences that are decentralized, verifiable, and transparent."[1]

AI, Blockchain, and Cyber Security work together in creating a powerful combination of advantages in the market place: Artory is an example of a use case that seeks to unlock art and collectibles as a credible asset class. "Artory is the leader in art and collectibles tokenization, accelerating the liquidity opportunities for the most trusted Real World Assets in art. Secured trusted information is collected from expert partners to tokenize physical art works and collectibles. These art works are incorporated into traditional financial instruments, next-gen digital first financial products, and other Web 3 opportunities.

This technological innovation promises to increase access to art investment while fostering trust and compliance in the market. Investors now experience an e-commerce-like platform, enabling them to directly and compliantly subscribe to, manage, and transfer digital funds, all while avoiding traditional barriers to entry. Similar to how the internet revolutionized information transfer, blockchain is revolutionizing value security and transfer.

Yet, one of the most significant changes is in fund distribution, which is set to unlock the liquidity of these assets. Once art funds are represented on a blockchain, digital funds can be distributed across any trading platform within the network."[2]

The future in now in the innovation of the ABC technologies and the advantages of the unique working combinations. Maturity of techniques will occur as additional research and best practices are developed over time, as Kong and team stated:

"Blockchain technology has the potential to disrupt various industries, including Artificial Intelligence (AI). In recent years, there has been increasing interest in the integration of Blockchain and AI, as it has the potential to create intelligent systems that are both trustworthy and secure. One of the main benefits of combining Blockchain and AI is the ability to ensure the integrity and provenance of the data used to train AI systems. Blockchain technology can be used to create a tamper-proof record of the data's origin and any modifications made to it, which can help to prevent data breaches and ensure that the AI systems are trustworthy and reliable." [3]

The future of ABC innovations will also need to deal with many ethical and legal considerations: "Several are listed:

**Privacy:** The use of AI and Blockchain can raise important privacy concerns, as both technologies have the potential to collect and analyze large amounts of personal data. It is important to ensure that data collection and processing is done in compliance with data protection laws and regulations, and that individuals have control over their personal data.

**Bias:** AI systems can perpetuate and amplify existing biases in the data used to train them, which can lead to discriminatory outcomes. It is important to ensure that AI systems are designed and trained in a way that minimizes bias and promotes fairness.

**Accountability:** AI and Blockchain systems can make decisions and execute actions autonomously, which can make it difficult to attribute responsibility for their outcomes. It is important to ensure that there are clear mechanisms for accountability and dispute resolution in place.

**Transparency:** The decentralized and distributed nature of Blockchain technology can make it difficult to understand how decisions are being made and data is being processed. It is important to ensure that AI and Blockchain systems are designed in a way that promotes transparency and explainability.

**Governance:** The integration of AI and Blockchain can raise important governance issues, such as how to regulate decentralized systems and ensure compliance with laws and regulations. It is important to ensure that there are clear governance mechanisms in place to address these issues.

**Jurisdiction:** The decentralized nature of blockchain can make it difficult to determine jurisdiction and enforce regulations, this has to be taken in consideration to prevent any legal ambiguity."[4]

It is currently a unique moment in the development of technologies that can make the world a better place for global civilizations. To be a part of these innovation cycles is truly a peak of experience of enlightenment.

## REFERENCES

1. Chenna, Sankalp, AI and Blockchain: Towards Trustworthy and Secure Intelligent Systems (January 14, 20230. Available at SSRN:https://ssrn.com/abstract=4324495, or http://dx.doi.org/ 10.2139/ssrn.4324495.

2. Artory, https://www.artory.com

3. R. Tian, L. Kong, X. Min, and Y. Qu, "Blockchain for AI: A Disruptive Integration", 2022 IEEE 25th International Conference on Computer Supported Cooperative Work in Design (CSCWD), May 2022, doi:10.1109/cscwd54268.2022.9776023.

4. B. K. Sharma and N. Jain, "An Integration of Blockchain and Artificial Intelligence: A Concept," 2019 International Conference on Intelligent Computing and Control Systems (ICCS), May 2019, doi: 10.1109/iccs45141.2019.9065555.

5. F. Xiaohua, C. Marc, E. Elias, and H. Khalid, "Artificial Intelligence and Blockchain for Future Cyber Security Application," 2021 IEEE Intl Conf on Dependable, Autonomic and Secure Computing, Intl Conf on Cloud and Big Data Computing, Intl Conf on Cyber Science and Technology Congress (DASC/PiCom/CBDCom/CyberSciTech), Oct. 2021, doi: 10.1109/dasc-picom-cbdcom-cyberscitech52372.2021.00133.

6. B. Chavali, S. K. Khatri, and S. A. Hossain, "AI and Blockchain Integration," 2020 8th international Conference on Reliability, Infocom Technologies and Optimization (Trends and Future Directions) (ICRITP), June. 2020, doi: 10.1109/icrito48877/2020.9197847

# Harry Pappas

I always get asked, who and what is the Intelligent Health Association? And we're kind of a unique association because we're focused on education and training. The IHA is an international social purpose entity technology-centric and focused on successful adoption of new technologies in healthcare and wellness medicine through vendor neutral educational programs that we have worked on with IEEE, HIMSS, and many other organizations. The Intelligent Health Association's International Summit stands as one of the largest and most comprehensive global events in the healthcare technology center that we know of.

What a Life changing, paradigm shift awaits us all as individuals, but also all industries and businesses globally, including health!

Are you /we ready for the transformation? Are we ready to get re-educated and change our lifestyles? I firmly believe that these three technologies along with other YET UNKNOWN Technologies will affect our lifestyles and work habits. Will these technologies enable us to live better, longer, safer, happier lives? The answer is, YES!

These technologies will certainly have a profound impact on all phases of health, wellness and wellbeing for all of us including,you the individual as well as the Health and wellness professionals of the world. How will AI impact the Local Hospital Operating room, your dentist, your eye doctor, or the Emergency Room? What about the appliances in your home and what about your new car?

I believe that these technologies will have a dramatic impact on the delivery of health and telehealth for ALL people. AI will be a REAL Health equity equalizer. These technologies will democratize healthcare for all.

Like all technologies, AI, Blockchain and Cybersecurity will touch us in so many ways that we have no clue today. We need to continuously get educated and retrained and be prepared to "Learn and Unlearn" to adjust our lives and our work environment on a regular basis.

There are POSITIVE and NEGATIVE forces with any new technology, just look at the transformation brought about globally by the WWW, Text messaging, email, or better yet the smartphone in your pocket?

Who ever thought that your phone would be a computer and what would you do with a camera in your phone? Have these technologies changed our lives? YES! But they also have wrought a negative impact on our daily lifestyles that I will not go into.

I am excited to be joining my associates in publishing this book so that all of us may "Learn and Unlearn" as we adopt and adjust to AI, Blockchain, and Cybersecurity not only in the health and wellness community but in our homes and places of business.

Are you ready to change for the better? Are we ready to set up a set of new rules and safeguards? OR will "HAL" from Space Odyssey run our lives?

Are we ready to use these technologies for "Social Good"?

# Chapter 2:

## The Evolution of AI in Healthcare: A Double-Edged Scalpel

**Dexter Hadley, MD, PhD**
*Chief of Artificial Intelligence*

*University of Central Florida, College of Medicine*

### *Editor's Note*

In this chapter, Dr. Hadley provides an overview of AI in the context of *ABC*. He describes both the past and what has changed in current technologies. his role as both a practicing physician and a researcher and head of Artificial Intelligence at UCF's College of Medicine. His unique perspective also provides personal examples of how AI can be used in healthcare research, as well as personal examples and perspective.

The 'Art of Medicine' has long relied on intuition and human experience to navigate healthy outcomes through the complex network of interacting cells, tissues, and organs that comprise human beings. More recently, Artificial Intelligence (AI) has been carving a path through the medical landscape, promising precision, efficiency, and perhaps a glimpse into the future of healthcare. However, as with any powerful tool, AI in healthcare comes with its own set of complexities and ethical dilemmas that have the significant potential for harm. The most recent scandal documenting this divide is a massive class action lawsuit against multiple insurance companies that use biased AI algorithms to illegally deny coverage and thus care for large swaths of minority patients[1]. This chapter delves into its evolution in healthcare including its promises and perils to explore how AI, complemented by Blockchain and Cybersecurity (ABC) may future proofs the technology to reduce the burden of disease and maintain health for all patient populations in the age of social networks. In so doing, we explore how ABC may make the 'Art of Medicine' much more scientific in building communities of patients that are healthier together.

## Early rules-based expert systems: The example of MYCIN

The history of AI in healthcare isn't a linear one, but rather a series of leaps and stumbles. The early days saw strict rule-based systems intended to function at the level of an expert, or so-called 'expert systems', mimicking human decision-making processes by analyzing specific criteria. These expert systems, while limited, found success in tasks like drug interaction checking and diagnosis support[2]. In the 1970s, a pioneer named MYCIN emerged, one of the first expert systems to tackle the complex reasoning of diagnosing and treating bacterial infections. MYCIN could analyze patient symptoms, laboratory results, and medical history, then suggest antibiotic regimens tailored to the specific bacteria culprits. Its cleverness went beyond picking a drug; it considered factors like patient allergies, potential drug interactions, and even adjusted dosages based on weight. Although limited by the technology of its time, MYCIN paved the way for modern AI in healthcare, proving the potential for machines to assist in crucial medical decisions.

While MYCIN was groundbreaking for its era, it came with its own set of limitations and shortcomings. Its knowledge base was human-encoded and therefore static, requiring continual expert input for updates. The rules-base also limited its scope to primarily bacterial infections, excluding other types of infections such as viruses and broader medical considerations. Furthermore, MYCIN struggled with uncertainty and ambiguity inherent in medical data, and its reliance on rigid rules couldn't fully account for nuances and exceptions, leading to potential inaccuracies in diagnoses and treatment recommendations. MYCIN was also plagued by a lack of explainability of its opaque process, and this lack of transparency hindered trust and acceptance by clinicians. Moreover, MYCIN was limited by the computing power and data availability of the 1970s with only limited access to electronic medical records. It couldn't analyze complex data like medical images, further hindering its accuracy and applicability.

Despite these shortcomings, however, MYCIN left a lasting impact, highlighting the potential of AI in healthcare and paving the way for more advanced, sophisticated systems. By learning from its limitations, modern AI approaches strive to address issues like transparency, broader scope, and adaptability, moving towards a future where AI can truly supplement and enhance human expertise in healthcare.

## The emergence of 'Big Data' in Healthcare: The beginning of 'Precision Medicine'

While the underlying mathematics of modern-day AI has been postulated since the 1950s, one of the biggest limitations of early AI systems in healthcare, like MYCIN, was the lack of enough compute combined with data required to train more sophisticated models. This is because early predictive machine learning, in healthcare or other domains, relied on simple rules and relatively underpowered statistical models with only a few possible parameters to tune. Today, modern AI is defined by complex 'deep' algorithms that rely on highly parameterized models that mandate large diverse datasets to accurately fine tune. For instance, the latest large language models from OpenAI, Google, Anthropic and others have billions and even trillions of parameters to estimate which mandates expensive training of on massive corpora of text for accurate performance. One of the most technical difficulties to overcome, that remained unsolved for decades, was to comprehensively optimize the parameterization space for these deep algorithms to perform accurately. However, the back propagation[3] computational method emerged to do just that which helped win its developers the Turing Award[4], the equivalent for a Nobel Prize in computer science. When combined with highly parallelized compute power now commonplace in modern GPUs, back propagation in deep learning motivated in the era of AI we are experiencing today across virtually all aspects of society. Moreover, the dawn of 'Big Data' accessible through vast troves of medical records served as the substrate to usher in the era of AI in healthcare we are living in today. Now, as opposed to standard statistical methods that have persisted relatively unchanged for many decades, there is continued development of deep algorithms to learn patterns from patients Big Data to uncover hidden correlations to predict disease risks, design drugs, etc. with ever increasing accuracy.

The quest for the initial Big Data in healthcare to satisfy these hungry deep learning algorithms in AI is punctuated by leaps and stumbles perhaps best illustrated by the initial sequencing of the human genome project (HGP) in 2003. The HGP was a global endeavor that interrogated 6 billion nucleotides that define our genome to provide the blueprint for inherited health and disease among the human population. Moreover, HGP catalyzed a domestic research program of 'Precision Medicine' federally mandated by President Barrack Obama to tailor treatments to individual patients based on their unique genetic and medical profiles[5]. However, the 2000s marked only the tip of the proverbial iceberg of leveraging Big Data of HGP in medicine because incessant genome-wide association studies (GWAS) leveraged only basic statistics, such as the chi-square test and meta-analysis, to define that first decade of research into Precision Medicine. As of 2023-11-23, the GWAS Catalog contained 6652 publications since then, the majority of which leverage only simple statistical methods to define 561,096 top genetic associated with hereditary disease or traits. Today, there is an abundance of true deep learning algorithms being applied to genomics Big Data from patients that is not only redefining the molecular landscape of disease and health, but also a multi-modal landscape across radiology, pathology, and almost all other clinical tests that can be used to improve the delivery of Precision Medicine.

Much like the insurance scandals of today, this early era of Precision Medicine tended to discriminate against large swaths of often minority patients because its recommendations were based on findings from small and biased datasets. These disparity patterns are not only evident in the clinical outcomes for patients, but they are also reflected in the Big Data underlying Precision Medicine. As late as 2013, which was at least a decade after the HGP was initially sequenced, up to 96% of all genetic sequence was still European derived which makes the majority of GWAS studies performed in that period inaccurate for most patients. Given disparate data and research, after at least a decade of Precision Medicine GWAS research, people of color (POC) continue to experience overall higher morbidities, earlier onset of morbidities and higher mortality rates when compared to non-Hispanic whites (NHW)[6,7]. COVID-19 laid bare how vulnerable / marginalized populations suffer higher rates of chronic and co-morbid conditions[8] that compounded the risks for contracting and dying from the disease[9–11]. These patterns hold across the board where compared to NHW, African Americans (AA) have significantly more morbidity and mortality from diabetes[12], heart disease[13], asthma[14], obesity[15], and HIV[16], despite comprising only 13% of the population. Similar trends hold for Latino/Latina (Latinx)[17–19] and American Indian/Alaska Native (AIAN)[20–22] when compared to NHW controls. Therefore, to ethically leverage medical data and to develop digital interventions that may improve these disparate outcomes, digital communities must actively incentivize a diverse recruitment of patients from the most vulnerable communities to identify this implicit bias across the healthcare data and ultimately correct for it with more finely tuned AI.

# The Dawn of AI in Medicine

It would take another decade or so for the true revolution in AI to occur with the arrival of 'deep' nested neural networks, a type of AI inspired by the human brain. Fueled by the ready availability of Big Data and cheap computation today, continually improving algorithms are making breakthroughs in AI more possible now than ever before[23]. As opposed to traditional computer programming that relies on human coding of rules, deep learning algorithms are capable of autonomously coding the rules by fine-tuning their parameters on accurate Big Data. Deep learning has been applied to a variety of tasks with extraordinary results[24–39], but the most remarkable progress has been made in the field of computer vision (CV). In just seven years, The annual ImageNet Large Scale Visual Recognition Challenge (ILSVRC) competition[40–43] showed the winning accuracy in classifying objects in the dataset rose from 71.8% to 97.3%, significantly surpassing human abilities and effectively proving that bigger data leads to better decisions.

In medicine today, deep neural networks can now process vast amounts of data which opens up new frontiers in medical imaging, diagnosis, and even drug discovery[44]. AI algorithms can now analyze medical scans with superhuman precision, identifying tumors and other abnormalities faster and more accurately than human radiologists, for instance. The potential benefits of AI are vast and include making healthcare more accurate, efficient and accessible for patients worldwide[45,46]. AI underlies the emerging new domains of digital health that can interpret a wealth of information from smart wearables towards improved diagnostics and disease prediction can lead to earlier interventions and better outcomes. AI-powered virtual assistants can provide 24/7 patient support, managing chronic conditions and monitoring vital signs[47] while robotic surgery, guided by AI algorithms, offers minimally invasive procedures with faster recovery times[48]. Undoubtable we are now seeing the tip of the proverbial iceberg of what AI-powered healthcare can be as this technology will undoubtable impact the healthcare landscape.

## The Promises and Pitfalls of AI: A Double-Edged Scalpel

The path to this utopian future that leverages AI in healthcare, however, is paved with potential pitfalls. The ever-increasing reliance on AI in general society raises concerns about the future of its impact on the healthcare workforce, with some jobs potentially being replaced by automation[49] which can paradoxically obstruct the acceptance of the technology in practice, but these fears remain relatively distant today. One major immediate concern is the significant bias resultant from AI algorithms trained on limited accessible patient data that may often reflect societal inequalities that exponentially perpetuate existing biases in healthcare, leading to discriminatory outcomes for certain demographics[50–53]. Indeed, both recent and future AI breakthroughs trained on small and limited datasets may be biased towards the populations on which they were trained[54,55] as evidenced by the numerous ongoing lawsuits alleging various insurance companies used AI to illegally deny claims serves as a stark reminder of the ethical implications of relying solely on AI for healthcare decisions. These and other scandals further expose the vulnerability of patients to opaque and potentially biased AI systems in healthcare billing, claims processing and all other aspects of processing patient's personal data. The lack of community provided data means that the bulk of AI in healthcare today is trained on limited datasets from which must inherently perform better on in-sample patient populations most like their training data than more diverse out-sample performance. AI exponentiating such biased recommendations are becoming a phenomenon playing out in deep learning models to detect pneumonia in chest radiographs using private data stores relative to open training data[56]. These incidents highlight the need for transparency and accountability in AI development and deployment, particularly in sensitive areas like healthcare.

Moving forward, the journey of AI in healthcare must be guided by a strong ethical framework which includes ensuring fairness and inclusivity of accessible Big Data to promote transparency and explainability of decisions to the community of patients and providers that may rely on AI as a service. For the current state-of-the-art deep learning frameworks that have come to dominate AI, generalized models must be pre-trained on massive, labeled datasets that require fine-tuning on smaller more curated datasets for accurate performance across more specialized applications. This fine tuning or so-called 'transfer learning' of a specialized models allows for Social Determinants of Health (SDH) and other drivers of the existing disparities in health outcomes to be directly incorporated into machine learning and as part of the experimental design. Therefore, the idea of *Community-Driven AI is to build interactive digital communities*[57] that can be more finely curated to include these and other features from patients directly 'in the loop' of the machine learning.

## Community Driven AI: The ABCs of a Healthier Future

The concept of Community-driven AI was catalyzed during the COVID-19 pandemic[57] which forced the virtualization of almost every aspect of modern life including our healthcare. However, it is a modern paradigm shift towards digital medicine, a term which emerged since 2007 when the iPhone was introduced as the first smart-phone[45] and is now used to describe any kind of mobile app-based intervention that served patients via smart phones or wearables. Since then, programs like the Patient-Centered Outcomes Research Institute (PCORI) have supported online patient engagement to recruit patients to share data and improve healthcare outcomes[58–67]. In perhaps one of the most impactful instances of digital health innovation, the Apple Heart Study[68] recruited 419,297 participants over 8 months to eventually develop an FDA approved real-time algorithm for Apple Watch to detect atrial fibrillation through its integrated EKG. The massive NIH sponsored AllOfUs[69] research program plans to enroll at least 1M participants to track medical records in order to accelerate research and improve health. These and many other programs all seek to build interactive diverse communities of patients to better predict risk and outcomes, but their results run the risk of propagating the existing data disparities that mirror disparate healthcare outcomes in underserved populations.

However, one of the most pressing challenges in healthcare today is the proliferation of misinformation on social media platforms[70]. This misinformation can have detrimental effects on patient health, often leading to delayed diagnoses, incorrect treatment choices, and even vaccine hesitancy. As AI systems become more sophisticated, they become increasingly susceptible to manipulation by malicious actors[71]. Generative AI algorithms, such as Generative Adversarial Networks (GANs) for images[72] and Generative Pre-Trained Transformers (GPTs) for text[73], can be used to flood AI systems with fake data, leading to inaccurate diagnoses and potentially harmful treatment decisions. Blockchain provides robust security features using distributed ledger technologies to create an immutable record of all transactions, making it nearly impossible to tamper with patient data or inject fake information[74]. However, AI algorithms can be trained to identify and flag inaccurate health information online as well as to offer accurate health guidance for most diseases today to both patients and clinicians. In our observational CovidImaging.US clinical trial[75] pioneering Community Driven AI, however, we documented significant recruitment bias using existing social networks such as Facebook[57] to identify patients willing to share their COVID-19 imaging. Therefore, ongoing research and development are crucial to address existing limitations and develop robust recruitment networks to develop AI tools that truly serve the needs of all patients and healthcare providers.

The idea of Community-driven AI encourages building networks of patients willing to share their medical data via such trustless algorithms in IRB-approved research that contributes toward that network's shared clinical intelligence of potential recommendations of interventions to improve outcomes. Moreover, the success of such AI recommendation systems, for both patients and providers, hinges on access to accurate and reliable clinical data. Indeed, health systems and data aggregators are doubtless already training such AI 'copilots' to improve clinical workflows and efficiencies in delivering healthcare and improved outcomes. However, patients are less able to share their valuable patient data with other patients or with AI algorithms across health systems due to health information blocking[76] where economic and market conditions create business incentives for some persons and entities to exercise control over electronic health information in ways that unreasonably limit its availability and use. In the CovidImaging.US case study we also propose that by providing a secure and transparent platform for sharing patient information, adhering to protocols like HL7 and FHIR, blockchain may empower patients to control and share their data seamlessly with authorized healthcare providers and researchers to facilitate Community-driven AI[57]. Therefore, the evolution of AI in healthcare is a story still being written, and it is a complex narrative with both triumphant chapters and cautionary tales. By acknowledging the challenges and embracing ethical considerations, we can ensure that Community-driven AI becomes a powerful ally, not a threat, in our quest for a healthier future for all patients.

# References:


1. Ledford H. Millions of black people affected by racial bias in health-care algorithms. Nature. 2019;574(7780):608-609. doi:10.1038/d41586-019-03228-6

2. Shortliffe EH, Buchanan BG, Feigenbaum EA. Knowledge engineering for medical decision making: A review of computer-based clinical decision aids. Proc IEEE. 1979;67(9):1207-1224. doi:10.1109/PROC.1979.11436

3. Rumelhart DE, Hinton GE, Williams RJ. Learning representations by back-propagating errors. Nature. 1986;323(6088):533-536. doi:10.1038/323533a0

4. Turing Award Won by 3 Pioneers in Artificial Intelligence - The New York Times. New York Times. https://www.nytimes.com/2019/03/27/technology/turing-award-ai.html#. Accessed December 21, 2023.

5. Ashley EA. Towards precision medicine. Nat Rev Genet. 2016;17(9):507-522. doi:10.1038/nrg.2016.86

6. Anderson KM. Roundtable on the Promotion of Health Equity and the Elimination of Health Disparities Board on Population Health and Public Health Practice. National Academies Press; 2012.

7. Cunningham TJ, Croft JB, Liu Y, Lu H, Eke PI, Giles WH. Vital signs: Racial disparities in age-specific mortality among blacks or African Americans — United States, 1999–2015. Morb Mortal Wkly Rep. Published online 2017. doi:10.15585/mmwr.mm6617e1

8. Report D. 2016 National Healthcare Quality and Disparities Report | Agency for Healthcare Research & Quality. Rockville, MD Agency Healthc Res Qual. Published online 2017.

9. People who are at higher risk for severe illness | CDC. US Centers Dis Control Prev. Published online 2020.

10. Williams DR. Stress and the Mental Health of Populations of Color: Advancing Our Understanding of Race-related Stressors. J Health Soc Behav. Published online 2018. doi:10.1177/0022146518814251

11. People who need extra precautions. U.S. Centers for Disease Control and Prevention (CDC). Published 2020. https://www.cdc.gov/coronavirus/2019-ncov/need-extra-precautions/

12. U.S. Department of Health and Human Services Office of Minority Health. Diabetes and African Americans.

13. U.S. Department of Health and Human Services Office of Minority Health. Heart Disease and African Americans.

14. Centers for Disease Control and Prevention. Most Recent National Asthma Data.

15. U.S. Department of Health and Human Services Office of Minority Health. Obesity and African Americans.

16. Centers for Disease Control and Prevention. HIV and African Americans. 2020.

17. Bandi P, Goldmann E, Parikh NS, Farsi P, Boden-Albala B. Age-related differences in antihypertensive medication adherence in hispanics: A cross-sectional community-based survey in New York City, 2011-2012. Prev Chronic Dis. Published online 2017. doi:10.5888/pcd14.160512

18. Foti K, Wang D, Appel LJ, Selvin E. Hypertension awareness, treatment, and control in US Adults: Trends in the hypertension control cascade by population subgroup (National Health and Nutrition Examination Survey, 1999-2016). Am J Epidemiol. Published online 2019. doi:10.1093/aje/kwz177

19. Ogden CL, Carroll MD, Fryar CD, Flegal KM. Prevalence of Obesity Among Adults and Youth: United States, 2011-2014. NCHS Data Brief. 2015;(219):1-8. http://www.ncbi.nlm.nih.gov/pubmed/26633046

20. U.S. Department of Health and Human Services Office of Minority Health. Diabetes and American Indians/Alaska Natives - The Office of Minority Health.

21. U.S. Department of Health and Human Services Office of Minority Health. Obesity and American Indians/Alaska Natives - The Office of Minority Health.

22. U.S. Department of Health and Human Services Office of Minority Health. Heart Disease and American Indians/Alaska Natives - The Office of Minority Health.

23. The Three Breakthroughs That Have Finally Unleashed AI on the World | WIRED. Accessed October 5, 2015. http://www.wired.com/2014/10/future-of-artificial-intelligence/

24. Ba J, Mnih V, Kavukcuoglu K. Multiple Object Recognition with Visual Attention. Iclr. Published online December 24, 2014:1-10. doi:10.48550/arXiv.1412.7755

25. Gonzalez-Dominguez J, Lopez-Moreno I, Moreno PJ, Gonzalez-Rodriguez J. Frame-by-frame language identification in short utterances using deep neural networks. Neural Networks. 2015;64:49-58. doi:10.1016/j.neunet.2014.08.006

26. Vinyals O, Kaiser L, Koo T, Petrov S, Sutskever I, Hinton G. Grammar as a Foreign Language. arXiv. Published online 2014:1-10. doi:10.1146/annurev.neuro.26.041002.131047

27. Mikolov T, Corrado G, Chen K, Dean J. Efficient Estimation of Word Representations in Vector Space. Proc Int Conf Learn Represent (ICLR 2013). Published online 2013:1-12. doi:10.1162/153244303322533223

28. Le Q V, Ranzato M, Monga R, et al. Building high-level features using large scale unsupervised learning. Int Conf Mach Learn. Published online 2011:38115. doi:10.1109/MSP.2011.940881

29. Ramsundar B, Kearnes S, Riley P, Webster D, Konerding D, Pande V. Massively Multitask Networks for Drug Discovery. Published online February 6, 2015. Accessed March 6, 2015. http://arxiv.org/abs/1502.02072

30. Lusci A, Pollastri G, Baldi P. Deep architectures and deep learning in chemoinformatics: the prediction of aqueous solubility for drug-like molecules. J Chem Inf Model. 2013;53(7):1563-1575. doi:10.1021/ci400187y

31. Alipanahi B, Delong A, Weirauch MT, Frey BJ. Predicting the sequence specificities of DNA- and RNA-binding proteins by deep learning. Nat Biotechnol. 2015;33(8):831-838. doi:10.1038/nbt.3300

32. Nair A, Srinivasan P, Blackwell S, et al. Massively Parallel Methods for Deep Reinforcement Learning. arXiv:150704296. Published online 2015:14. http://arxiv.org/abs/1507.04296

33. Angelova A, Krizhevsky A, Vanhoucke V. Pedestrian detection with a Large-Field-Of-View deep network. In: Proceedings - IEEE International Conference on Robotics and Automation. Vol 2015-June. ; 2015:704-711. doi:10.1109/ICRA.2015.7139256

34. Heigold G, Vanhoucke V, Senior A, et al. Multilingual Acoustic Models using Distributed Deep Neural Networks. In: Icassp. ; 2013:8619-8623. doi:10.1109/ICASSP.2013.6639348

35. Hinton G, Deng L, Yu D, et al. Deep Neural Networks for Acoustic Modeling in Speech Recognition. IEEE Signal Process Mag. 2012;(November):82-97. doi:10.1109/MSP.2012.2205597

36. Zeiler MD, Ranzato M, Monga R, et al. On rectified linear units for speech processing. In: ICASSP, IEEE International Conference on Acoustics, Speech and Signal Processing - Proceedings. ; 2013:3517-3521. doi:10.1109/ICASSP.2013.6638312

37. Karpathy A, Toderici G, Shetty S, Leung T, Sukthankar R, Li FF. Large-scale video classification with convolutional neural networks. In: Proceedings of the IEEE Computer Society Conference on Computer Vision and Pattern Recognition. ; 2014:1725-1732. doi:10.1109/CVPR.2014.223

38. Szegedy C, Liu W, Jia Y, et al. Going Deeper with Convolutions. In: Proceedings of the IEEE Computer Society Conference on Computer Vision and Pattern Recognition. Vol 07-12-June. ; 2014:1-9. doi:10.1109/CVPR.2015.7298594

39. Frome A, Corrado G, Shlens J. Devise: A deep visual-semantic embedding model. Adv Neural .... Published online 2013:1-11. http://papers.nips.cc/paper/5204-devise-a-deep-visual-semantic-embedding-model

40. Deng JDJ, Dong WDW, Socher R, Li L-JLL-J, Li KLK, Fei-Fei LF-FL. ImageNet: A large-scale hierarchical image database. 2009 IEEE Conf Comput Vis Pattern Recognit. Published online 2009:2-9. doi:10.1109/CVPR.2009.5206848

41. Russakovsky O, Deng J, Su H, et al. ImageNet Large Scale Visual Recognition Challenge. Int J Comput Vis. 2015;115(3):211-252. doi:10.1007/s11263-015-0816-y

42. Krizhevsky A, Sutskever I, Hinton GE. ImageNet Classification with Deep Convolutional Neural Networks. In: Advances in Neural Information Processing Systems. ; 2012:1097-1105. Accessed September 19, 2015. http://papers.nips.cc/paper/4824-imagenet-classification-with-deep-

43. Google AI Blog: Using Machine Learning to Explore Neural Network Architecture. Accessed January 24, 2019. https://ai.googleblog.com/2017/05/using-machine-learning-to-explore.html

44. Miotto R, Wang F, Wang S, Jiang X, Dudley JT. Deep learning for healthcare: review, opportunities and challenges. Brief Bioinform. 2018;19(6):1236-1246. doi:10.1093/bib/bbx044

45. Topol EJ. A decade of digital medicine innovation. Sci Transl Med. 2019;11(498). doi:10.1126/scitranslmed.aaw7610

46. Rajpurkar P, Chen E, Banerjee O, Topol EJ. AI in health and medicine. Nat Med. 2022;28(1):31-38. doi:10.1038/s41591-021-01614-0

47. Tian S, Yang W, Grange JM Le, Wang P, Huang W, Ye Z. Smart healthcare: making medical care more intelligent. Glob Heal J. 2019;3(3):62-65. doi:10.1016/j.glohj.2019.07.001

48. Zemmar A, Lozano AM, Nelson BJ. The rise of robots in surgical environments during COVID-19. Nat Mach Intell. 2020;2(10):566-572. doi:10.1038/s42256-020-00238-2

49. Shuaib A, Arian H, Shuaib A. The Increasing Role of Artificial Intelligence in Health Care: Will Robots Replace Doctors in the Future? Int J Gen Med. 2020;13:891-896. doi:10.2147/IJGM.S268093

50. Panahiazar M, Bishara AM, Chern Y, et al. Gender-based time discrepancy in diagnosis of coronary artery disease based on data analytics of electronic medical records. Front Cardiovasc Med. 2022;9:969325. doi:10.3389/fcvm.2022.969325

51. O'Reilly-Shah VN, Gentry KR, Walters AM, Zivot J, Anderson CT, Tighe PJ. Bias and ethical considerations in machine learning and the automation of perioperative risk assessment. Br J Anaesth. 2020;125(6):843-846. doi:10.1016/j.bja.2020.07.040

52. Chen IY, Szolovits P, Ghassemi M. Can AI help reduce disparities in general medical and mental health care? AMA J Ethics. Published online 2019. doi:10.1001/amajethics.2019.167

53. Panahiazar M, Baygoui R, Hadley D. A Multidimensional Gender-Based Study on UCSF Electronic Medical Record to Improve Women Health. In: Journal of Womens Health. Vol 28. ; 2019:19.

54. Rajpurkar P, Irvin J, Zhu K, et al. CheXNet: Radiologist-Level Pneumonia Detection on Chest X-Rays with Deep Learning. Published online 2017:3-9. doi:1711.05225

55. Esteva A, Kuprel B, Novoa RA, et al. Dermatologist-level classification of skin cancer with deep neural networks. Nature. Published online January 25, 2017. doi:10.1038/nature21056

56. Zech JR, Badgeley MA, Liu M, Costa AB, Titano JJ, Oermann EK. Variable generalization performance of a deep learning model to detect pneumonia in chest radiographs: A cross-sectional study. PLoS Med. Published online 2018. doi:10.1371/journal.pmed.1002683

57. Hadley D, Kyin C, Sannegowda R, Nedimyer Horner J, Cyrus E, Metcalf D. How COVID-19 Catalyzed Community-Driven AI in the Metaverse of Medical Data. In: Harry P. Pappas PHF, ed. Leveraging Technology as a Response to the COVID Pandemic. 1st ed. Taylor & Francis; 2022:151-180. doi:10.4324/b23264-10

58. Manchikanti L, Falco FJE, Benyamin R, Helm S, Parr AT, Hirsch JA. The impact of comparative effectiveness research on interventional pain management: Evolution from Medicare modernization act to patient protection and affordable care act and the patient-centered outcomes research institute. Pain Physician. 2011;14(3):E249-82. Accessed June 18, 2020. http://www.ncbi.nlm.nih.gov/pubmed/21587337

59. Franck LS, McLemore MR, Williams S, et al. Research priorities of women at risk for preterm birth: Findings and a call to action. BMC Pregnancy Childbirth. 2020;20(1):10. doi:10.1186/s12884-019-2664-1

60. Lo B, Zhang T, Leung K, et al. Identifying best approaches for engaging patients and family members in health informatics initiatives: A case study of the Group Priority Sort technique. Res Involv Engagem. 2020;6(1):25. doi:10.1186/s40900-020-00203-8

61. Andress L, Hall T, Davis S, Levine J, Cripps K, Guinn D. Addressing power dynamics in community-engaged research partnerships. J Patient-Reported Outcomes. 2020;4(1):24. doi:10.1186/s41687-020-00191-z

62. Esmail L, Moore E, Rein A. Evaluating patient and stakeholder engagement in research: Moving from theory to practice. J Comp Eff Res. 2015;4(2):133-145. doi:10.2217/cer.14.79

63. Forsythe L, Heckert A, Margolis MK, Schrandt S, Frank L. Methods and impact of engagement in research, from theory to practice and back again: early findings from the Patient-Centered Outcomes Research Institute. Qual Life Res. 2018;27(1):17-31. doi:10.1007/s11136-017-1581-x

64. Kraft SA, McMullen C, Lindberg NM, et al. Integrating stakeholder feedback in translational genomics research: an ethnographic analysis of a study protocol's evolution. Genet Med. 2020;22(6):1094-1101. doi:10.1038/s41436-020-0763-z

65. Forsythe LP, Ellis LE, Edmundson L, et al. Patient and Stakeholder Engagement in the PCORI Pilot Projects: Description and Lessons Learned. J Gen Intern Med. 2016;31(1):13-21. doi:10.1007/s11606-015-3450-z

66. Hemphill R, Forsythe LP, Heckert AL, et al. What motivates patients and caregivers to engage in health research and how engagement affects their lives: Qualitative survey findings. Heal Expect. 2020;23(2):328-336. doi:10.1111/hex.12979

67. Forsythe LP, Carman KL, Szydlowski V, et al. Patient engagement in research: Early findings from the patient-centered outcomes research institute. Health Aff. 2019;38(3):359-367. doi:10.1377/hlthaff.2018.05067

68. Turakhia MP, Desai M, Hedlin H, et al. Rationale and design of a large-scale, app-based study to identify cardiac arrhythmias using a smartwatch: The Apple Heart Study. Am Heart J. 2019;207:66-75. doi:10.1016/J.AHJ.2018.09.002

69. Murray J. The "All of Us" Research Program. N Engl J Med. 2019;381(19):1884. doi:10.1056/NEJMc1912496

70. Health Misinformation — Current Priorities of the U.S. Surgeon General. Accessed January 23, 2024. https://www.hhs.gov/surgeongeneral/priorities/health-misinformation/index.html#:~:text=How health misinformation spreads,well as via search engines.

71. Artificial Intelligence (AI) in Cyber Security | FDM Group | UK. Accessed January 23, 2024. https://www.fdmgroup.com/blog/ai-in-cybersecurity/#:~:text=In the context of cybersecurity,information or making incorrect decisions.

72. Goodfellow I, Pouget-Abadie J, Mirza M, et al. Generative Adversarial Nets. Adv Neural Inf Process Syst 27. Published online 2014:2672-2680. http://papers.nips.cc/paper/5423-generative-adversarial-nets.pdf

73. Radford A, Narasimhan K, Salimans T, Sutskever I. Improving language understanding by generative pre-training. Published online 2018. Accessed January 23, 2024. https://www.mikecaptain.com/resources/pdf/GPT-1.pdf

74. Mehta S, Grant K, Ackery A. Future of blockchain in healthcare: potential to improve the accessibility, security and interoperability of electronic health records. BMJ Heal care informatics. 2020;27(3). doi:10.1136/bmjhci-2020-100217

75. Dexter Hadley. Study Details | Crowdsourcing an Open COVID-19 Imaging Repository for AI Research | ClinicalTrials.gov. Accessed January 8, 2024. https://clinicaltrials.gov/study/NCT05384912

76. (ONC) O of the NC for HIT. Report on Health Information Blocking. Published online 2015:1-39.

# Chapter 3:

# Blockchain Fundamentals and Advanced Applications

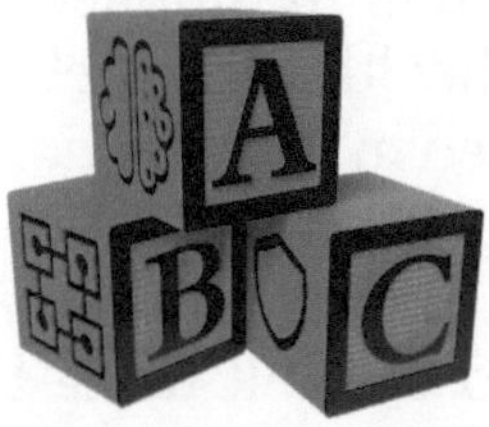


**Vikram Dhillon, MD**
*Clinical Fellow in Hematology/Oncology*

*Houston Methodist Neal Cancer Center*

## *Editor's Note*

In this chapter, Dr. Dhillon shares his expertise in the baseline technology for blockchain and how it can be used in various aspects of healthcare, with particular emphasis on privacy, trust, and privacy. Smart contracts can also add intelligence to records and ensure interoperability.

# Introduction

The genesis of blockchain can be traced to 2008, with the advent of Bitcoin, the inaugural successful cryptocurrency application. Satoshi Nakamoto, an enigmatic figure, proposed a framework for safe, decentralized digital payments, laying the groundwork for contemporary blockchain. Emerging from the niche realm of cryptocurrencies, blockchain technology has transcended its original use-case of providing a mechanism to transfer value between two users in a network. Since then, its promise of allowing trustless transactions and between two parties in a synchronous manner has caught the imagination of developers across diverse industries.

The blockchain constitutes a distributed ledger system positioned to revolutionize various industries from finance to digital health, supply chain management to voting frameworks. Its potential is rooted in its exceptional capacity to generate a secure, transparent, and tamper-resistant record of transactions, cultivating trust and accountability in a world replete with digital interactions. Ethereum, the first project to be built using the blockchain paradigm, expanded its capabilities to sustain programmatic smart contracts, paving the way for a new wave of decentralized applications. Presently, blockchain research and development is proceeding at a very rapid pace and focused on building the infrastructure necessary to enable collaboration, transactions, and new forms of governance in a digital era.

This chapter starts with defining the core components of a blockchain and the major types of blockchain implementations currently available. Then, we dive into the concept of privacy on the blockchain and technologies that are making it possible. After that, we delve into consensus mechanisms that are heavily being researched and deployed. We then discuss features available in next generation blockchains such as smart contracts, decentralized applications, Decentralized Autonomous Organizations. We showcase large-scale applications built on newer blockchains such as DeFi and Stablecoins. Finally, we conclude with an outlook of what the future holds for the blockchain world.

# Defining the Blockchain

Imagine a digital ledger, not nestled within an isolated server but replicated across a global network of computers. Each entry, or "block," retains data timestamped (in the form of addresses) and cryptographic signature linked to the preceding one, configuring a succession of blocks in a chain. This constitutes the essence of a blockchain: a communal, immutable archive of each transaction, verifiable by any network constituent. At the most fundamental level, a blockchain validates a trade between two addresses (entities on the blockchain) in a trustless fashion. Users rely on software called a wallet to interact with the blockchain, create transactions and broadcast the transactions for verification to the network. Once verified, the transactions are cryptographically mined, compiled into a block and added to the blockchain.

Creating new blocks involves three key steps: minting, hashing, and chaining. Minting begins with miners competing to solve a cryptographic puzzle for a reward. The victor earns the right to "mint" a new block, encapsulating recent transactions from the network. These transactions are time stamped and cryptographically signed, resembling data parcels waiting for secure delivery. Hashing safeguards the newly minted block. A unique fingerprint, generated by feeding the block's data (including the prior block's hash) into a cryptographic hashing function, acts as an immutable seal. Any attempts to modify the block's contents will lead to a new hash that does not resemble the original hash at time of block creation. This property makes the blocks tamper evident. Finally, chaining integrates the new block into the existing blockchain and announces it to the network. This process of adding new blocks creates chronological order with a history available to every user of the network, and over time, longstanding histories allow for more reliable transactions.

## The Blockchain Quartet

The following four principles are crucial to any blockchain implementation, and we will refer to them throughout the chapter:

**Decentralization:** No central body controls the blockchain. All network-based decisions are bound to a consensus mechanism distributed among network nodes, constituting a system resistant to manipulation and isolated points of failure.

**Transparency:** All transactions are perceptible to any participant on the network, encouraging trust and accountability. Blockchain explorers allow a user possessing appropriate knowledge to examine the entire open volume and even trace transactions if necessary. In certain deployments, users may need appropriate cryptographic keys to trace transactions.

**Immutability:** Once inscribed within a block, data cannot be modified or erased. Discrepancies can only be rectified by incorporating new blocks, preserving the chain's integrity and factual precision. Deviations in the network, called forks, are all available as version history of the blockchain for inspection.

**Security:** Cryptography is crucial in maintaining blockchain security. Each block is hashed, producing a unique digital imprint connected to the preceding block. Any tampering endeavor would perturb the entire chain, alerting the network. Given the high amount of computational power necessary to break the cryptographic hashes, an attacker would have to control 51% of the network.

While the core principles of decentralization and immutability are common denominators, modern blockchains come in distinct flavors, each catering to varying application vertical and access privileges. To navigate the blockchain landscape, we can broadly classify most implementations into three categories:

**Public Blockchains:** The original implementation of a blockchain. Anyone can participate as a network member or host a node. Public blockchains power Bitcoin and Ethereum, where transactions are transparent, and consensus is achieved through open competition among miners. Their strength lies in unparalleled security and trust, but scalability and privacy concerns can limit broader applicability, especially in the context of building regulatory applications.

**Private Blockchains:** Implementations of a blockchain where user privileges and access control lists are necessary and maintained by a trusted single entity. Network participants are pre-approved, this allows more granular control over who has access to advanced features such as creating new smart contracts, on-chain contract execution and voting. Businesses seeking secure, customized platforms for internal operations or supply chain management often favor private blockchains. While governance remains centralized, transaction confidentiality and efficient performance benefit all network participants.

**Consortium Blockchains:** This is a hybrid between the two previous implementations. A public/private interface between individual users, groups of organizations such as banks or healthcare providers represented by users and policy makers who may be observers or validators on the network. All entities on the network are categorized into user-groups where each group has well-defined access privileges. This allows for open governance and shared responsibility on the network, as well as an avenue to onboard new members from the public-facing side. These hybrid chains combine the security and control of private networks with the transparency and partial decentralization of public ones. Ideal for large consortia projects requiring both trust and accountability.

Choosing the appropriate blockchain implementation depends on specific applications, types of users as well as balancing governance needs. Let's reapply the blockchain quartet in order to clarify these decisions:

- **Accessibility:** Public networks offer open access, while private and consortium chains involve permissioned participation.
- **Security:** Decentralization of public chains enhances security, while private and consortium models offer additional roles and user-group provisions.
- **Scalability:** Public chains may face scalability challenges and rely on publicly available nodes, while private and consortium networks will often have dedicated infrastructure that can be optimized for specific use cases.
- **Transparency:** Public chains offer full transparency, while private and consortium blockchains will need to agree upon what can be shared completely publicly and data will be internally approved by independent validators, however, the details may be sensitive business operations and cannot be shared.

# Privacy and Security on the Blockchain: Striking a Balance

While newer blockchain implementations have made significant strides in enhancing user privacy and security, inherent limitations in public blockchains and their wallet-based transaction systems persist. These limitations primarily concern the pseudonymous nature of public addresses, the lack of full anonymity for wallets, and the inherent traceability of transactions. Public blockchains maintain a high degree of transparency via the availability of transaction histories associated with blockchain addresses. This transparency can compromise user privacy as transactions are visible to anyone and given the appropriate circumstances, advanced statistical analysis techniques can link multiple transactions to a single entity, de-anonymize the users and further attach wallet addresses to track the flow of transactions. Newer cryptographic mechanisms are being developed to enhance privacy that we will discuss next.

## Privacy Enhancement via Zero-Knowledge Proofs and Ring Signatures

In addressing the need for privacy on blockchain networks, advanced cryptographic techniques have been developed to bolster the confidentiality of transactions and obfuscate user identities. Two noteworthy methods are zero-knowledge proofs and ring signatures. Zero-knowledge proofs (ZKPs) allow two parties to prove the authenticity of a statement without revealing any underlying information. In the context of blockchain, ZKPs enable the verification of transactions without disclosing the sender, recipient, or transaction amount. This technology ensures that only the necessary information is divulged to maintain the integrity of a blockchain, while preserving the sensitive data.

Let's walk through an example: Imagine Alice wants to convince Bob she has access to a specific block on the blockchain without revealing its location. In a ZKP, Alice acts as the "prover" and Bob as the "verifier." Here's how it unfolds:

1. **Commitment:** Alice commits to the block's location by applying a cryptographic function, creating a unique "commitment" like a sealed box.

2. **Challenge:** Bob sends random challenges, asking Alice to prove knowledge of the block without revealing its location. Think of Bob peeking into the box without opening it.

3. **Proof Generation:** Alice uses her knowledge of the block's location to generate a "proof" using mathematical algorithms. This proof acts as a key that unlocks the "commitment" box without revealing its contents.

4. **Verification:** Bob verifies the proof against the commitment. If valid, Bob gains confidence that Alice knows the block's location without learning its specific details.

The proof systems in ZKPs are technically backbone that enable development of applications and come in two flavors: Interactive and non-interactive. In interactive proof systems, a prover and verifier engage in a series of challenges and responses, ensuring proof validity through probabilistic verification (for instance, Schnorr signatures in Bitcoin). On the other hand, in non-Interactive proof systems such as ZK-SNARKs (Zero-Knowledge Succinct Non-interactive ARguments of Knowledge), the proofs are pre-computed offline and efficient verification on-chain written in libraries such as Marlin ZK protocol. SNARKs often utilize SNARK-friendly circuits to encode computations and verify their execution without divulging details. Circuits are then compiled into low-level arithmetic circuits for proof generation and verification. Specialized libraries like ZoKrate facilitate circuit creation and proof generation in languages like Solidity. Then, dedicated verification circuits are deployed on-chain, enabling lightweight execution of proof validation. Once a proof-system, statement validation mechanism, as well as a prover and validator construct is deployed, a smart contract can use these lower-level circuits to trigger actions based on the verified proof. ZKPs hold immense potential for enhancing blockchain privacy in specific domains:

- **Blockchain-based loans:** Users can prove they meet financial requirements for a loan without revealing their account balances.
- **Identity Management:** Users can verify their name/institutional affiliation for access to sensitive content without disclosing all personal details.
- **Medical Records:** Patients can grant access to specific medical data to healthcare providers without sharing their entire medical history.

Implementations of ZKPs have a few unique challenges:

- **Computational burden:** Complex ZKPs can require significant computational resources that can impact transaction speed and increase the overhead.
- **Implementation complexity:** Developing and integrating ZKPs into existing blockchain systems can be complex and require developers with specialized expertise.
- **Circuit design complexity:** Encoding complex computations into SNARK-friendly circuits can be challenging.
- **Verification costs:** On-chain verification incur gas costs and restrain larger on-chain verification operations.

Despite these challenges, ZKPs are an active area of research and development with regards to enhancing privacy on the blockchain. With more sophisticated libraries handling lower-level implementation, ZKPs can showcase how blockchains enable privacy-derived transactions.

Another privacy-enhancing measure for transactions is the concept of ring signatures. Here, a cryptographic signature allows a user to sign a transaction using their own private key along with a ring of other public keys belonging to other network members. This makes the search for the original user from the ring very computationally expensive, effectively obscuring the source of the transaction. Here's a breakdown of how it works between Bob and Alice:

1. **Building the Ring:** Bob will be the signing user in our case, and he wants to send a transaction to Alice. His wallet uses his private key, combines it with several public keys of other users to create a ring. These public keys can be chosen at random from the blockchain or follow specified rules.

2. **Creating the Signature:** Bob's wallet then uses the ring as well as his private key to create a signature for the transaction. This signature mathematically guarantees the validity of the transaction without revealing any identities.

3. **Verification on the Blockchain:** The signed transaction is broadcast to the blockchain network. Anyone on the network can verify the signature using the combined public keys of the ring, but they cannot isolate the specific keys used to sign or build the ring.

A prominent example of implementing ring signatures is the cryptocurrency Monero. Although ring signatures create "bulky transactions" due to the additional public key data added to a transaction, the enhanced privacy and resistance to transaction tracking are reasonable trade-offs for users.

# Consensus mechanisms on a blockchain

One of the most striking features of a blockchain is the consensus mechanism. A mathematical construct by which nodes in a distributed system agree upon a single version of events or transactions. This ensures that all nodes in the network have a consistent view of the state of the system, even when they are operating asynchronously. In other words, it enables nodes to reach agreement on the order of events without relying on a central authority. For a blockchain to function in a trustless manner, consensus mechanisms are a key innovation. There are four general consensus mechanisms in use at present:

1. **Proof of Work (PoW):** The most widely used consensus mechanism in blockchain networks. Nodes compete with each other to solve complex mathematical puzzles to validate transactions and create new blocks. The node that solves the puzzle first gets to add a new block to the chain and is rewarded with cryptocurrency. PoW is energy-intensive but provides strong security against malicious actors.

2. **Proof of Stake (PoS):** In proof of stake (PoS), validators are chosen to create blocks based on the amount of cryptocurrency they hold (i.e., their "stake"). The idea behind PoS is that those who have more at stake in the network will be more motivated to act honestly and maintain its integrity. PoS is typically seen as a more energy-efficientand less wasteful alternative to proof of work (PoW), as it doesn't require expensive hardware to mine blocks. PoS consensus algorithms power some of the most technically innovative blockchain projects and may become the de facto consensus mechanism in the near future.

3. **Delegated Proof of Stake (DPoS):** A type of proof of stake (PoS) consensus that allows users to vote for validators who can propose new blocks. Validators with more votes have higher chances of being selected to create new blocks. DPoS is faster than PoW and reduces the carbon footprint associated with mining. DPoS, in comparison to PoS, is a more democratic way of choosing who verifies the next block, allowing a diverse group of people to participate in the process since it's based on earned reputation as a lawful staker and not overall token ownership. Additionally, because there are a limited number of validators, DPoS allows the network to reach consensus more quickly.

4. **Proof of Elapsed Time (PoET):** Proof of elapsed time (PoET) is a type of proof of stake (PoS) algorithm that utilizes a timer to determine when a transaction is added to the blockchain. Each transaction is time stamped with the current time, and the next transaction cannot be processed until a certain amount of time has passed since the last transaction was recorded. This helps to prevent double-spending attacks and ensures that transactions are processed in a predictable manner. PoET implementations have been used in permissioned blockchain networks, where the validators are pre-approved and the network operates under a fixed set of rules.

5. **Byzantine Fault Tolerance (BFT):** A consensus algorithm designed

to handle faulty or malicious nodes in a decentralized system. BFT requires nodes to communicate with each other to ensure that all nodes agree on the state of the system. Therefore, BFT-based systems are more resilient to network failure and can tolerate a certain percentage of faulty nodes. It is often used in private blockchain networks and more popular implementations include PBFT (Practical Byzantine Fault Tolerance) and RAFT (Reliable Asynchronous Fault-Tolerant).

Although the earlier blockchain implementations relied heavily on PoW algorithms, there are several limitations to PoW. The computational intensity of PoW leads to significant amounts of electricity usage and for networks at scale, for instance, at the height of Bitcoin, energy usage was becoming a very relevant issue. To design consensus algorithms with sustainability in mind, newer generation mechanisms such as PoS gained popularity. The time necessary to create hashes, sign the blocks and propagate to a network within PoW consensus also becomes a hurdle as the network scales. Efficient consensus such as DPoS focus on node-based voting of validators which are much smaller in number, can approve transactions more rapidly and reduce latency for the network overall. In private or consortia blockchains, any consensus scheme that fits the requirements of the organization and goals of the participants can be chosen. A blockchain network with scalable consensus becomes a robust platform for on-chain application development. In the next sections, we will discuss this phenomenon in-depth.

# Smart contracts and on-chain capabilities

Smart contracts are self-executing contracts between two parties where the contract terms are written directly as lines of code. Once deployed on a blockchain, the contract carries out its specified obligations autonomously and immutably, without the need for intermediaries. Although the theoretical concept dates back to the mid-90s, it was first deployed in a decentralized context on the Ethereum blockchain in 2015. Since then, writing sophisticated smart contracts with better data abstraction and virtual- runtime environments for executing a contract on-chain have become the cornerstone of next generation blockchains. The process of creating and executing smart contracts requires eight components as described below:

**State:** Represents the terms of contract written in a programmatic language. This includes the current status of the agreement, state variables such as payment amounts, item ownership details, completion terms, terms of contract revocation or partial completion.

**Storage:** A mechanism for the contract to store data beyond the blockchain state including sensitive participant information and results from off-chain computations

**Triggers and Events:** Smart contracts can be programmed to execute based on specific triggers or pre-specified events on the blockchain such as transfer of funds, new transactions by a user or a fork in the chain itself. These triggers can lead to auto-execution of the code defined in the contract without the need for a third-party.

**Functions:** Actions defined in a smart contract that can be programmatically carried out on the blockchain once triggered by a participant, by participant interactions, or a pre-defined event.

**Rules:** The logic that all functions written in a smart contrast must follow. The rules provide an abstraction layer for how a contract must execute functions, the scope of those functions and how changes in blockchain state should be recorded by the contract. These rules are written in contract-specific language (for instance Solidity for Ethereum) and understood by the executing mechanism on the chain.

**Execution environment:** Smart contracts are executed in an isolated and secure environment that interfaces with the underlying blockchain. Such environments allow for programmatic execution and state manipulation to happen in sync with the whole network. In Ethereum, the Ethereum Virtual Machine (EVM) is responsible for smart-contract execution.

**Gas:** Computational resources are scarce on a blockchain, therefore, smart contracts must be written in a resource-aware manner. To implement this fundamental rule, each contrast must pay gas, a measure of computational effort on a blockchain to execute the contract. For each blockchain, gas is paid in native currency prior to execution, such as Ether for Ethereum.

**Oracles:** In some cases, a smart contract may require access to external data or the outcomes of real-world events that are not accessible to a blockchain. An oracle is a trusted, semi-autonomous agent that can bring in external sources of data and verify off-chain events for the smart contract to execute and react to real-events.

# Decentralized applications (dApps)

A decentralized application (dApp) is the decentralized equivalent of a traditional mobile or web application, operating on a blockchain network. Unlike traditional web applications that rely on a centralized server to manage requests and responses, dApps use a decentralized architecture to distribute processing tasks among peers on the network.

A dApp stack is composed of various layers and tools that work together to provide a seamless experience for users. At the base layer is the blockchain, which serves as the foundation for the dApp's decentralized architecture. Popular blockchain platforms for dApp development include Ethereum, Cardano, and EOS. The dApp's backend is typically built using a combination of smart contracts and decentralized storage solutions. The smart contract is a critical component of a dApp, as it acts as the governing logic for the application. It specifies the rules and constraints that govern the behavior of the dApp, and it is responsible for executing the desired actions and updates to the back-end database. Popular smart contract platforms include Solidity for Ethereum and Chaincode for Hyperledger Fabric. Decentralized storage solutions, such as InterPlanetary File System (IPFS) and Swarm, are used to store and retrieve data in a decentralized manner. IPFS is a content-addressed file system that allows for the distribution of files across a network of nodes, making it ideal for storing large datasets. Swarm is a decentralized storage solution that uses a honeycomb-shaped data structure to store and retrieve data. The middleware layer of the dApp stack is responsible for handling communication between the frontend and backend. Web3.js is a JavaScript library that enables the interaction between web browsers and decentralized applications. It provides a simple and consistent API for building decentralized applications. The frontend of the dApp stack is built using modern web frameworks such as React, Angular, and Vue.js. These frameworks provide a robust set of features for building responsive and interactive user interfaces. The UI is designed to be intuitive and user-friendly, allowing users to easily interact with the decentralized application and ignore the inner-workings of the application.

Overall, the architecture of a dApp is designed to be modular, flexible, and highly scalable. By distributing processing tasks among peers on the network, dApps can achieve greater security, transparency, and resilience, while also offering the potential for greater performance and scalability. Collections of dApps are being curated and organized into blockchain-specific app-stores, and eventually, dApps will become platform agnostic to run on any blockchain.

Marketplaces for dApps are platforms that enable the discovery, sale, and exchange of dApps. These marketplaces provide a central location for users to find and acquire dApps, simplifying the process of accessing and utilizing them. Some examples of dApp marketplaces include:

- **Dappstore:** A decentralized marketplace for dApps, built on the Ethereum blockchain. Users can browse and download dApps, and developers can list their dApps for sale.
- **State of the Dapps:** A directory of dApps, featuring a curated selection of high-quality dApps across various categories.
- **Dappradar:** A comprehensive directory of dApps, with detailed information on each dApp, including ratings, reviews, and usage statistics.
- **Dapphub:** A decentralized marketplace for dApps, allowing developers to showcase and sell their dApps.
- **Superfluid:** A decentralized marketplace for streaming media, allowing creators to monetize their content through micropayments.

These marketplaces provide a valuable service to the dApp ecosystem by aggregating and organizing dApps in one place, making it easier for users to discover and access them. They also serve as a platform for developers to showcase their work and reach a wider audience, ultimately driving growth and innovation in the field of dApps.

# Decentralized autonomous organizations (DAOs)

Decentralized autonomous organizations (DAOs) emerged in 2016 as a novel form of blockchain-based organization created and executed by smart contracts on next generation blockchains like Ethereum. When compared to traditional organizations, DAOs rely on an open governance structure: All members can propose new ideas, debate issues, and vote on topics that directly impact the DAO's direction. DAOs rely on blockchain technology to provide the underlying consensus mechanism and establish a transparent, auditable record of all actions and decisions made by the organization according to agreed-upon mechanisms by the members. Participation rights like voting and access to the organization assets are managed based on possession of governance or voting tokens on the underlying blockchain. The incentives for all members of a DAO and the rules they abide by are encoded in the smart contract and participants can propose changes using the DAOs tokenization system.

The first versions of DAOs were designed to have a set of smart contracts that managed assets contributed by participants in exchange for voting rights. The rules of governance were encoded in those smart contracts that also allowed voting decisions on the stored assets and monetary transfers. A high profile exploit of the first public DAO on Ethereum led to a revision in the base-layer of security for smart contracts that coordinate DAO creation, decision making mechanisms and participation rights. Now, there are more sophisticated and well-tested smart contract frameworks dedicated to DAOs. Early DAOs adopted simple majority vote-based governance where proposals were open for token holders to vote on with their allocation of tokens equating to voting power. This follows a one-token-one-vote system where distributed stakeholders signal preferences on token distributions, protocol changes, and DAO-spending. As DAOs have evolved, governance has grown more advanced, moving beyond simple majoritarian voting to account for voter apathy, enable representative structures, and manage different classes of stakeholders. Variations include liquid democracy systems enabling proxy voting, reputation-weighted voting where participation and contribution boost influence, prediction voting for gauging sentiment, and quadratic voting to privilege minority stakeholders. As DAOs expand to encompass larger consortia, more complex governing structures are being incorporated. Multi-chamber governance resembles representative democracy, incorporating different branches for executive, legislative, and judicial functions to provide checks and balances. Tokenized voting power can also be managed through locked staking, vesting schedules, and reputation systems to reduce sybil attacks and encourage long-term alignment. Similarly, new proposal processes specific to the industry are also being used such as varying consensus thresholds, voting durations, mechanisms to manage proposals, and spacetime voting.

## StableCoins

Stablecoins are a type of cryptocurrency whose value is pegged to a stable asset, such as the US dollar or gold, in order to mitigate the volatility inherent in other cryptocurrencies. The goal of stablecoins is to provide a more stable and reliable means of conducting transactions and storing value in the cryptocurrency space. There are several types of stablecoins, each with its own underlying asset and method of stabilization. Some common examples of stablecoins include:

- **Fiat-collateralized stablecoins:** These stablecoins are collateralized by fiat currencies, such as the US dollar or euro. Examples of fiat-collateralized stablecoins include USDC (US Dollar Coin), TUSD (TrueUSD), and GUSD (Gemini Dollar).

- **Cryptocurrency-collateralized stablecoins:** These stablecoins are collateralized by other cryptocurrencies, such as Bitcoin or Ether. Examples of cryptocurrency-collateralized stablecoins include PAXOS Standard (PAX), and Binance USD (BUSD).

- **Gold-backed stablecoins:** These stablecoins are collateralized by physical gold. Examples of gold-backed stablecoins include Perpetual Protocol (PERP) and Aurora DAO (AURA).

- **Hybrid stablecoins:** These stablecoins combine two or more different types of collateral, such as both fiat currency and cryptocurrency. Examples of hybrid stablecoins include DAI (Multi-Collateral Dai) and KNC (Kyber Network Crystal).

Stablecoins have several potential benefits, including:

- **Price stability:** Stablecoins are designed to maintain a stable value relative to a stable asset, reducing the volatility often seen in other cryptocurrencies.

- **Improved usability:** Stablecoins can make it easier for non-technical users to adopt and use cryptocurrencies, as they are less susceptible to volatility of cryptomarkets.

- **Increased adoption:** By providing a more stable and reliable means of conducting transactions, stablecoins may encourage greater adoption of cryptocurrencies in a wider range of applications.

At present, stablecoins face regulatory uncertainty and currently, there is a lack of clear guidance from the SEC and other organizations on adoption and use of stablecoins. Additionally, if stablecoins do become heavily regulated given their reliance on fiat currency, the centralization process can compromise the stability of the coin.

# Decentralized Finance

DeFi, short for Decentralized Finance, refers to the practice of using decentralized technologies such as blockchain and smart contracts to build financial systems. These systems aim to provide financial services that are more accessible, transparent, and equitable than their traditional counterparts. DeFi also offers opportunities for lending and borrowing in a decentralized manner. A few popular DeFi platforms are presented below:

**MakerDAO:** MakerDAO is a decentralized lending platform that allows users to generate a stablecoin called DAI by locking up their cryptocurrencies as collateral. The interest rate on this loan is determined by a decentralized oracle based on the collateral and the total amount of debt in the system, rather than by a centralized institution. This creates a dynamic and adaptive interest rate mechanism that responds to market forces. For example, if the value of BTC increases, the interest rate on DAI generated from BTC as collateral would decrease, encouraging more people to lock up their BTC and mint DAI.

**Compound:** Compound is a decentralized lending platform that allows users to earn interest on their cryptocurrencies by supplying them as collateral. The platform uses an algorithmic interest rate model that takes into account the current market conditions and the risk associated with the supplied assets. For example, if the price of ETH increases, the interest rate on ETH supplied as collateral would increase, attracting more users to supply their ETH and earn higher returns.

**Aave:** Aave is a decentralized lending platform that allows users to borrow and lend a variety of assets, including cryptocurrencies. The platform uses a reputation-based credit scoring system to evaluate the creditworthiness of borrowers and sets interest rates accordingly. For example, if a borrower has a good reputation and a strong track record of repayment, they may be eligible for lower interest rates compared to a borrower with a poor reputation.

**Uniswap:** Uniswap is a decentralized exchange that allows users to trade a variety of assets, including ERC-20 tokens. The platform uses a unique pricing mechanism that is based on the ratio of the reserve assets held in the liquidity pool. For example, if the reserve asset is USDC and the trading asset is ETH, the price of ETH would be determined by the ratio of the number of USDC to ETH in the liquidity pool. Through Uniswap, participants can swap tokens with one another, benefiting from the pool's depth and liquidity. Additionally, Uniswap offers a feature known as "liquidity providers," which allows users to earn a share of transaction fees in exchange for providing liquidity to the pool. These pools act as a shared resource for participants, allowing them to engage in peer-to-peer trades without relying on traditional centralized exchanges.

**SushiSwap:** Another prominent decentralized exchange that operates on the Ethereum blockchain. Similar to Uniswap, SushiSwap provides a liquidity pool for a variety of assets, however, SushiSwap differs in that it charges a small fee on all trades, which goes toward funding the development of new features and improvements to the platform.

**Yearn Finance:** Yearn Finance is a decentralized investment management platform that allows users to invest in a variety of assets, including cryptocurrencies. The platform uses a suite of algorithms to optimize the allocation of assets within the portfolio, taking into account factors such as risk tolerance, return expectations, and diversification. For example, if a user has a high risk tolerance and expects higher returns, the platform might allocate a larger percentage of their portfolio to risky assets such as Bitcoin.

**Curve:** A decentralized liquidity pool that offers a novel yield farming (generating additional income by lending or staking assets in a decentralized system) approach by allowing participants to earn interest on their assets without the need for complex mathematical calculations. Curve achieves this by automatically adjusting the interest rates offered to borrowers based on the volume of assets in the pool. This approach helps to maintain a stable balance between supply and demand, resulting in more predictable yields for participating lenders.

Overall, DeFi represents a significant shift towards decentralized financial systems, which have the potential to increase efficiency, reduce costs, and provide greater autonomy and control for individuals and organizations alike.

## Future Outlook

To conclude on the potential of blockchain technology, we present an outlook on the future of blockchain technology and the new developments happening in the blockchain world:

- **Layer 1 and 2 Scalability Solutions:** Scalability remains a crucial hurdle for wider blockchain adoption. Layer 1 advancements like sharding, blockchains with efficient consensus mechanisms, and Layer 2 scaling solutions like sidechains and rollups will continue to be actively developed and implemented, fostering higher transaction throughput and lower fees.

- **Interoperability and Cross-Chain Communication:** Fragmented blockchain ecosystems hinder data and asset flow. Cross-chain bridges and interoperable protocols are actively under development to better connect isolated blockchain networks using techniques like atomic swaps and distributed message relays. This will enable seamless communication and value transfer between different chains, creating decentralized economies at scale.

- **Quantum-Resistant Cryptography:** With the looming threat of quantum computers, migrating to post-quantum cryptography schemes will be vital for securing blockchain networks and safeguarding digital assets. Research in lattice-based and multivariate cryptography holds significant promise in this regard.

- **Privacy-Preserving Technologies:** Balancing blockchain's transparency with user privacy is crucial for real-world adoption. Zero-knowledge proofs, ring signatures, and homomorphic encryption are actively being developed to enable confidential transactions and computation while maintaining the benefits of blockchain's immutability and auditability.

- **Artificial Intelligence and Machine Learning Integration:** Integrating AI and ML into blockchain systems can enhance performance, optimize resource allocation, and automate decision-making. This opens doors for intelligent contract execution, predictive analytics, and dynamic fee adjustments.

- **Decentralized Identity and Reputation Management:** Blockchain-based self-sovereign identity (SSI) solutions empower individuals to control their personal data and online identity. Verifiable credentials and reputation systems on blockchains can revolutionize data ownership, access control, and trust in online interactions.

- **Metaverse and Web3 Integration:** Blockchain technology will play a fundamental role in powering the decentralized infrastructure for the metaverse. Secure digital ownership, asset management, and interoperable token economies will be crucial for building immersive and interactive virtual worlds.

- **Supply Chain Management:** Blockchain's ability to track provenance and establish trust can revolutionize supply chain management. Tracking goods, verifying provenance, and automating logistics processes will optimize efficiency and transparency across industries. The integration of blockchain technology with IoT devices has the potential to make supply chain management even more efficient.

- **Energy Consumption:** One of the major criticisms of blockchain technology is its energy consumption, which can be quite high due to the computational requirements of mining and validation. To address this issue, researchers are exploring alternative consensus mechanisms, such as proof of stake and delegated proof of stake, which require significantly less energy to operate.

- **Enterprise Adoption:** Blockchain technology is expected to gain widespread adoption in enterprises, particularly in industries such as banking, healthcare, and supply chain management. As more businesses recognize the benefits of blockchain, such as transparency, traceability, and immutability, they will begin to implement it in their operations.

- **Regulatory Landscape and Legal Considerations:** Developing a clear and adaptable regulatory framework for blockchain and digital assets is critical for enabling responsible innovation and fostering mass adoption. Addressing concerns around consumer protection, anti-money laundering, and taxation will be crucial for mainstream adoption.

In conclusion, this chapter has covered the fundamental concepts and advanced features of blockchain technology. We began by discussing the basics of blockchain, including distributed ledger technology, consensus mechanisms, and the importance of decentralization. From there, we delved deeper into the topic, covering more advanced features such as smart contracts, decentralized applications, DAOs and blockchain-based applications such as DeFi and Stablecoins. Each of these topics was discussed in detail, highlighting their significance and potential impact on various industries. Overall, this chapter aims to provide a reader with a comprehensive understanding of the core principles and cutting-edge capabilities of blockchain technology.

# References


1. Attaran, M., 2022. Blockchain technology in healthcare: Challenges and opportunities. International Journal of Healthcare Management, 15(1), pp.70-83.

2. Bhutta, M.N.M., Khwaja, A.A., Nadeem, A., Ahmad, H.F., Khan, M.K., Hanif, M.A., Song, H., Alshamari, M. and Cao, Y., 2021. A survey on blockchain technology: Evolution, architecture and security. Ieee Access, 9, pp.61048-61073.

3. Dutta, P., Choi, T.M., Somani, S. and Butala, R., 2020. Blockchain technology in supply chain operations: Applications, challenges and research opportunities. Transportation research part e: Logistics and transportation review, 142, p.102067.

4. Fernandez-Carames, T.M. and Fraga-Lamas, P., 2020. Towards post-quantum blockchain: A review on blockchain cryptography resistant to quantum computing attacks. IEEE access, 8, pp.21091-21116.

5. Fiedler, I. and Ante, L., 2023. Stablecoins. In The Emerald Handbook on Cryptoassets: Investment Opportunities and Challenges (pp. 93-105). Emerald Publishing Limited.

6. Ghosh, A., Gupta, S., Dua, A. and Kumar, N., 2020. Security of Cryptocurrencies in blockchain technology: State-of-art, challenges and future prospects. Journal of Network and Computer Applications, 163, p.102635.

7. Guo, H. and Yu, X., 2022. A survey on blockchain technology and its security. Blockchain: research and applications, 3(2), p.100067.

8. Harvey, C.R., Ramachandran, A. and Santoro, J., 2021. DeFi and the Future of Finance. John Wiley & Sons.

9. Hussain, A.A. and Al-Turjman, F., 2021. Artificial intelligence and blockchain: A review. Transactions on emerging telecommunications technologies, 32(9), p.e4268.

10. Javaid, M., Haleem, A., Singh, R.P., Khan, S. and Suman, R., 2021. Blockchain technology applications for Industry 4.0: A literature-based review. Blockchain: Research and Applications, 2(4), p.100027.

11. Pop, C., Cioara, T., Anghel, I., Antal, M. and Salomie, I., 2020. Blockchain based decentralized applications: Technology review and development guidelines. arXiv preprint arXiv:2003.07131.

12. Sanka, A.I., Irfan, M., Huang, I. and Cheung, R.C., 2021. A survey of breakthrough in blockchain technology: Adoptions, applications, challenges and future research. Computer communications, 169, pp.179-201.

13. Tagde, P., Tagde, S., Bhattacharya, T., Tagde, P., Chopra, H., Akter, R., Kaushik, D. and Rahman, M.H., 2021. Blockchain and artificial intelligence technology in e-Health. Environmental Science and Pollution Research, 28, pp.52810-52831.

14. Wang, Q. and Su, M., 2020. Integrating blockchain technology into the energy sector—from theory of blockchain to research and application of energy blockchain. Computer Science Review, 37, p.100275.

# Chapter 4:

## Enabling Trust, Identity, Privacy, Protection, Safety, and Security: IEEE/UL TIPPSS for Clinical IoT

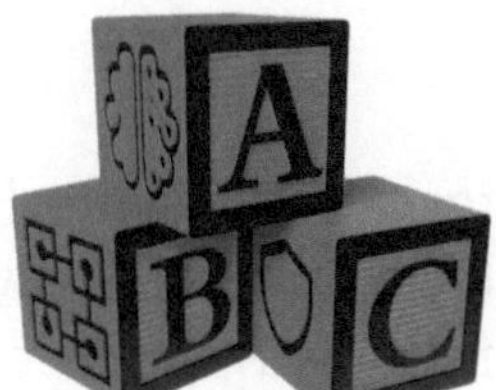


**Florence Hudson**
*Executive Director & Principal Investigator*

*US NSF, NIH and Department of Transportation*

**Ken Fuchs**
*Director Standards and Process Management*

*Dräger*

**William Harding, PhD**
*Distinguished Techincal Fellow & Professor*

### *Editor's Note*

At the Intelligent Health Summit, our authors presented an excellent overview of some of the latest cybersecurity practices and emerging standards that will meet the coming challenges of ABC. Fundamentals of AI, blockchain, and cybersecurity will be enabled because of emerging standards like TIPPSS and the efforts to advance standards that can unlock the power and potential of these technologies for healthcare applications. Focus on privacy, security, and interoperability will drive the utility and adoption. The following is a transcript of their excellent presentation.

## Florence Hudson

I've been a VP at IBM so, you know, we can hang with the executives and the geeks, William and I. My name is Florence Hudson. I'm Executive director and Principal Investigator for the Big Data Innovation Hub at Columbia University, funded by the US National Science Foundation, National Institutes of Health, and Department of Transportation. And I'll be moderating our panel today. But basically, William and I are going to be going back and forth because we both bring a lot of knowledge and passion to this whole area. And so, I'd like William to introduce himself next.

## William Harding, Ph.D.

Sure. So, I'm William Harding, a PhD in technology integration, formerly just recently retired from Medtronic as a Distinguished Technical Fellow, and presently a Full Professor at Trine University and Graduate Studies

## Florence Hudson

Wonderful. And William just brings so much knowledge. Not only in designing and manufacturing, but using some of these devices, and he's probably going to share some of those stories with you which makes it very real.

Ken Fuchs can't be with us today. He's one of the other officers we have at the IEEE/Underwriters Laboratories working group that we're leading. Ken is Director of Standards and Process Management at Dräeger Medical Systems. And the other person who can't be with us today, was the other officer, the Co-Vice Chair for our working group, Mitch Parker from Indiana University Health, and he can't be here today either, but they're both with us in spirit because we actually talk every week, whether we need it or not as we've been developing this standard. So, what we're going to talk about today is enabling TIPPSS (Trust, Identity, Privacy, Protection, Safety and Security). And our first application is for clinical IoT devices, clinical Internet of Things devices. And so, we're gonna go into why we're doing this and how we're doing it and how it affects you. And we're also gonna be putting a few little links in the chat in case anybody wants to click on any of the cool publications that we're gonna be talking about. So, let's get started.

So, our discussion topics today are going to be first starting with the emerging threat landscape.

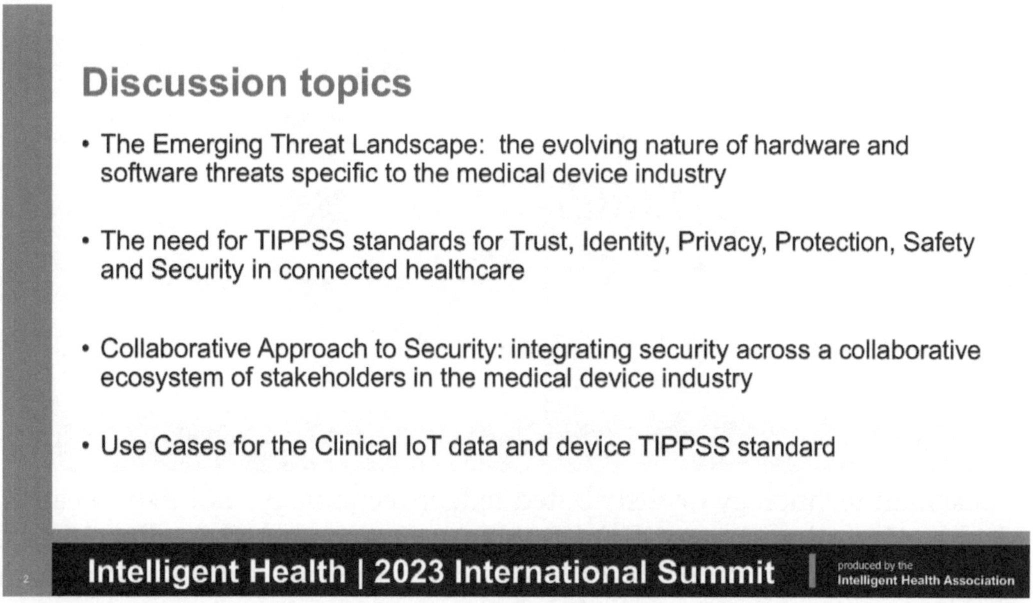


The evolving nature of hardware and software threats specific to the medical device industry. And there are so many new technologies as we know, and William and I will both be talking about those, the benefits that they bring, but also the threats and the risks that are associated with them. The need for this TIPPSS standard for Trust, Identity, Privacy, Protection, Safety and Security and connected healthcare. And we see this as the first step in a longer series of potential standards across different cyber-physical infrastructures whether it could be energy grids or autonomous vehicles, or all sorts of things. And we're actually talking with IEEE and NIST about doing that. Then we're going to talk about the collaborative approach needed for security to integrate security across the whole ecosystem of stakeholders in the medical device industry. And then we're going to talk about use cases for the clinical IoT data and device TIPPSS standard. We also are giving you extra credit today. We are going to be going deep into all of the elements of trust and identity, privacy, protection, safety, and security. So, we hope you get a whole lot out of this.

So, let's start with the bigger picture. This is something you can say to anybody in a boardroom, you know. So, this is something you can take with you wherever you go. And the advanced technologies that we're enabling these days are so powerful. They're enabling digital transformation, Internet of Things, gathering data anywhere, sensing and actuating. You know, sensing what's going on and then actuating, changing something, making something happen.

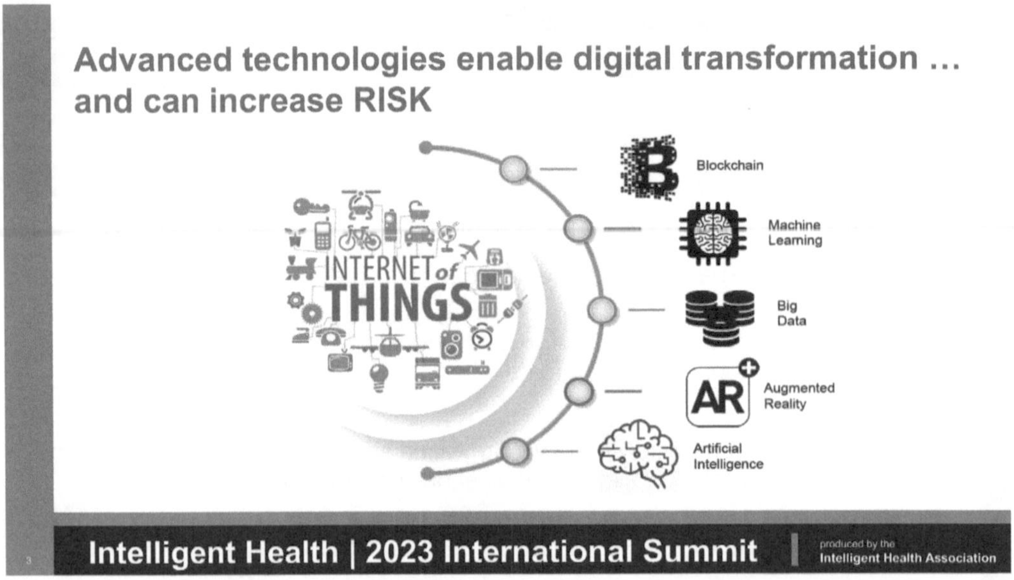


Blockchain technology or distributed ledger technology, as I like to call it, Machine Learning and Artificial Intelligence, Augmented Reality, Virtual Reality, and big data. Or, as we used to say when we were working with ARM, a lot of little data that makes big data. So, and that's what happens with IoT. And so, with all of this, we're gaining so much more insight and so much more connectivity and the opportunity for more interoperability if the standards allow us to do that. But at the same time, it's a little tricky because it can actually create a lot of risk.

So, what we want to talk a little bit about today is the connected healthcare solutions and the value side of it. So why do we do this? Well, we can leverage these advanced technologies to enable precision healthcare, improving insights and outcomes. We can use connected healthcare devices and data. They could be implanted devices, wearable devices in home devices in hospital devices, all these different connected healthcare devices. The clinical care data that they access that they get from devices on you devices near you. That's more from the clinical side, as compared to in the wild. Environmental data which could be more in the wild, you know I think about, you know, I have asthma, and when there were fires in Canada and the smoke was coming down here, I could smell it in my living room in New York. I'm like what the heck, right? But when you're going into the hospital or the doctor, and you're having problems breathing, what's going on in your environment is important to your health. Patient lifestyle data. Do you exercise, do you not? What do you eat? What do you drink? How often? You know, all of that information and clinical and fundamental research data. And what's so exciting is that there's so much more going on in clinical and fundamental research that we can access more easily because we can share data. And we can share metadata. So, you have this compendium of healthcare data. So, there's so much upside to this, so much positive opportunity.

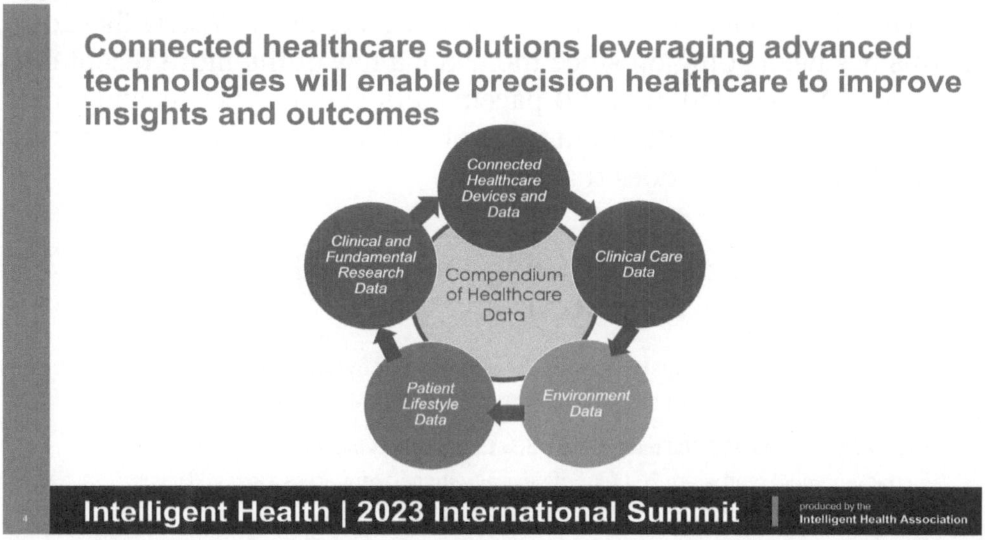


But on the other side of it any medical device connected to a communications network like Wi-fi or public or home Internet may have cybersecurity vulnerabilities that could be exploited by unauthorized users. But at the same time, as we just said, remember that the increased use of this technology and medical devices, hardware and software and services, I'd like to say, can also offer safe and more convenient and timely healthcare delivery. And this is as spoken by the US FDA, the Food and Drug Administration. So, some people will say to me, well, why are we using the technology if there's risk? Because there's a lot of benefit. You know, and that's what we want to do is enable the benefit while reducing the risk.

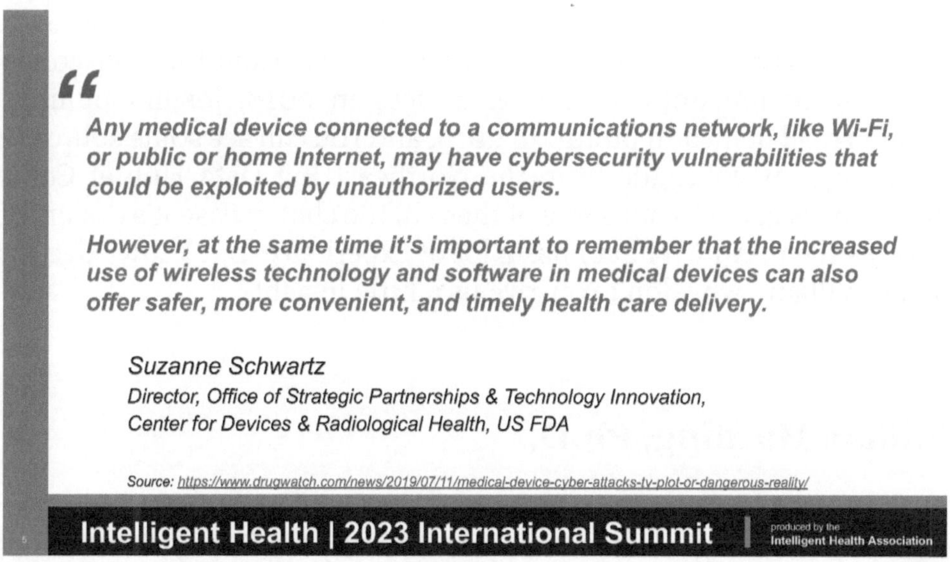

So, we say, increased connectivity brings increased risk. So, what could possibly go wrong? Well, things can go wrong. So, the US FDA has actually identified software vulnerabilities that could let hackers take advantage of personal medical device devices dating back as far as 2008. You're like 2008, really this has been going on since then? So, a few of the more recent ones in 2017 the FDA recalled 465,000 pacemakers due to cyber hacking fears. They could reprogram 20 different types of devices with adjacent access and a low skill level. So, what does that mean?

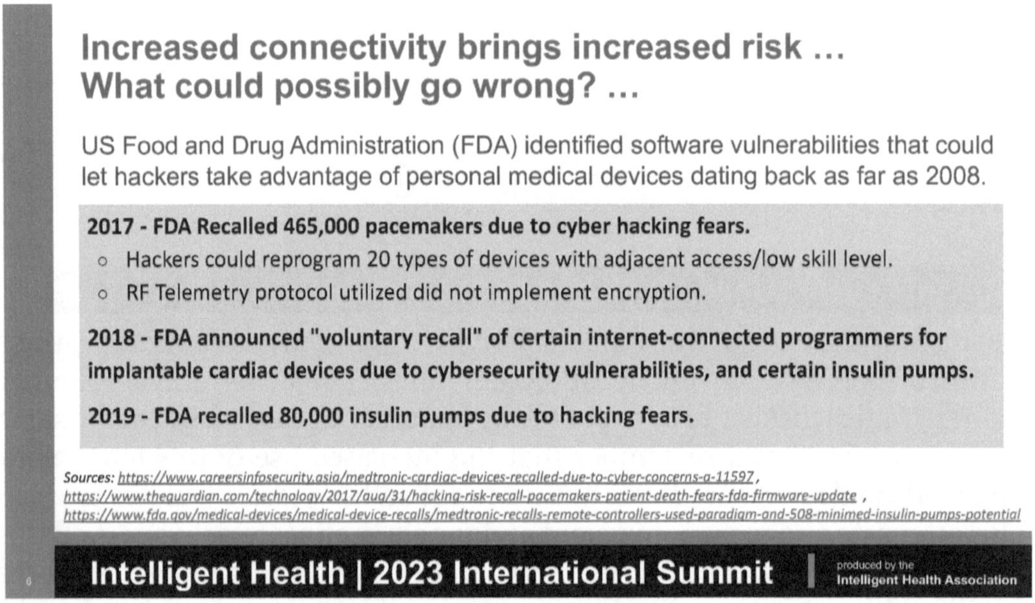
Increased connectivity brings increased risk …
What could possibly go wrong? …
US Food and Drug Administration (FDA) identified software vulnerabilities that could let hackers take advantage of personal medical devices dating back as far as 2008.
2017 - FDA Recalled 465,000 pacemakers due to cyber hacking fears.
Hackers could reprogram 20 types of devices with adjacent access/low skill level.
RF Telemetry protocol utilized did not implement encryption.
2018 - FDA announced "voluntary recall" of certain internet-connected programmers for implantable cardiac devices due to cybersecurity vulnerabilities, and certain insulin pumps.
2019 - FDA recalled 80,000 insulin pumps due to hacking fears.
Sources: https://www.careersinfosecurity.asia/medtronic-cardiac-devices-recalled-due-to-cyber-concerns-a-11597,
https://www.theguardian.com/technology/2017/aug/31/hacking-risk-recall-pacemakers-patient-death-fears-fda-firmware-update ,
https://www.fda.gov/medical-devices/medical-device-recalls/medtronic-recalls-remote-controllers-used-paradigm-and-508-minimed-insulin-pumps-potential
Intelligent Health | 2023 International Summit
produced by the Intelligent Health Association

I tell people well, like when you're in a movie theater or you're in airplane, or you're at a concert, or you're in a mall, how many people are within, like, you know, 50 feet of you, which is the adjacent access? A lot. How many of them do you know you can trust? None. And with a low skill level, there's really a lot of risk. There was also a voluntary recall of certain Internet-connected programs for implantable cardiac devices in 2018, insulin pumps, and another recall of insulin pumps in 2019, and you can see some sources here. And Emily, my colleague from the Northeast Big Data Hub at Columbia University, is going to put some of these in the chat in case it's easier for you to access them. And William has a lot of experience and knowledge in this, too. So William, why don't you give us a little insight?

## William Harding, Ph.D.

Oh, perfect and great introduction to all this and even as a little backtrack on some of the things relative to environmental, you know, as it even applies to some of the end devices you've got here, as well as even things like AR, VR, and XR, is the interconnectivity of these, the interoperability of these devices with other devices is what we often overlook when it comes to, how do we protect the data, how we protect the patient, how we predict the device? Speaking from my own personal perspective, I actually have an implanted therapy therapeutic device for pain control, and it involves a handheld controller and involves a charger, involves the implanted device itself. I can actually interrogate and see it with just an innocent Bluetooth device looking for signals. So, though I haven't personally tried to hack my own device, I know what's in it, and I know how to do that, but the concern is that maybe somebody can't really necessarily control my device, but could they cause an adverse stimulation? Could they shut it down when I need it? And though it's just there for pain therapy, think about that, use that as an example or a muse toward a pacemaker, a neuro device, deep brain stimulation a pacemaker or a defibrillator that's keeping a patient alive. To think that even if it interfered with its functionality, then what could be the devastating impact on the device and ultimately the patient.

So, when we think we need, when we think about protecting devices, it isn't always about, oh, they hacked it, they reprogrammed it, they did something, but did they block its function? Did they decrease its battery capability? Did they impact it and inject some data that might cause confusion. Think about going to an airport and somebody, a TSA person's key in radio? Will the interference impact that device. So, when we think about, you know, why these devices were recalled, you know, why we need to protect them, we need to think more deeply beyond the fact of even just the patient, you know. It could come down to loss of IP, and even a company's, well say branding. You know, not that that's any more important than human. But you start to see exactly the elements that influence us when, you know, developing the standard round TIPPSS.

## Florence Hudson

Absolutely. So, that makes it very real. And you know, honestly, when I started working on this when I was a VP and a Director in Corporate Strategy at IBM and ARM actually came to us, and they make, you know, they make the IP for the design of a lot of the chips that go in a lot of these cute little devices, as I say, cute little chips, very powerful though, and one of the gentlemen I was working with came running into my into my cubicle and said, they keep me alive. I was like Whoa! Where did that come from? I was in the middle of a PowerPoint slide deck, and he wears the Medtronic insulin pump. And so,

I was like, whoa, so end to end trust and security became very real for me at that moment, you know. And so, he was very interested in this project. And so, we've been working on it, you know, basically, ever since. And it affects people you love, and it can even affect you. And so, what we're trying to do is basically keep the humans alive.

So, the way we look at this, we must secure connected healthcare devices and data while enabling interoperability. You know, if you lock everything down and then we can get to anything. And how are we going to get to precision medicine? How are we going to have this context and content to help protect the human? So, the top concerns we have are connected healthcare devices and data. The way we look at it. You could immediately kill somebody if you hack one of those immediately sensing, actuating, changing the reading, actuating and delivering a medication that's not needed, over delivering it, under delivering it, changing the delivery. There are all sorts of things. So, connected healthcare is our first. Then we're looking at the broader cyber, physical infrastructure, space, as I was talking about. Connected hospitals, campuses, cities, vehicles, energy grids. So, we see this expanding into that in the future. And then also clinical, scientific and research device and data integrity.

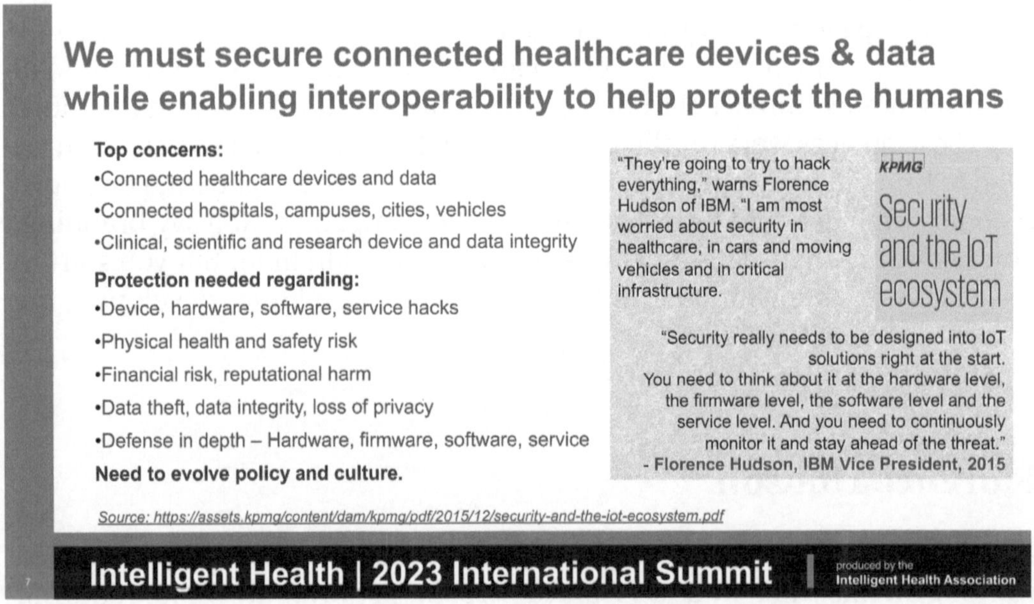
We must secure connected healthcare devices & data
while enabling interoperability to help protect the humans
Top concerns:
•Connected healthcare devices and data
•Connected hospitals, campuses, cities, vehicles
•Clinical, scientific and research device and data integrity
Protection needed regarding:
•Device, hardware, software, service hacks
•Physical health and safety risk
•Financial risk, reputational harm
•Data theft, data integrity, loss of privacy
•Defense in depth – Hardware, firmware, software, service
Need to evolve policy and culture.
"They're going to try to hack everything," warns Florence Hudson of IBM. "I am most worried about security in healthcare, in cars and moving vehicles and in critical infrastructure.
KPMG
Security and the IoT ecosystem
"Security really needs to be designed into IoT solutions right at the start. You need to think about it at the hardware level, the firmware level, the software level and the service level. And you need to continuously monitor it and stay ahead of the threat."
- Florence Hudson, IBM Vice President, 2015
Source: https://assets.kpmg/content/dam/kpmg/pdf/2015/12/security-and-the-iot-ecosystem.pdf
Intelligent Health | 2023 International Summit
produced by the Intelligent Health Association

I also run a COVID Information Commons for the US Government that has over 10,000 NSF and NIH-funded awards in it, and you may recall, or you may not have known that one of the large research universities their research data was actually hacked during COVID. So, what happens when you hack research data? Well, hmm, so you could be changing the information about what the research is actually showing, and then people could be making decisions based on bad information. So, it's really important that we protect all of this data. We need protection at the device level, the hardware software and service level, we need to reduce the risk for physical health and safety, financial risk, and reputational harm. You know, when the brand is known to have been hacked that doesn't look good. I guess the good and bad news is so many have been hacked by now. It's like you're just one of them, unfortunately. But what we wanna do is really reduce the risk to the people, the financial and reputational harm. We want to protect against data theft, improve data integrity, reduce veracity or uncertainty about the data, reduce loss of privacy, and do this at a defense in depth level, hardware, firmware software and service level. And very honestly, since there are geeks in the room, as Harry was saying, you know, some people don't think about firmware anymore. And actually, I've had colleges, I've gone to where I go to the dean of the engineering school and say, why don't you teach firmware anymore? Like, Oh, gosh, firmware. Yeah, like they forgot, they forgot their bag, like on the train. I'm like, are you kidding me? So, what we need to do is use all these pieces as a defense in-depth strategy. And that's part of what you'll see in the standard. And then we need to evolve policy and culture which includes standards to expect TIPPSS. And this was from 2015, this quote. So, I've been working about on this for a while, as I said, they're gonna try to hack everything. And as I mentioned then, I'm most worried about security and healthcare cars, moving vehicles and critical infrastructure. And so, we need to stay ahead of it, you know, really needs to be designed in security and TIPPSS into the solutions right at the start. At all these hardware firmware software and service levels. And you need to continually monitor it and stay ahead of the threat. So, what you'll see as we talk more about the standard is that that's what we have in the standard draft.

## William Harding, Ph.D.

And Florence, if you don't mind on that previous side, you just had. I thought you had a really good point especially around healthcare and other devices. The things that we don't expect, the things we don't anticipate is being associated with healthcare, is something we also, as you talked about hardware and firmware, you know, a lot of people talked about firmware, and they thought, it's just something different. You know, it's still software. It's still programming language. But one of the big things you hit on is, think about in sensors, you say, well, if I'm doing glucose sensing, SpO2 sensing, or an EMG sensing, that's obvious health sensing. But often when we think about particulate count, humidity and heat index, these types of things inform, if you were an asthmatic patient or other patients, these would inform your decisions, or whether you go outside. They affect your health. So, the TIPPSS team really took a deep dive into things that may not be obvious.

## Florence Hudson

Totally agree. Thank you for sharing that, William, and that's what we're going to try. Our goal, too, is to teach everybody about TIPPSS. So once, God willing, the standard comes out the door, it's gotten through the initial vote, we passed the initial vote, we're going through comment resolution right now, we're praying it comes out by next year sometime, you know, there's a whole process. You know, eventually, what we want to do is teach everybody, teach all the patients about it, and we made it something anybody could say TIPPSS. It's like Q-tips, or TIPPSS and techniques, you know, easy to remember. And as William knows, I often say, we're doing this between IEEE and Underwriters Laboratories. When I was a little girl, being a geek, I used to crawl around looking for the UL tag on the electric cords because I knew it was safer. And so that's what we're trying to do is teach people working with IEEE and UL to create the standard, to make it safer. And some 3 to 5 years from now, maybe sooner, when this is totally deployed, there'll be a little girl at the doctor with her grandmother and the doctor's gonna try to give one of them an insulin pump and the doctor's going to look up at them and say, does it have TIPPSS.

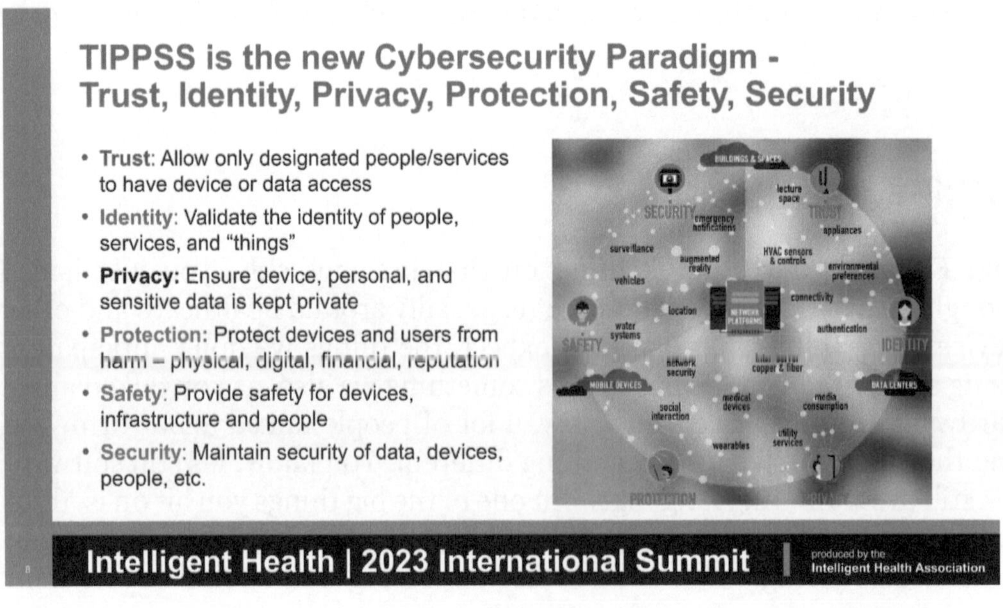
TIPPSS is the new Cybersecurity Paradigm -
Trust, Identity, Privacy, Protection, Safety, Security
Trust: Allow only designated people/services to have device or data access
Identity: Validate the identity of people, services, and "things"
Privacy: Ensure device, personal, and sensitive data is kept private
Protection: Protect devices and users from harm – physical, digital, financial, reputation
Safety: Provide safety for devices, infrastructure and people
Security: Maintain security of data, devices, people, etc.
Intelligent Health | 2023 International Summit
produced by the Intelligent Health Association

So that's how we see this is, we want to work with the manufacturers, the payers, the providers to everyone, get focused on this to deploy it and then teach the humans to ask for it.

So that's our strategy. So, hop on board. So, thinking through all that, we created this TIPPSS idea, and it was originally created, I was speaking with a gentleman that worked a lot with IEEE when I was still at IBM, I believe, and then at Internet 2, we were on the Cisco IoT world Forum steering committee. We were at one of these meetings and saying, nobody's worrying about end-to-end trust and security on this stuff, you know, nobody. And we said, let's do it. So, we actually got a small grant from NSF at the time, and then IEEE hosted it, and we had a meeting in Washington and we talked about this whole idea. We had NSF there, we had different government agencies there, we had the Department of Homeland Security, I think we might have had the CIA, we had researchers, industry people, and talked about, what are we gonna do about this? And we came up with this TIPPSS framework. So, we look at it as the new cybersecurity paradigm. The CIA cybersecurity paradigm is the one that many of you may know if you're in security, confidentiality, integrity, and availability. When that was created it was really created at the Enterprise Nation-State security level, how to keep information safe from people who shouldn't see it. But now what we're talking about is technology inside humans and humans inside technology. And we have to really worry about human safety, protecting them, security of their data, privacy of their data, and the trust and identity aspects of devices trying to talk to each other and humans trying to get into devices all the time and making sure we really are validating the identity of that thing or that human or that service, and then deciding, if it could be trusted or not. If the human can trust it, if the device can trust it, if the software can trust it, if the service can trust it.

So that's kind of this, that's the scope of TIPPSS. So, trust means allowing only designated people or services to have device or data, access. Identity validates the identity of the people, services and things so you know you can trust it. It's like if somebody comes to your door and says, you know, I'm a policeman let me in. You go, prove it. They say, I just am, and you're like, prove it. Where's your badge? I'm going to call the cops, you know. You have to make sure. And that's really critical in these situations. Privacy is ensuring device, personal, and sensitive data is kept private. Protection is protecting devices and users from harm (physical, digital financial reputational). Safety is providing safety for the devices, infrastructure, and the people and security of data devices and people. And, as you can see, there are many different areas that are connected in here. There are many different aspects of this and that's what we're working on as a team.

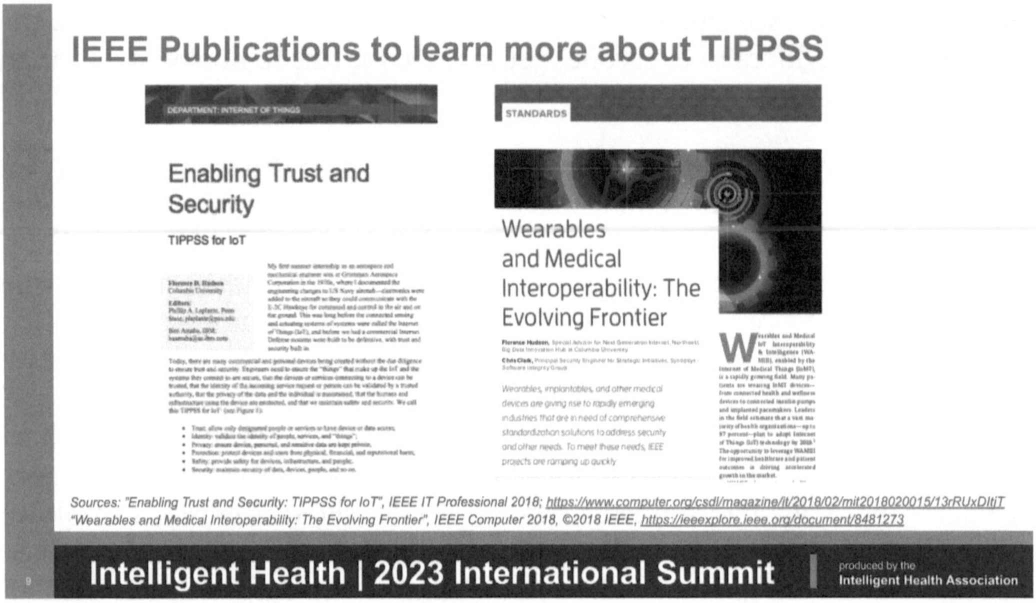


So, we've been building this idea since around 2015, I guess, when I was quoted in that article we just showed you, then 2016 for this TIPPSS meeting we had in DC, and then we started a drumbeat. I used to be a VP of marketing to boom, boom, boom, get the word out! So, we did a couple of articles which you can read. I think my colleague, Emily Rothenberg, from the Northeast Big data Hub at Columbia University is adding things to the chat. Thank you, Emily. So, these are, I believe they're still all open and available. You might have to log in to IEEE and create an account to see them because they like to see how many people are looking at them, but I think they're all still free. So, enabling trust and security TIPPSS for IoT, and then wearables and medical interoperability, the evolving frontier, both published in 2018. And then we had a lot of fun, and this is when William and I met.

So, there was a pre-standards effort we started working on with IEEE with their industry connections group. And this is when, they're not sure if it's gonna be a standard effort yet, but we wanna try to figure that out. So, one of our colleagues and good friends, Maria Palombini, who leads the Healthcare and Life Sciences practice at IEEE. She started working with us and said, you know, introduce us to the team at IEEE and said, let's create this pre-standards effort. And at the time we were looking at blockchain, honestly. So, you can see the report that came out is the Pre-Standards Workstream Report: Clinical IoT data Validation and Interoperability with Blockchain. But as we were going through the process, we said, you know, blockchain, isn't the answer. It could be one of the pieces. But that's also a risk. So, what is really the scope of this right, William, do you wanna say anything before we go into?

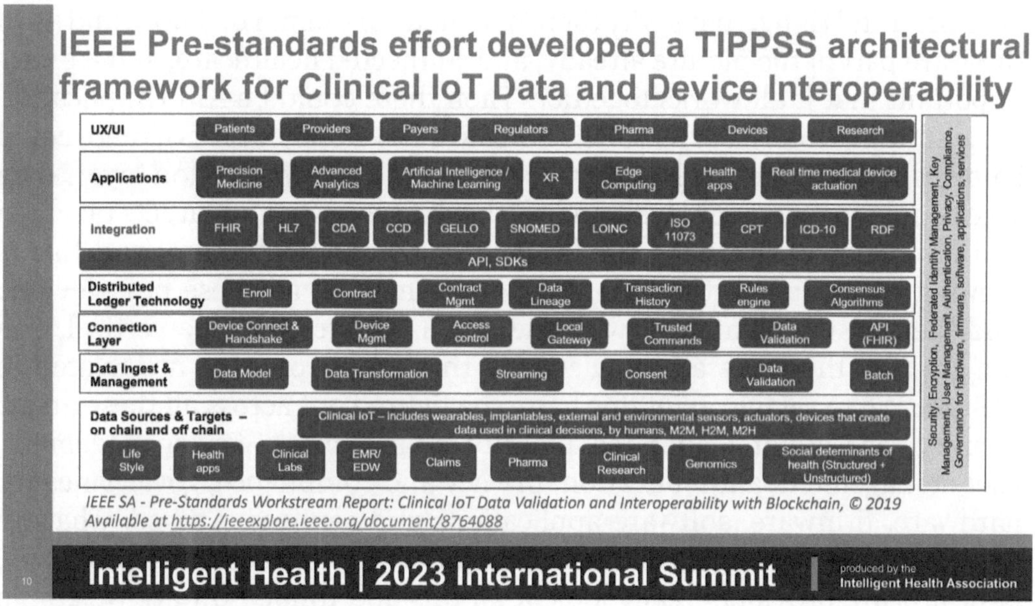


## William Harding, Ph.D.

No, that was, I love the fact that you said that because in the beginning we really were all about distributed ledger systems. And you know things about blockchain. And we literally came up with the flat fact that it wasn't enough. You know, and as we started exploring this, I think I love this image here because it really represents all the explorations we did with a huge team when we think of HL7 for any of the different methods of data exchanges. But even as we, as you implied on the previous one about wearables, we started realizing it's not just an external that even the human as a platform was something we started to consider so as devices and interconnections and enter bodies and meshes. These things started developing. We realized we had to really look forward. And this was a good example of a lot of the things we were considering as we move forward.

## Florence Hudson

Exactly. And so, it's very comprehensive. This isn't something you would show in a boardroom unless it's like, you know AMD or something, maybe. But so, we start at the top with the user experience / user interface and actually, devices can be users if you think about it, you know, if devices are trying to decide if they can trust other things. So, we have, like a broad range of things in here from the UX and UI perspective, the different applications, integration through different standards, you know, as they say, standards are a beautiful thing, that's why there's so many of them. You know, and all of these are part of the picture already, and connected healthcare, and it's very important that it all works together. Then there could be API (Application Programming Interfaces) or SDK (Software Development Kits), there could be distributed ledger technology. There could be a connection layer, data ingest and management layer, and all the data sources and targets on chain and off chain. We're using the blockchain terminology there, and this is growing every day all the time. People are making all these new devices. And then on the right, and with the green background, the vertical, you can see that these are all the elements that cut across that are related to TIPPSS. We're saying, all of this has to be figured out across all these areas: security, encryption, federated identity management, key management, user management, authentication, privacy and compliance, governance for hardware, firmware, software applications and services. And so, what we want is that all the technical teams at manufacturers, at solution providers, at healthcare providers really look at all this and think, how are we gonna put this all together? And how are we going to apply these TIPPSS elements to it? And that's really what the standard tries to do.

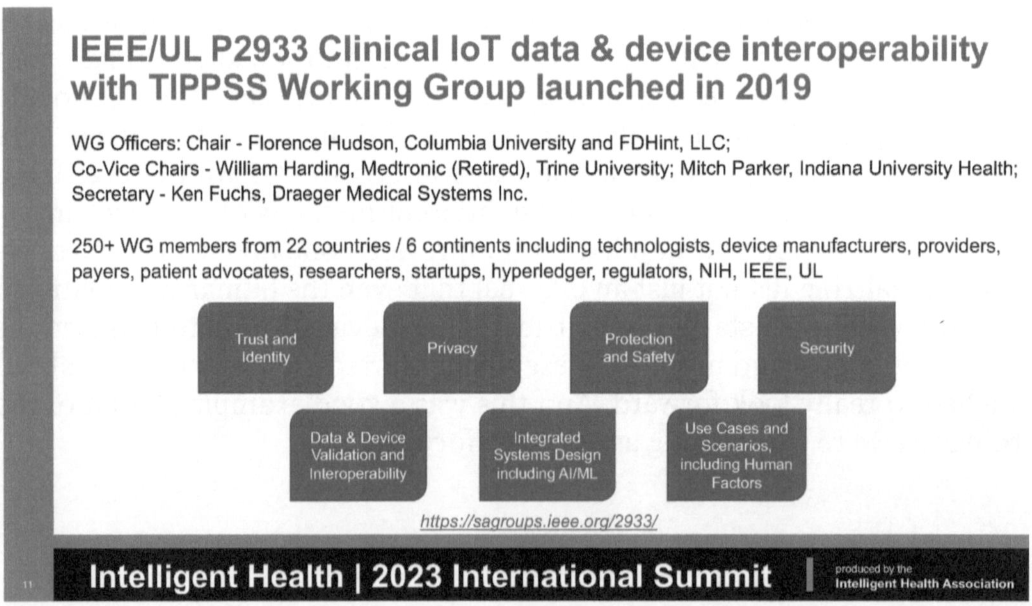
IEEE/UL P2933 Clinical IoT data & device interoperability with TIPPSS Working Group launched in 2019
WG Officers: Chair - Florence Hudson, Columbia University and FDHint, LLC;
Co-Vice Chairs - William Harding, Medtronic (Retired), Trine University; Mitch Parker, Indiana University Health;
Secretary - Ken Fuchs, Draeger Medical Systems Inc.
250+ WG members from 22 countries / 6 continents including technologists, device manufacturers, providers, payers, patient advocates, researchers, startups, hyperledger, regulators, NIH, IEEE, UL
Trust and Identity
Privacy
Protection and Safety
Security
Data & Device Validation and Interoperability
Integrated Systems Design including AI/ML
Use Cases and Scenarios, including Human Factors
https://sagroups.ieee.org/2933/
11
Intelligent Health | 2023 International Summit
produced by the Intelligent Health Association

So, what we did is we created out of the Pre-Standards Working Group. We said, okay, we think this should be a Standards Working Group now and so we were very fortunate that William agreed to be one of the Co-Vice Chairs. And at the time he was a distinguished Technical Fellow, recently retired. And now he's at Trine University, too, as a professor, as he was mentioning. Mitch Parker was also very involved, and he and I were working together already. Cause when I was at another firm Internet 2, he's at Indiana University, and we work very closely with them. And so, he is the Chief Information Security Officer at Indiana University Health or their health system, and our secretary is, Ken Fuchs at Dräeger Medical Systems. So, these are people that are in it. We all know, and this is like, you know, if you know, you know, if you say to somebody you're really trying to like, lock this down hardware firmware software and service level, end-to-end trust and security. They look at you with laser beyond being behind as they go, I'm in. Because they know nobody is doing it. And so interestingly, when we first created this, we had to create a PAR. It's called a Project Authorization Request with IEEE. This is the beginning of the process. So, we'll tell you a little bit process, too. And they asked you in there, what's the scope? Who are the stakeholders? How many people will be involved in this? And so, I said, maybe 25 like if I invite my best friends. And now there are over 250 people in this working group. Once again, if you know, you know. And they're from 22 countries, 6 continents. Technologists, device manufacturers, healthcare providers, solution providers, payers, patient advocates, researchers, startups, Hyperledger folks, regulators, NIH, IEEE Underwriters Laboratories. So, there's a whole slew of us. And when we created this, we had so many people. We're like, how are we going to organize this? So, we decided to break up into little subgroups. And so, we have a Trust and Identity subgroup, because trust and identity go together. And that's a very important topic. And I think William and I will both talk about that. Some people try to rip those apart. But the whole point is that you need identity and access management, including the trust and identity elements. What's their identity? Who validated their identity, and can you trust them? If you can trust them, then you give them access? If not, you don't. The Privacy group, which was led by somebody in the EU, because they were way ahead of us for the US, Protection and Safety, and Security. We also had a Data and Device Validation and Interoperability team led by somebody from NIH and our working group, and Integrated Systems Design group, including Artificial Intelligence and Machine Learning. But for the first version, you know, this version of the standard that we're working on, we're not doing a lot with AI and ML, because there's so much change going on in that space. And I work at the Northeast Big Data Innovation Hub at Columbia University. I live in this space, AI/ML. There's a lot of change, a lot of new regulation being created. You know, the EU just created a new AI regulation I was reading about. So, we're talking about integrated system design, how all these hardware firmware software service pieces work together and all the different types of devices. And we'll get to AI and ML. And they're actually some IEEE AI and ML standards efforts now I'm involved in those for healthcare. So, I'm keeping an eye on that, and then we'll see how it comes together. And then Use Cases and Scenarios, including Human Factors, which was a very important group that was led by Ken Fuchs, the Secretary of the working group, and, William, you were very involved in that.

## William Harding, Ph.D.

Exactly what I like also, and I love your introduction on the how the team was formed, and stuff, and one thing I cannot ever say enough about is this core team of offices, of course. But I have to always do perfect shout out to Ken, because you may see Secretary, but if you don't see the word superstar there, it should be known for sure. He is definitely our superstar.

But yeah, I like what you've covered here, especially, like you were saying, one of the neat offshoots that came from this is the teams here have had generated a number of books already of the published material. Some of this material is already actually been influencing patents that have been awarded. So, to me, this, even before we finalized our standards, and so on. Just the positive output of this is amazing. And then, like you said with Trust and Identity, there was a lot of contention back and forth. But what is it? Is it Identity first, or Trust first, you know? And we don't want you, when you look at this, when you look at TIPPSS, and you think of Trust, Identity, Privacy, Protection, Safety, Security. The order is there in the form that we created. But it is not something that states and says, hey you, this is the sequence you follow. This is that you jump in. You have to attack a security at the last, or whatever. So, the fact that we discuss Trust and Identity in that sequence, it's not necessarily order dependent. And you'll hear more about that as we talk.

## Florence Hudson

Yeah, and on the other side, it is kind of the tip of the arrow because you can't have Privacy, and Identity, you can't have Protection and Safety. So, it's the tip of the arrow, but not everybody is responsible for every piece of this as William is saying. So, what we want to make sure is that, like the Chief Privacy Officer is focusing on privacy, right? The CISO is focusing on Security, and they care about all these other things. So, when we created the standard draft, we have different chapters for these different groups. So, if that's who you are, you can go deep in your chapter, and you'll care about the others, but you can focus on that. So, I appreciate your seeing that

William is that, you know, people can start in different places here, but all of it does go together.

## William Harding, Ph.D.

100%

## Florence Hudson

Great. Yeah. And anybody can join our working group if you want to. This is the website [https://sagroups.ieee.org/2933], and Emily will graciously put it in the chat. It's easy to find, IEEE, 2933, you know, Standard, you know, Working Group. You'll find it. And it's free. You do not have to be an IEEE member. We specifically made it free and open so that we could get smart people who care to work on this with us. You know, there's a different version of entity-based where the organization, a company signs up, but we didn't wanna do it that way. It could be an independent consultant. It could be a researcher that could bring a lot of it value someone who's retired. That is part of an institution that's fine. We really want them on board.

## William Harding, Ph.D.

I like what you just said there, because it really also gets to the core of how we appreciate input and diversity, literally we always, we've made comments of, you know, it could be an HR person, could be regulatory, could be quality, it could be engineering, it could be IT. You know, those diverse perspectives really enrich the results of this.

## Florence Hudson

Exactly. And for those of you who are thinking, what about all the other standards organizations? So, we brought UL in already. And actually, this is the first standard in history being created from the beginning between IEEE and UL. We actually had an MOU signed between IEEE and Underwriters Laboratories to do this. Usually one standards organization will say, well, we'll work this out, and then we'll let you know where we get. And then they throw it over the transom and say, okay, it's ready. You guys can use it, too, if you want. But we decided to do this together from the beginning, and we've also already reached out to ISO-IEC about, you know, having them involved. But one standards organization has to kind of take the lead of publishing and so that's how we're doing it. And so, we're very excited about that.

Okay, so that's the working group. So now, what I think we'll do is jump into the use cases if that sounds okay.

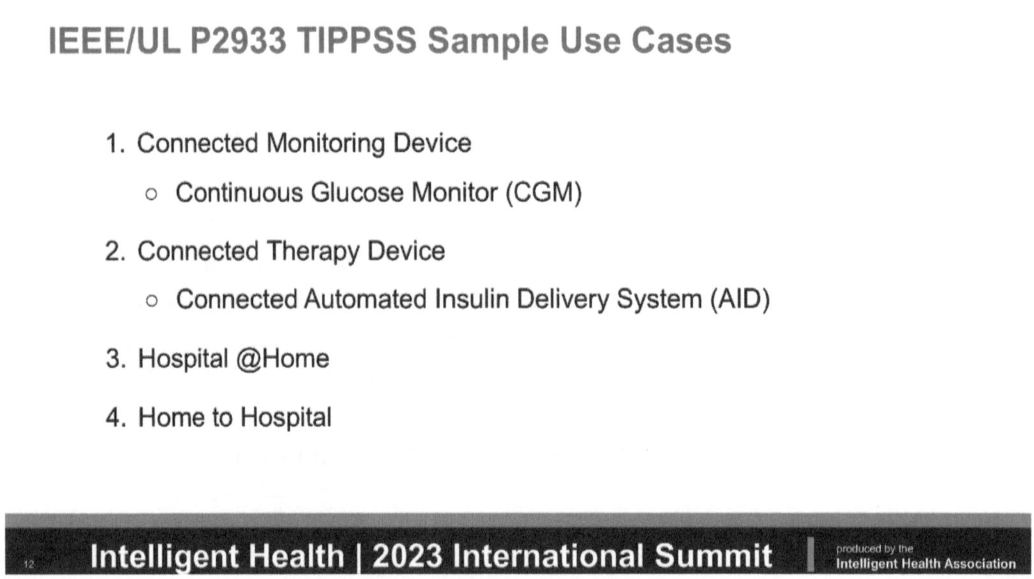


So, what we wanted to do is come up with some sample use cases to make this real.

So, you know you have this theoretical trust, identity, hardware, firmware, all this stuff and you're like, oh my goodness, right? But what we wanted to do is come up with real use cases. And we decided that the Continuous Glucose Monitors, very important for a couple of reasons. One is a lot of people know people that are diabetic that might need this. Very honestly we also work on social determinants of health, and some of the underserved communities tend to have higher rates of Diabetes. So, this actually helps those communities, too. And so, we felt it was a very inclusive way to really have an example that applied to many people.

So, we have the continuous glucose monitor. Then the Connected Therapy Device, the Connected Automated Insulin Delivery System (AID). Then the hospital at home use case which was happening a lot during COVID when there wasn't room in the hospitals. How sad is that! But also now, as humans are living so long and more of them are trying to get into hospitals. But there's more hospital home going on, cause there isn't as much room, or they're trying to reduce their cost of care, and then home to hospital, when you have to go back into the hospital, go into the hospital. So, these are all very real situations, and we thought they were rather helpful to look at it. But these are just sample use cases. We presented this at him last HIMSS last year, the Healthcare Information and Management System Society, and somebody actually said, are those the only use cases? Like oh, no, everything, right? I was like, oh, no, I'm sorry you said that, so I use the word sample on every slide, now. These are just sample use cases. But for any use case, what we suggest is that you look at your use case, and you kind of draw a picture of how does it work? Where are the attack vectors? Where am I worried about Trust and Identity? Where am I worried about Privacy? Where am I worried about Security? And that will help you develop a plan.

So, since you helped create a lot of these devices and use cases, William, maybe you'd like to talk about the different use cases for us.

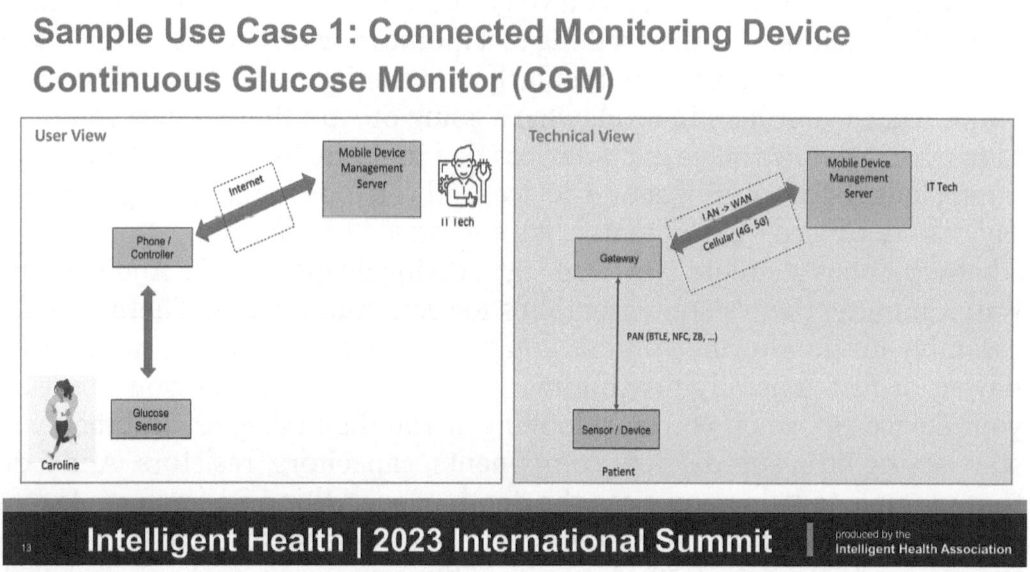


## William Harding, Ph.D.

I would love to. And I love that introduction to the different use cases, because, as we were exploring, you know, I'll use an example. When you're doing design thinking or doing different methods to work on a problem statement it's always helpful that maybe you talk to a patient, a caregiver, or you know, the end customer. So, it gives you a better story, gives you a construction of a story of the elements that you need to address, and it helps expose areas of pain points and things that you need to resolve or solve for. So, when we look at systems, we said, well, we could go with an SpO2 sensor. Oh, yeah, that's a simple device. What's its connectivity? What does it work with? How do we monitor? How do we collect data? How do we charge it? And we started exploring. We said, you know what a really perfect use case would be Continuous Glucose Monitoring for diabetics and anyone with insulin's issues, effectively. But we look at it. Because, and if you think about, to give you a better feel for why we picked it, if you think about a patient, and this is the story we talk about, a patient using these devices. They're going to have a sensor. Most likely, if you look at a Medtronic one, it will be a sensor on the skin, a small needle under the skin. It's collecting information, chemical information about the patient. It's then transmitting Bluetooth to a pump that the individual has, and it might be collecting information to another monitor, like a caregiver. So, if you were a 6 year old child, you may not know what to do with the device or information, so it might be going to your parents' wristwatch. It's giving them information. So now you've incorporated 3 devices. You've got a sensor, a wearable, and 2 wearables, and then the pump included. But then you've got a vial that goes into the pump with your insulin in it. You've got batteries they're working on that. You look at that person then talking to a monitoring device that might be in your house to tell, you know, to regularly communicate with your doctor. You know, what's your insulin level, what's going on, are there issues you need to resolve? So now you've got 4 devices tied in there. Now, if you look at the pump, let's go to look at just one device, and you look at that pump, and you say, it's comprised of an actuator, it's comprised of communications, it has a battery, it has a circuit. Now you start, diving deeper into it. And you say, wait a minute, there's sub-assemblies for communications. There's a sub-assembly for monitoring volume, you know. There's things for monitoring power, or just generally programming according to the way you've set up your device. So, when you start looking at you dig in deeper, and then you start seeing little sub-discrete components, capacitors, resistors. And I do that example to help people see the depth of everything we analyze. And at what point could there be a failure? At what point could there be a risk to the patient, to the data, to the integrity of the company, even as an example?

So, when we started exploring it, that's why we picked that as one of our first. It was such a rich format. Now as you now dive into, and I've already inferred to things like at the home type scenarios. And as we go to next slide, you'll see how that becomes part of a bigger picture, systems of systems. And so, when we look at all that, those are the obvious elements.

But also, what if you're the manufacturer of that Continuous Glucose Monitoring device, the bill of material, the information that's around it, the vendors you deal with? What is the other information you might need to protect, you know, proprietary trade secrets and patents? So, there's much more to it than just the obviousness of that single device. And it really goes into all the things of data transformation, interoperability. Even if we start to apply AI and ML type processes to it, you'll start to see, how does this device predict that I might need some sort of therapy? So, it's a much deeper and richer environment to explore from the perspective of data security, data protection, and all the elements of TIPPSS.

## Florence Hudson

Absolutely. Thank you so much, William, that was super helpful. So, what we've done through these sample use cases is show that there's a user view. And so Caroline just sees she has a sensor, right? God bless Caroline. And then we have a technical view. So once again, we're looking at how the users and the humans are interacting with this. And so, you can see here, she has her glucose sensor through her phone control over the Internet to a mobile device management server and IT tech on the back end. And then a technical view. So, there are no humans on this one. This is just technology. So, you can see, we have a personal area network (Bluetooth low energy, NFC (Near Field Communications), Zigbee), all these different things that they might be using, that they need to architect, LAN/WAN, going to mobile device management server.

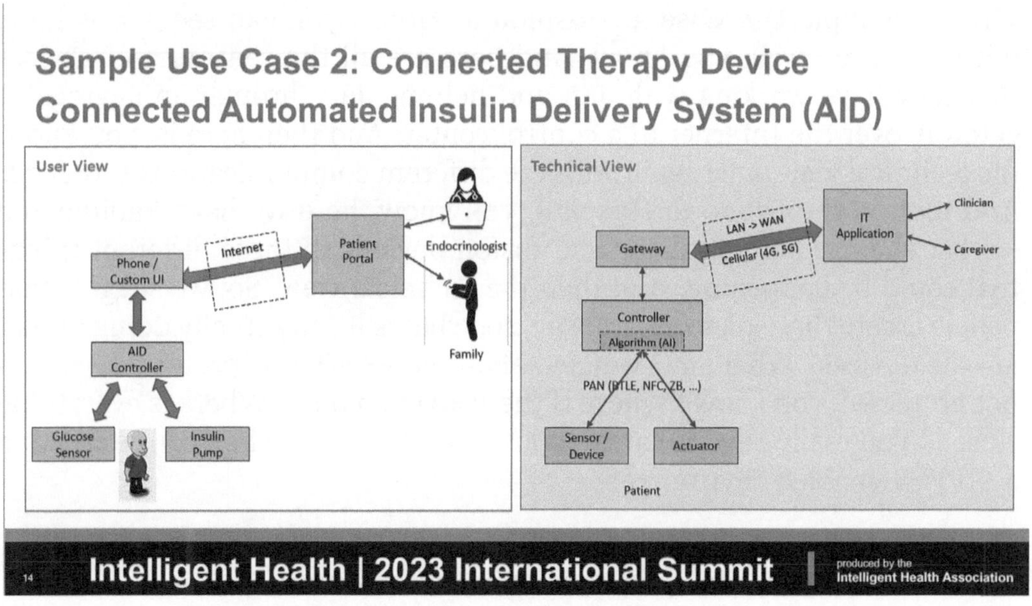

And then in the other ones you'll see this one, the Connected Automated Insulin Delivery System, here we have John. And, you know, here he has the AID controller going over the Internet, endocrinologist can see the information, family can keep track of what's going on, and then the technical view that goes along with that. So, what we wanted to do is show it this way so every person who tries to deploy this says, so, how are the users interacting with this stuff? And what's the technical view of how we enable it and support it with all the TIPPSS elements.

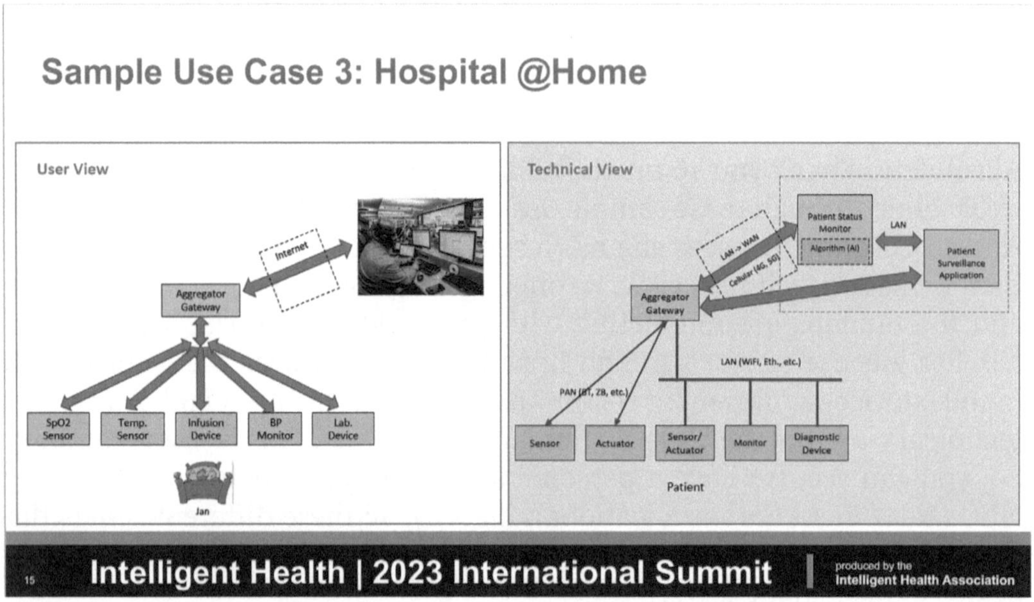


Then in Sample Use Case 3, Hospital at Home, you can see Jan is here, not feeling too well, you know. And here are all the sensors and devices that they have working with Jan and helping Jan through an aggregator gateway over the Internet to a control center. And then here is, you know, the technical view once again with the different communications protocols. And then in the Home to Hospital, you know, here we have Pauline and so that she has her ventilator and fusion devices all these different things that could be happening. And then the technical view. So, we suggest that people create these pictures and say, so, what is it I'm actually doing? What are the devices? What am I worried about here? What is protected, what is not protected, you know? Where is there an open port? Where is everything closed? You really have to think about all these things when you're creating a TIPPSS-enabled environment.

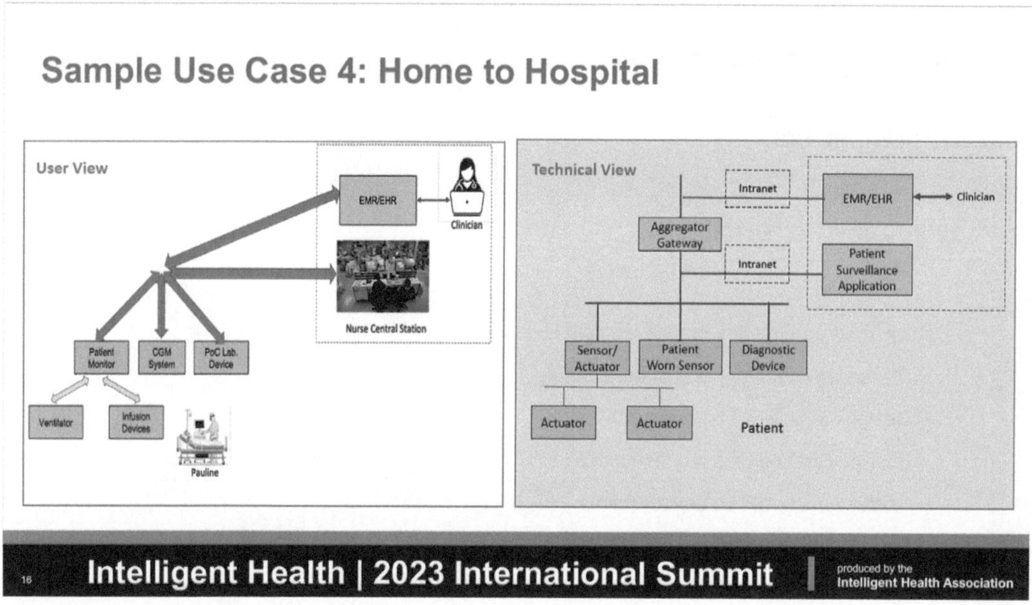


## William Harding, Ph.D.

If you don't mind, Florence, back on that one, and like what you emphasize is important is when we start thinking about Hospital to Home or Home and Hospital type scenarios, and everybody thinks about IoT and interconnection, you know, and as Harry and the rest of my already said, and we know we're super geeks. So, you look at ourselves, and you got an SpO2, blood pressure, EKG, you've got all these things at home that you're helping monitor your own health data. And they're interacting with each other. And they're interacting with your home system. So, when you're starting to build these type of systems out, smart mirrors, you know, at home monitoring post operative type assessments we need to be aware of these potential risks associated with to the patient, to the data, to the devices

## Florence Hudson

Constantly. That's wonderful. Thank you, William, so maybe what we can do now, I think we have about, I don't know, maybe 20 min left. I know, Harry, you can tell us. Maybe we can dive into some of the details of Trust and Identity, Privacy, Protection, Safety, and Security, and how we all bring it together with our integrated systems view. How does that sound, William?

## William Harding, Ph.D.

That sounds perfect.

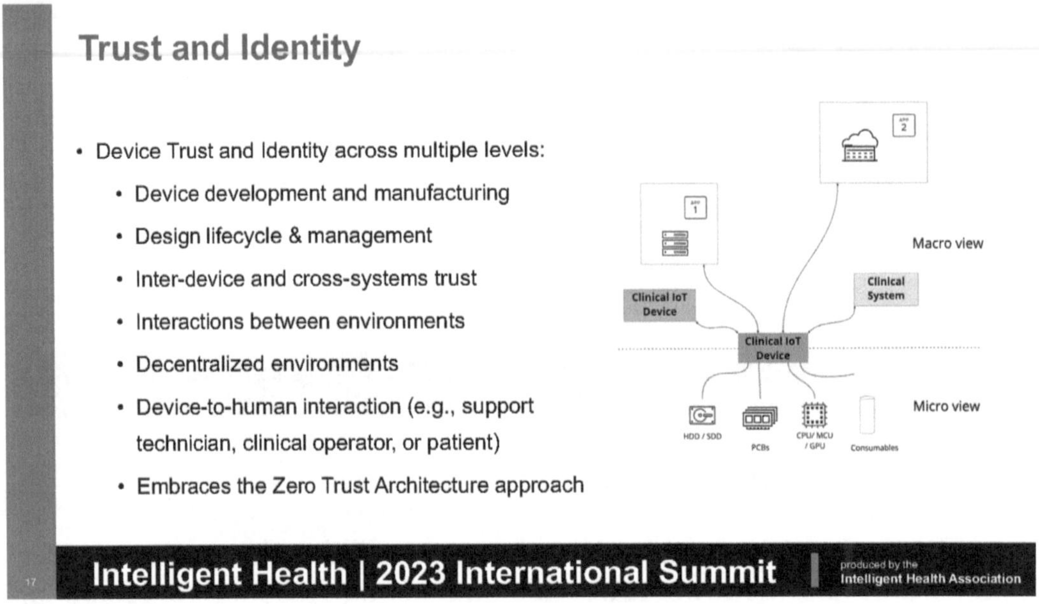


## Florence Hudson

Okay, so we looked at Trust and Identity across multiple levels at the device development and manufacturing level. As an example, you know, when William was at Medtronic or Ken is at Dräeger, you know, when they're designing the device, the life cycle and the management of the device, they're manufacturing the device, they're considering inter-device and cross-systems, trust, interactions between different environments like William was just talking about, decentralized environments, hospital at home, human in the wild, farmer Joe in the field, you know, people all over the place, device to human interaction, support technicians, clinical operators, and patients. How do they use it, you know? Can the patient unlock? What if it locks it up? There's a problem with the security. How do they make sure they can get their insulin? How are we doing all these things? And we embrace the Zero Trust Architecture approach.

And Zero Trust Architecture, I'll just, you know, I started out with Department of Defense work when I was working at Grumman as an aerospace engineer, and I was working on navy aircraft. So, the whole point about cybersecurity is Zero Trust, you don't trust anybody. So, we call it Zero Trust, the Zero Trust Architecture approach. That's always really the plan. But now, as people are looking at interoperability, and can things connect to other things, and can I trust it? We have this term which actually helps us focus on it, which is great. But we look at it and we embrace the Zero Trust Architecture. And then we have different Trust and Identity elements underneath that we provide.

## William Harding, Ph.D.

I like what you said here, Florence, in particular. As you indicated here, and we think about device development and manufacturing is what this points out is a lot of people, a lot of organizations in the past really didn't consider the protection we're talking about until it was what we call the adoption phase, the integration phase. But during this time, we really realize that, you know, for instance, if we think of technology integration life cycle phases, we really need to start thinking about TIPPSS right from the beginning. And that meant from relevant stakeholders, and specifically, to 9 phases, basically what we call technology integration which would be exploration, decision making, design, development, adoption, testing, deployment, validation, sustainability and even end of life or decommissioning. So, when we started thinking this way, we couldn't just produce a device and put it out in the field and say, oh, now we need to figure out how to protect it all the way down, like I said earlier, to the discrete component. If I'm not even putting a high quality resistor, or a shield, or some sort of something around an oscillator or an antenna, think about what my device might be radiating, how it could be, actually, you know, misused, or intercepted. We had to start thinking from that level before, even from the concept of how far this was going to go. And beyond that even the tools we use to make it. So, we mentioned AR/VR. In our company we used to use what we call Extended Reality (XR), which is Augmented Virtual Reality, Mixed Reality devices for manufacturing, design, and so on, but we found that devices themselves we were using weren't shielded, and here they were actually into injecting or influencing us through electromagnetic fields. The devices. So, we couldn't have them safely near our devices. Could they be chemically releasing chemicals that affect our devices? We really had to start breaking it down to the nth level to find out exactly where the points first emerge that could cause, you know, our devices be at risk. So, when we think of any sort of design, this is why TIPPSS is important for medical device manufacturers, for individuals, for designers and inventors is to start thinking of it literally from the beginning.

## Florence Hudson

Absolutely. And, as William said, it's established companies that you would expect know all this already. And it's in brand new startups like, oh, my gosh I have this great idea, but they haven't had to work in a structured environment like this before. Everybody has to worry about this, because all the attack surfaces are just exploding all the time. There are so many new vectors that you can get attacked through, and you have to really plan on thinking about that right up front and continuously worrying about it. As I say, my name is ABS (Always Be Suspicious), you know, if something is trying to connect. Why?

## William Harding, Ph.D.

Well, yeah. And you think, even add that BYOD (Bring Your Own Device) into that element. Think of convolutional neural networks, decentralized data. When we start thinking of ways that we crowdsource, how we could create collaborative partnerships, all those things for third party to vendors, to whatever it all represents these elements, the TIPPSS organization, the tip standard team had to really evaluate.

## Florence Hudson

Absolutely, and so hopefully what you're feeling, as we were saying, we have to evolve policy standards and culture. You can hear from William and myself, I think, that we're trying to create this culture. You know, that we really care all the way, Soup to nuts, end to end all the time. So, within the Trust and Identity area, we also have the macro view which you may have seen in the last slide, and the micro view. So, there's user manage software. There are the different Trust and Identity layers, identity authentication, context, authorization, audit and accounting, onboarding all the way to deprovisioning and then the micro view, the discrete components that William was talking about, the sub-assemblies, the device software, the finished product, the device registry, and decommissioning. And all of this is part of the Trust and Identity picture.

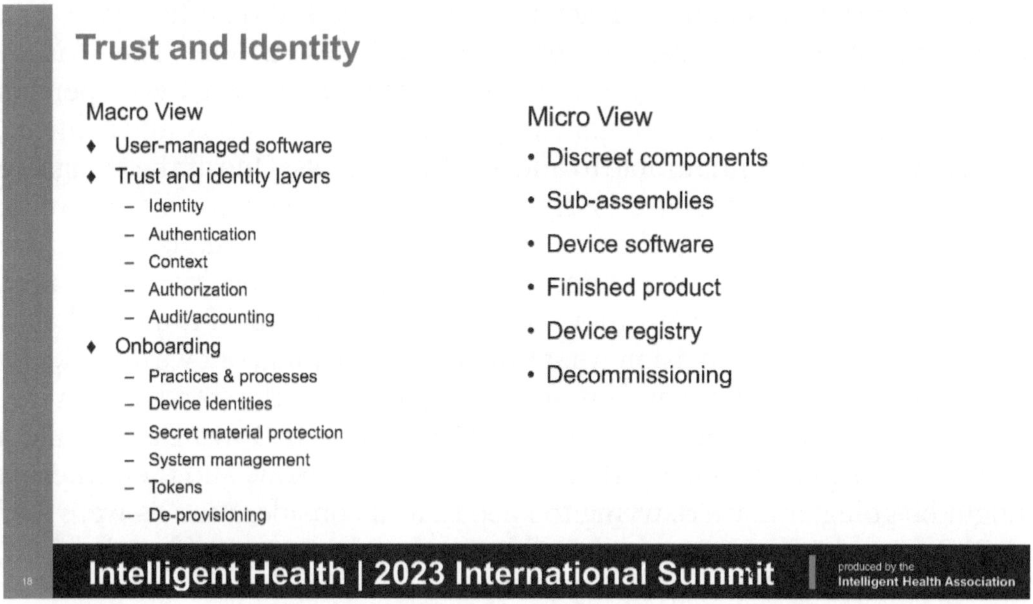
Trust and Identity
Macro View
User-managed software
Trust and identity layers
Identity
Authentication
Context
Authorization
Audit/accounting
Onboarding
Practices & processes
Device identities
Secret material protection
System management
Tokens
De-provisioning
Micro View
Discreet components
Sub-assemblies
Device software
Finished product
Device registry
Decommissioning
18
Intelligent Health | 2023 International Summit
produced by the
Intelligent Health Association

Then we get into Privacy, and there are a number of interrelated privacy elements that we include Data Protection Frameworks from around the world. And we have samples of those in the in the backup, the appendix of the standard, because you have to be careful in the standard. What you're supposed to do is say you shall do this, meaning everybody has to do it. But when there's separate governance it doesn't apply everywhere. So, some of these are frameworks we refer to. We say, make sure you know what's going on in your jurisdiction. Privacy by Design throughout the design and operational life cycle, just like William, was talking about at the beginning of the design and development phase.

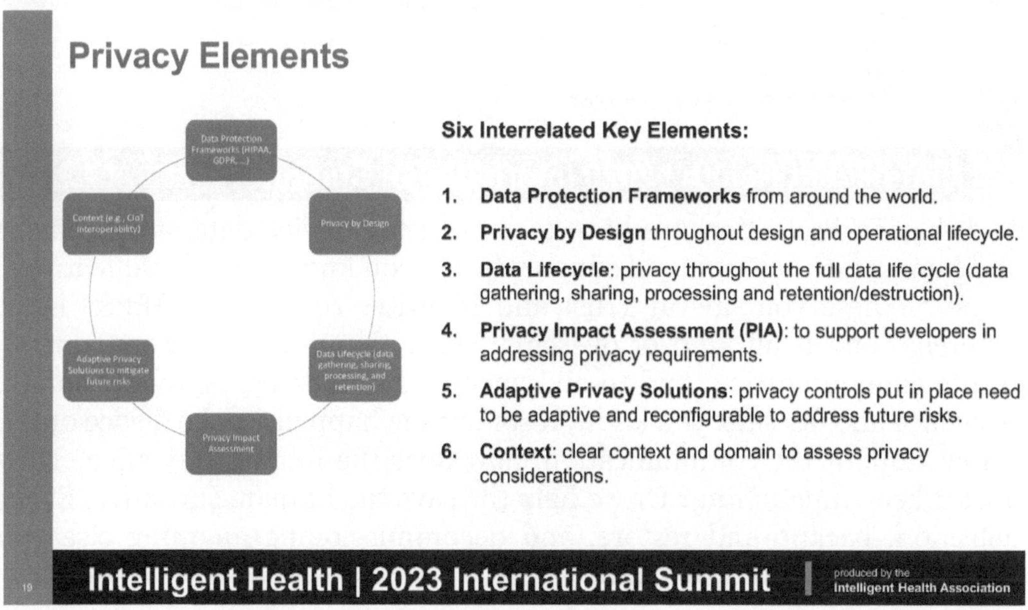

During the Data Lifecycle, privacy throughout the full data life cycle data gathering, sharing processing, retention, and destruction. The Privacy Impact Assessment. We suggest that's created to support developers in addressing privacy, requirements. Adaptive Privacy, Solutions, and controls, so that it can be reconfigurable to address future risks. One of the things we talk about with the standard is that we want it to be extensible, meaning that as we get to future technologies, like William was talking about, you know, Virtual Reality, Augmented Reality, Extended Reality, any reality, non-reality, whatever. You know, as we move into the future and new technologies. We can envision what might be happening, but we don't know exactly what's gonna happen, but we're trying to create the standard in a way that, as an aerospace engineer, I'd say there's a Heads Down Display and a Heads Up Display. You know there's what we have today, and then where it might be going, and we're trying to keep that in consideration as well. And then having clear context and domain to assess privacy considerations. So, all this is explained in the Privacy section.

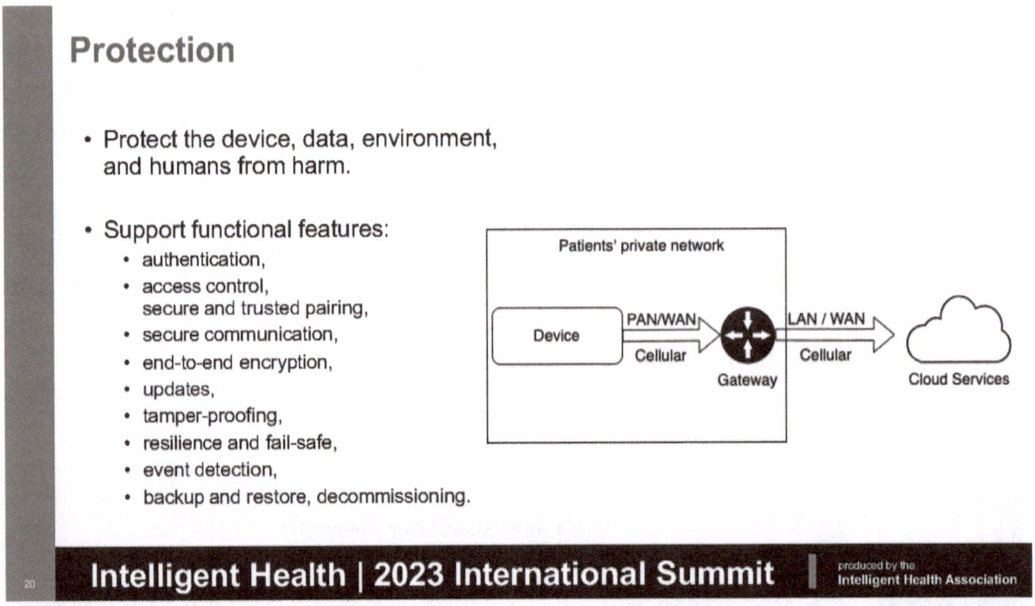


And then in Protection, we have to protect the device data, environment and humans from harm, and support these, you know, functional features. Some of these you saw in Trust and Identity. You know, TIPPSS is an umbrella, and it all kind of overlaps. So, authentication, access control, secure communication, end-to-end encryption, updates, tamper proofing, resilience and fail safe, you know, if something happens to the device or the connection, or the communication, how does the human stay alive? How does it keep functioning? Or we help the save the human, stay alive. Event detection, backup and restore, and decommissioning anything else you want to say about this, William?

## William Harding, Ph.D.

No, I think that's a mouthful for sure.

## Florence Hudson

And then, of course, safety, which is, an element of all medical devices already that have a governance structure like the FDA that we have here in the US. And then also consideration of direct and indirect patient safety, like disruption of clinical data flows. You know, if you're not getting new clinical information and clinical data about a patient, can you be making a poor assessment? Disruption of patient engagement, inability to use clinical devices. God forbid, there's a ransomware attack which we see on TV all the time, and unfortunately, it's real. Addressing risk due to regulatory constraints and unavailability of supporting systems. You know, central monitoring, interpretation, analysis, prescription that can actually impede, you know, proper care. And operational impacts that can compromise safety, environmental disruption, workflow and business disruption, loss of sensitive data or intellectual property, and compromise of user and network credentials. So, all of these are safety elements. So, what you'll see in the standard, God willing, when it comes out in the draft, you could see is that we have technical elements all the way down to like trusted platform modules and chips, and then also process elements. You know, how you should be approaching this.

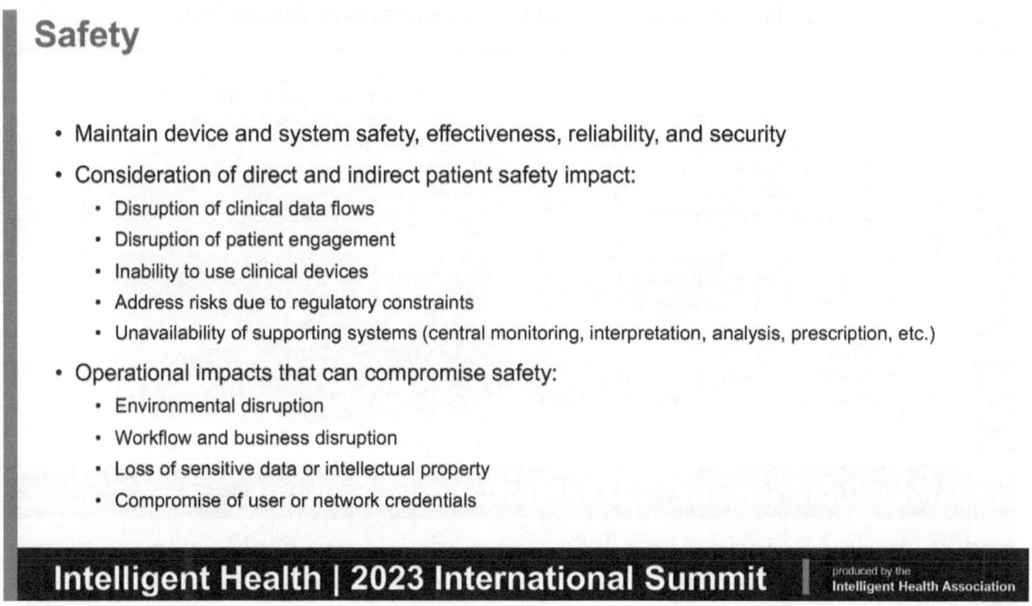

## William Harding, Ph.D.

And I like what you said on that portion there, because in looking at that slide it really talks beyond just direct attacks. You know, brute force, or whatever type of attacks. It talks about disruption that may not even look like it's even associated with the devices. And then, actually, when we think unavailable support, we thought about central monitor monitoring analysis, and so on down the line. But, speed, and that all really came to, you know, when we think of designing our systems is, we have to be able to make sure that the inner process of getting data back and forth between caregivers and patients has to be addressed. So, even the just the effectiveness of transferring data or transforming data. Was one thing, but it had to be done in a timely fashion.

## Florence Hudson

Exactly. And we have a whole analysis we did. And I wanna bore you with the details. It's a very, it looks like little finite element model for those of us who are in aerospace engineering. You and I both worked in aerospace before. And it has a lot of detail on what exactly would you do in these different situations?

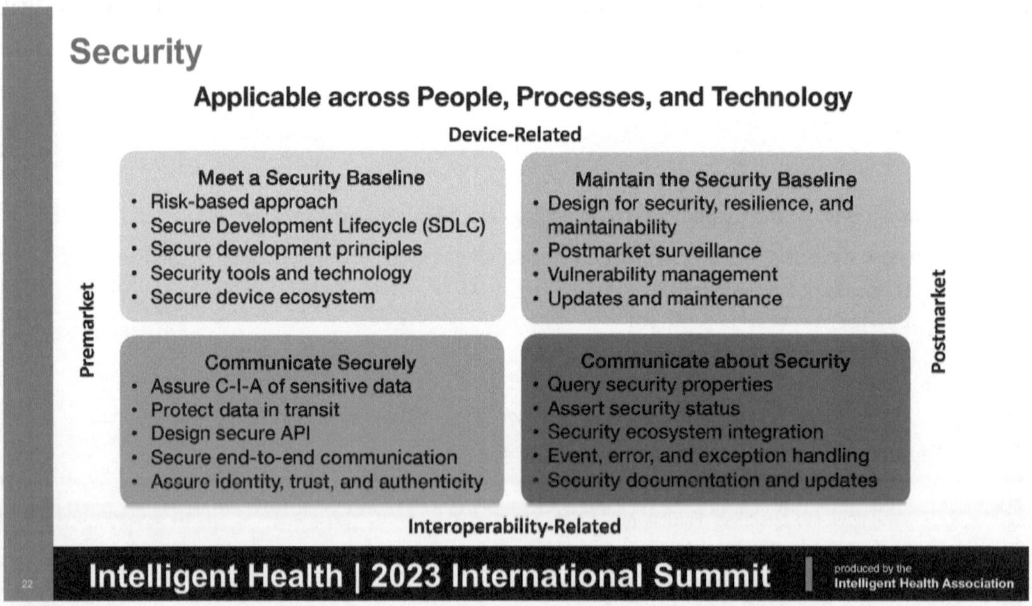
Security
Applicable across People, Processes, and Technology
Device-Related
Meet a Security Baseline
• Risk-based approach
• Secure Development Lifecycle (SDLC)
• Secure development principles
• Security tools and technology
• Secure device ecosystem
Maintain the Security Baseline
• Design for security, resilience, and maintainability
• Postmarket surveillance
• Vulnerability management
• Updates and maintenance
Communicate Securely
• Assure C-I-A of sensitive data
• Protect data in transit
• Design secure API
• Secure end-to-end communication
• Assure identity, trust, and authenticity
Communicate about Security
• Query security properties
• Assert security status
• Security ecosystem integration
• Event, error, and exception handling
• Security documentation and updates
Premarket
Postmarket
Interoperability-Related
22
Intelligent Health | 2023 International Summit
produced by the
Intelligent Health Association

And then, for Security, you know, Security is applicable across people, processes, and technology. And someday, God willing, when you get to see the standard, you'll see that we have those 3 different things. And actually, we have this thing called Tripod, which is People, Organizations, and Technology, and how all of them are part of the system of systems that we're talking about. And so, there are different elements that we need to look at, meeting a security baseline, having a risk based approach, communicating securely. You can see CIA is still part of the picture, sharing confidentiality, integrity, availability of sent sensitive data. Maintaining the security baseline and communicating about security. And all of these are important elements, pre-market and post-market.

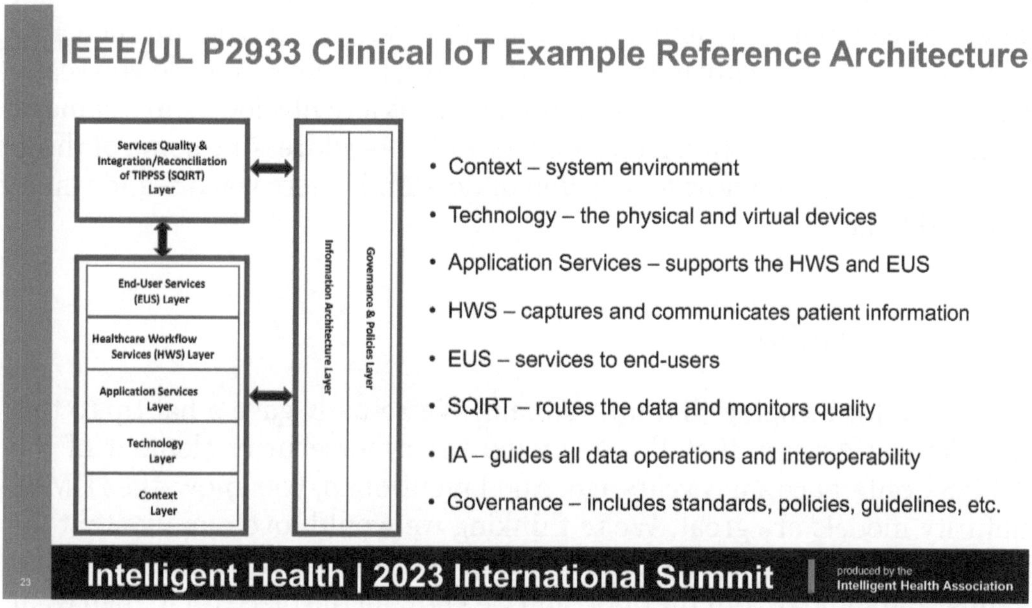


Then what we did is we pull this all together. We had the integrated system design team that did a great job. And they created this example reference architecture. So, it's not a required reference architecture, because everybody is different, but it's an example of a reference architecture that could be leveraged. And so, when we first started this, we gave the team opportunity. So, we actually gave the team liberty to say, you know, maybe you want to create a new word, you know, because we're doing something that hasn't been done before. So don't be limited. So, they did. And they created this SQIRT layer, which is Services Quality & Integration/Reconciliation of TIPPSS. Very interesting. And so, what they look at here is that there are different layers. There's Context, which is the system environment, the Technology layer, which is the physical and virtual devices, Application Services layer supporting the Healthcare Workflow Services, and End User Services, and then SQIRT that routes the data and monitors quality for the TIPPSS elements. And then we have the Information Architecture layer and the Governance and policy layer. And so, what I imagine, if I were the CTO or CIO or CISO, I would take this and I would put it on a wall. And I would say, okay, what is ours gonna look like? You know, what goes in here? And so that's the idea here. That's why they're like big white boxes, you know, so they can be customized by organization and application. Is there anything you wanted to add?

## William Harding, Ph.D.

No, that's perfect. I love it. And, in fact, in some ways it starts to form what we would call maturity model. Are you there yet? So, as you are the CISO or individual that's really managing it, your organization, how do you really determine if you're there yet? And though this is a really good start, some of the next follow ups to things that we'll be doing is addressing some of those maturity models, and how to help you understand where you are and where you need to be.

## Florence Hudson

Thank you for bringing that up, William. We actually gave a hat tip to this idea the last 2 years that I've keynoted the cybersecurity element of the HIMSS Conference a few years ago. And I mentioned, you know, the HIMSS maturity models are great. We're thinking we would love one like that for TIPPSS and then we talked about it again last year. So, after we have, God willing, the standard out the door, and we know all the pieces of it, then what we'd like to do is create like a working group to create a maturity model. A TIPPSS maturity model.

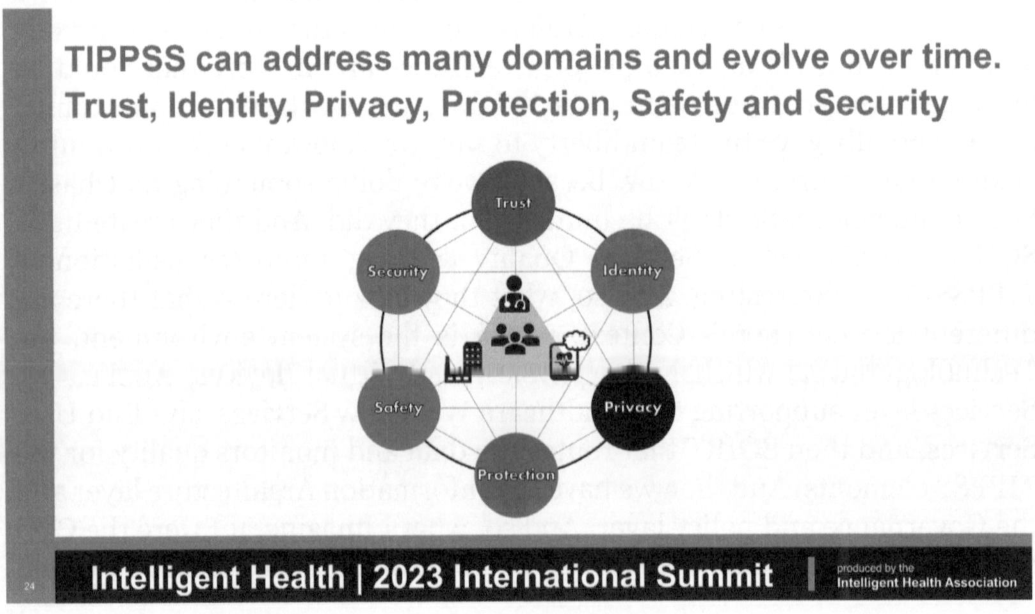
TIPPSS can address many domains and evolve over time.
Trust, Identity, Privacy, Protection, Safety and Security
Trust
Identity
Privacy
Protection
Safety
Security
24
Intelligent Health | 2023 International Summit
produced by the Intelligent Health Association

And as we look at this, TIPPSS can address many domains and evolve over time. You know, as I was saying, as we were both saying, there are future technologies that will come out. There are future use cases that will come out. There are other domain areas that we're already talking to. We're actually on November first of this year, 2023 we actually had a meeting in Boston with a decentralized clinical trials team, and they want to create a TIPPSS working group for decentralized clinical trials specific to that environment. I presented it at a National Cancer Institute in Us. Department of Energy co-hosted Virtual Human Global Summit about a month or two ago. And they're very interested in how this applies to biomedical digital twins. You know, those could be hacked. What a problem that would be, God forbid, right? And so, what we're doing is taking this, like, you know, TIPPSS lens and applying it in new areas. I've already started talking to the smart grid people. I'm actually on an advisory board for some smart grid research and we're talking about that. And I already presented about this in Berlin in December of 2019, right before everything shut down at an autonomous vehicle discussion with a lot of the European manufacturers in the automotive space. And so, there's a lot of opportunity to apply this across many domains. And when NIST the National Institute of Standards Technology had me present this a year ago, they said, so can we apply this to all the other domains? I said, absolutely, let's get the first one done so we know what we're talking about, and then see how we could evolve it.

## William Harding, Ph.D.

I love it, cause that means we're not trying to bite off more than we can chew. We're really trying to hit the impactful areas. And I like how that you characterize, you know, where we're trying to get accomplished right now, what we will be moving to when we think of artificial intelligence, superposition of data, quantum computing, and AI and so on, like, I've said, so it let the teams and people who are watching this understand we have a group and we have been evaluating these elements and we're trying to get the most impactful, the most direct elements out, the foundations established, and then continue to work on those efforts.

## Florence Hudson

Absolutely. And our role model for people who follow standards is 802 like, you might know 802.11, you know, Wi-fi standards. So, they created it years ago. Now there are all these different forks? It's like a big blockchain, you know, and they went in all different directions. It could be different applications for different communication speeds for different whatever, different devices, you know. So that's what we're thinking to create a base TIPPSS standard. And then hopefully, it can apply in multiple domains. And we look forward to working on that, and we'll be looking for experts in any of those areas who want to jump in. Right now, we're developing the Decentralized Clinical Trials Group. If you have knowledge in that area and you let me know here's our contact information and thank you for having us. We're very grateful and so emails, and you can always connect with us on LinkedIn. And here's Twitter, X, I like the birdie better, but I put X there, too. And these are the organizations, FDHint is my consulting organization. Then the Northeast Big Data Hub is where we work for real my day job. And then IEEE Standard Association. We're very grateful that they're supporting the working group and UL, Underwriters Laboratories that is partnering with us for this whole thing. So that was our plan today.

And so that's what we wanted to share. And I think that if people have access to the chat. We have a lot of information in there. Thank you, Emily, for putting it in there. And things you can look at.

So, I think that's it. William, any other comments you'd like to make?

## William Harding, Ph.D.

That’s good for me. It was wonderful partnering with you as always.

# Chapter 5:

## ABC in Action: AI, Blockchain, and Cybersecurity from Lab to Launch

**David Metcalf, PhD**
*Director, METIL*

*University of Central Florida, Institute for Simulation & Training*

### *Editor's Note*

David Metcalf pulls together concepts of ABC and examples from projects and programs that are leveraging AI, Blockchain and Cybersecurity. The spectrum of development from "Lab to Launch" is even evident in the process of developing published materials, studies, reports and books. Whether in industry, academia, military/government or nonprofits, benefits as well as cautions exist. Which segments will benefit most? How can technologies from other sectors improve healthcare?

I'm David Metcalf at the University of Central Florida's Institute for Simulation and Training. And getting to sit at a large public and very diverse university gives us an opportunity to see a lot of these technologies in action and to get to experience them firsthand. And that's what's been great to be able to do in adjacent technology areas like cybersecurity. How can we make sure that we have the proper protections and privacy on these new systems? We heard a lot about that, about the ethics of this, and the underpinnings of this from a technology standpoint. Building on that stack is technologies like blockchain, which you think of as for Bitcoin and other areas like that too, but it's more than that. And even some of the front end interfaces, leveraging from areas like game design. How can we build upon that? It really takes a whole interdisciplinary team. That's what we've established at a laboratory that I run called the Mixed Emerging Technology Integration Lab (METIL).

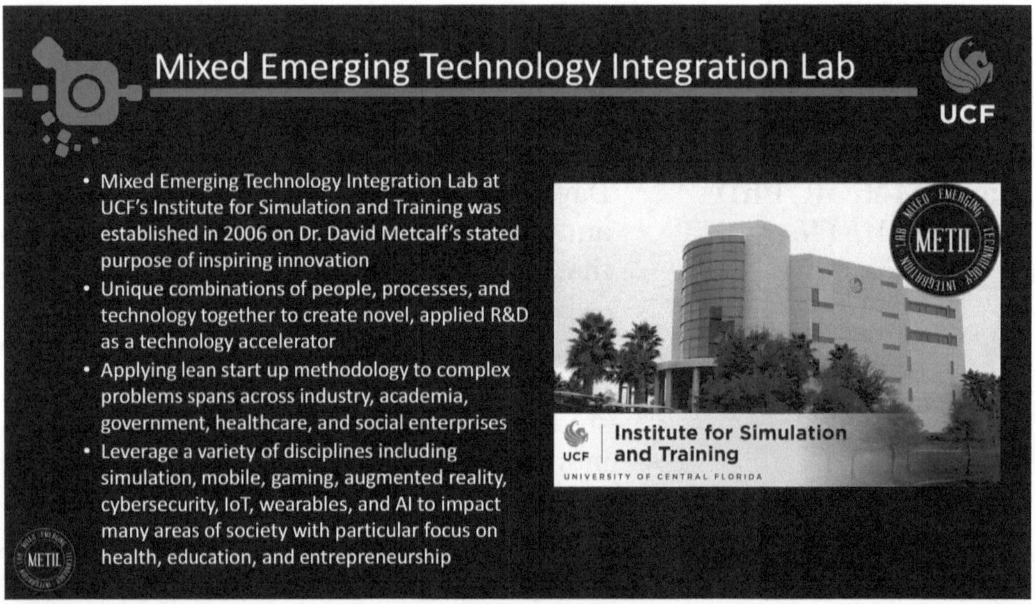


We get to have a lot of fun with people like Dexter and people like Val doing some of these different projects and doing the technology below them too across a wide variety of industry segments. Of course, a major one of those is healthcare too. We sit at that epicenter of research in these areas of simulation and how simulation cuts across all these different areas and includes things like artificial intelligence, blockchain, cybersecurity, some of the advances in Augmented and Virtual Reality for smart cities, and the Internet of Medical Things. We get to sit at the epicenter for that for really the world. One of the things we have to ask ourselves early in the Design Thinking process is, how do we go and build some of those components that are going to survive the test of time and really be practical, pragmatic, and able to be rolled out? Innovation management is a key part of that.

The National Science Foundation and National Institutes of Health have been using a program called I-Corps, Hacking4Defense, Hacking4Diplomacy or Disaster, or other techniques that look at this innovation life cycle. I wanna set a big picture context that doesn't just narrowly focus only on AI but also takes us down the pathway of what other emerging technologies will make AI better, what other emerging technologies can secure AI, what other emerging technologies can be put together in a meaningful way to form those building blocks for the next generation of enterprise solutions and information architecture.

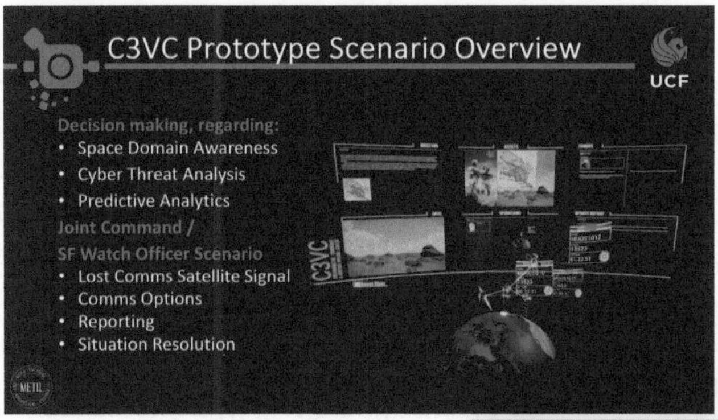


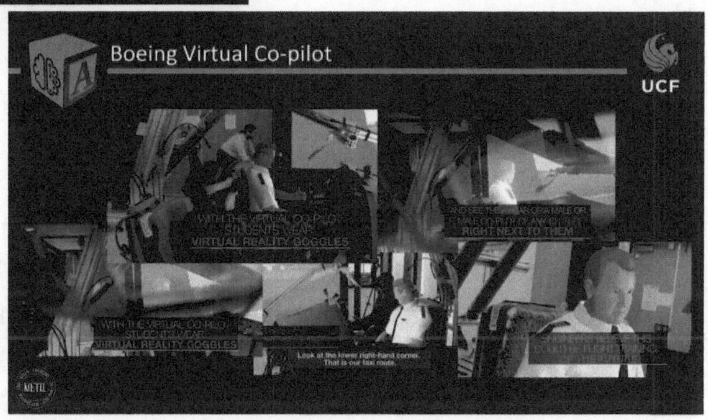


A very wise Colonel, Colonel Wilson Ariza came up to me one day when we were looking at our research portfolio and all the different things we were doing. He said, really over the next 10 to 20 years, you should keep it simple. Look at *ABC*, AI, blockchain, and cyber. And looking at cybersecurity and all of these technologies within the post-quantum era, and what happens within quantum computing. Those are the types of projects that seem to be coming more and more to laboratories like ours and really having a profound effect on how we plan for the next generation of these solutions. This is evident in things like work we've done on the health front with Defense Health Agency and the Navy working together. They have a big picture view of the training that has to be done and every single rating and role, including those within the health professions, and opportunities to go and build an architecture that a few years ago, even we were planning on, how would you fundamentally have this structure to be able to keep track of from recruit to retire? The health and learning records of the individuals who are not only providers, but also the patients too, within these health systems. We were adamant when we were doing this project work that we needed to make sure we had space for even something as simple as a recommendation engine to try and personalize the learning and personalize the health experience, but also the Artificial Intelligence that might be used. We were kind of mistaken in thinking about what might be used say in 2030, many, many years from now. It was interesting to see that all of that technology came to bear in such a short period of time.

We've been able to start to integrate those things into these large scale programs of record that are going to last for a really long time. The ability to leverage this within large scale deployments of medical information and medical informatics. Having this at your fingertips, new systems that are coming out across the Army Future Command and the Army partnership with the University of Miami, University of Central Florida, to even do these types of Deployed Medicine activities across trauma and triage care for the globe has been instrumental. Not only during the time of COVID, but any major natural disaster, any conflict, all of those areas are very important to the practical, pragmatic view of medicine. Using AI, using blockchain, and using the best in cybersecurity methods is a fundamental capability that needs to be there for any type of large scalable system that's going to go to 500,000+ like this one.

We've also had an opportunity to think about what this means in terms of the patient experience and having a little bit of intelligence, a little bit of humanity, if we can call it that, embedded into things like robotic systems that might take the scare out of going for a cancer diagnosis. Orlando Health has their Betty Project that some of the docs came up with and we helped build the first couple of prototypes that had the ability to tell simple jokes, to start to do patient intake, and to have some intelligence almost like smart electronic health records. Those are the types of things that we're starting to see. AI being integrated so much so that you may not even say the words Artificial Intelligence. It's just going to be the way that systems are in a very short order.

That's also true of other interventions within the learning space, saving lives through the use of advanced personalization of learning within the field of medicine. How can we have humans learn as fast as these machines are learning? Those are the types of things that we're trying to make sure that we have a way to keep pace within these different areas. We've also been building whole digital twins of facilities and locations. This gives us an opportunity to have a preview of what a building is going to be like before it's there, to define all of the different flow and dynamics of workflow, and plan all of that out using AI, Virtual Reality, and Augmented Reality techniques. We've done that at the places like the Veterans Administration. What you're seeing over on the right side of the screen is actually showing one of the state-of-the-art digital studios for Department of Energy to deal with a radiological element within something like blood irradiator.

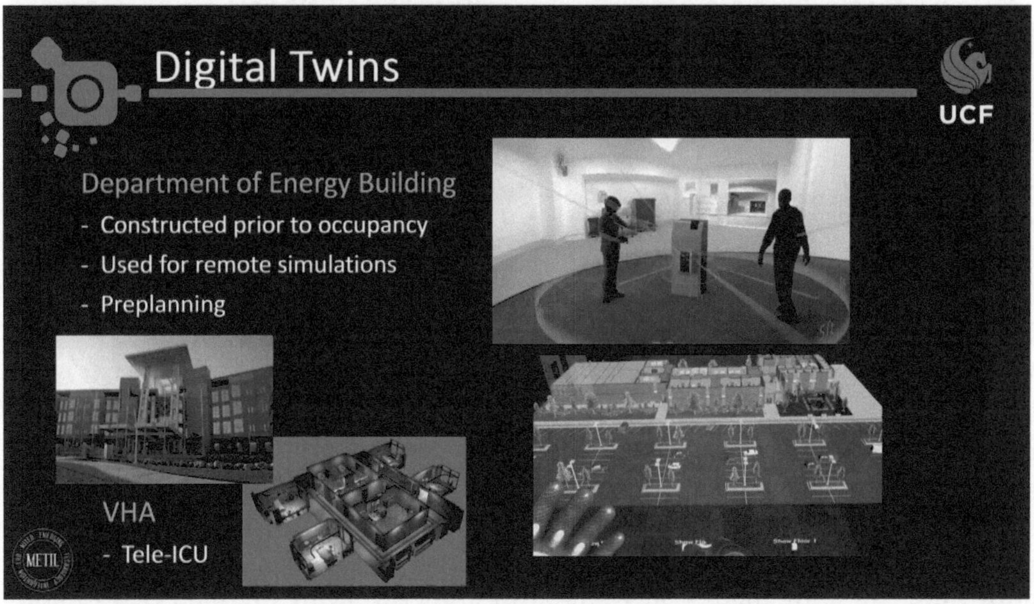


We're building these things on top of an infrastructure. You may have thought of large-scale computing clusters. Well, we're looking at putting together some of the next generation of those. Thanks to a grant from Army Research Office, we've had an opportunity to build the world's first Blockchain and Quantum Defense Simulator. You can simulate taking AI projects like Dr. Hadley's and having a blockchain to have an immutable record of whatever different technologies and whatever different medical records you need to have access to, whether that's medical imaging or some other area. Having the ability to also have part of this array be retuned to Artificial Intelligence has given us opportunity to look at ways that we can combine the best of cybersecurity. Asking questions such as, can we keep the records safe from future quantum attacks where every one can be a zero, every zero can be a one? All of a sudden, you may have a big issue, almost like having a skeleton key to those health records. And of course, with HIPAA and other GDPR and TECFA different standards, we need to make sure that we are following through with that by leveraging some of the best thinking from places like what's going on at the Linux Foundation with the Open Voice Network and TrustMark. Those are examples of some of the different types of processes and standards that need to be put in place.

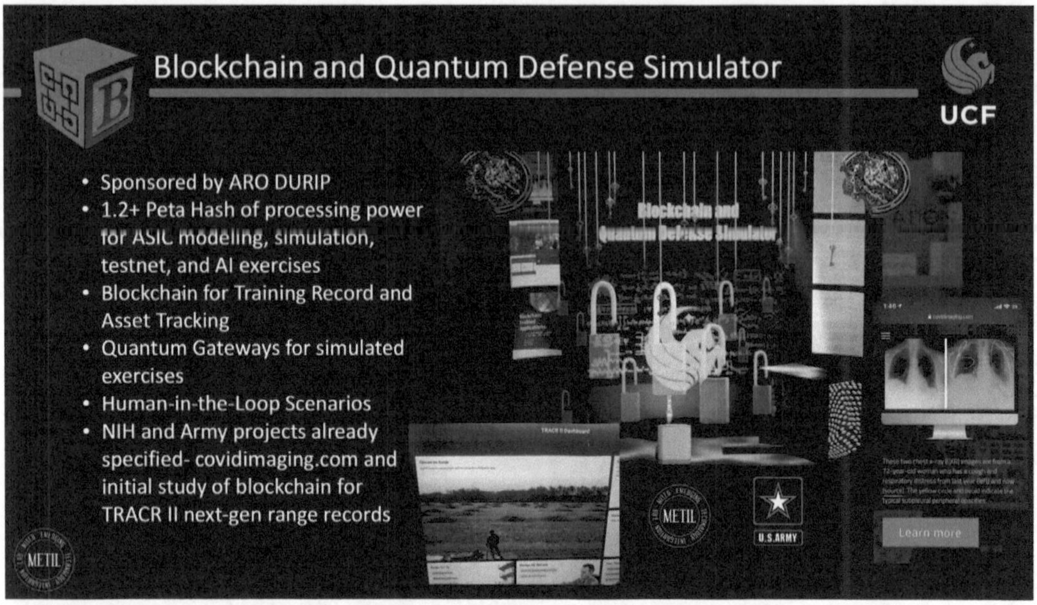


We're getting a chance to have test beds set up to see if these work in real-life settings and have these as separate examples. A number of different use cases over the course of time that we've been able to look at in other areas, but particularly in healthcare in this case, is to look at 5G and IoT technologies along with AI, blockchain, and cyber and how you might defend against some of the potential types of attacks that you can have on your data, on your health systems, and your different medical technology that's in place within a hospital. Those are all important areas.

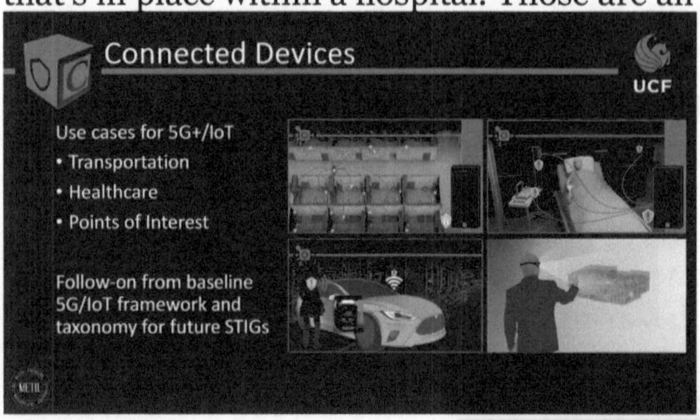


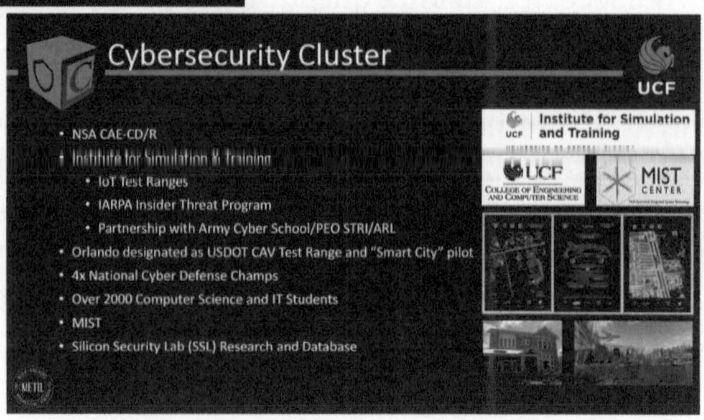

Having a wide variety of backgrounds has helped, but also having the cybersecurity teams that include even our students that are able to help with some of the application and development of the next generation defenses. They're 4x National Cyber Defense champs as of right now. And we're quite proud of those types of things with the students that we have that are an integral part of how we train up the next generation of leaders in healthcare and in technology that are going to look at these solutions and help us build them out.

These are the types of things that we're also getting to do again with the Navy and with other groups. We are working on some of the ways that the next generation of data handling happens for the front end interfaces to show recruit to retire across all of the different roles that you have within the military. Putting some of these pieces together with various projects and having something that could be an out-of-the-box capability. Your own AI as a service to be able to go and test these things is part of what we're doing as a public university to make sure that we can meet the needs of both private industry, government organizations, and nonprofits that want to be able to test out their technology in advance. Whether that's speeding up their whole production process for creating learning materials, in this case for health educators, or having the actual diagnosis, operations, and decision support tools that we hear about so often within the medical community so that you can have that secondary consult.

How do we keep those systems safe? How do we make sure that we have good records that you can keep track of across time? Those are the types of things that we're doing with a number of different tools. We're also able to test out the latest and greatest tools and put this into practice with real-world applications, such as a range where you're shooting targets and, on those targets, you would normally have a range officer that would give you access to a regular physical scorecard at the end that shows you how you did. Now you've got AI-driven computer vision on those ranges and the ability to bring those back and put them together in a sort of showcase, a digital twin of that person's record from recruit to retire. That can be across any discipline. It could be across your medical education, like what Dexter was talking about. These are the types of things that we're seeing in education and in simulation and in the health field.

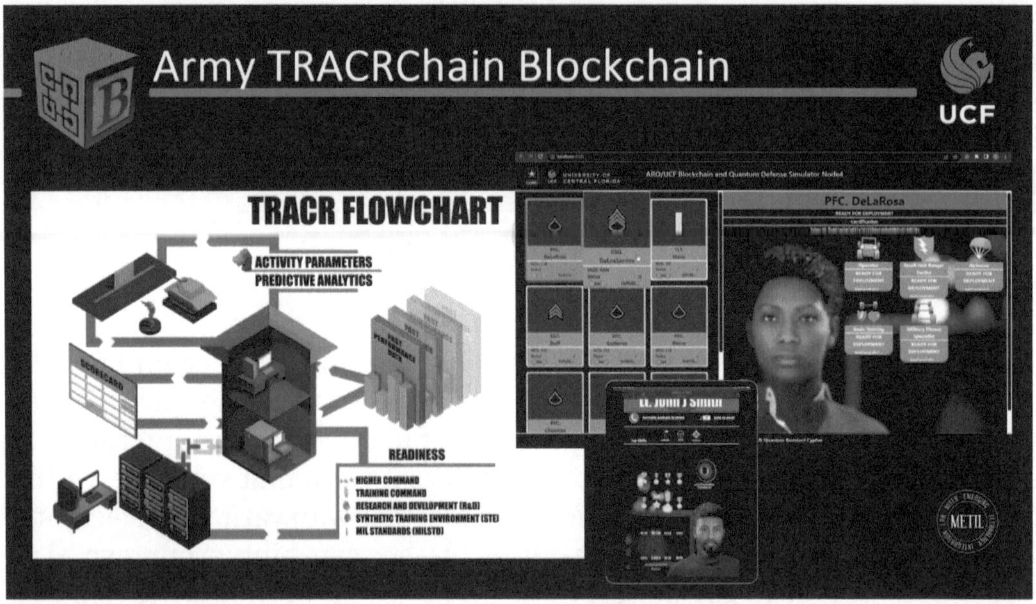


Every agency is going to have to meet the standards for HR 7535, a new law that came into effect that said every agency had to have quantum computing cybersecurity preparedness and have a plan for that by 2025. This includes private industry, hospitals, every aspect of society. We're trying to put together some of the tools to be able to do that. Again, where cybersecurity, AI, and blockchain for some of the verification that come together.

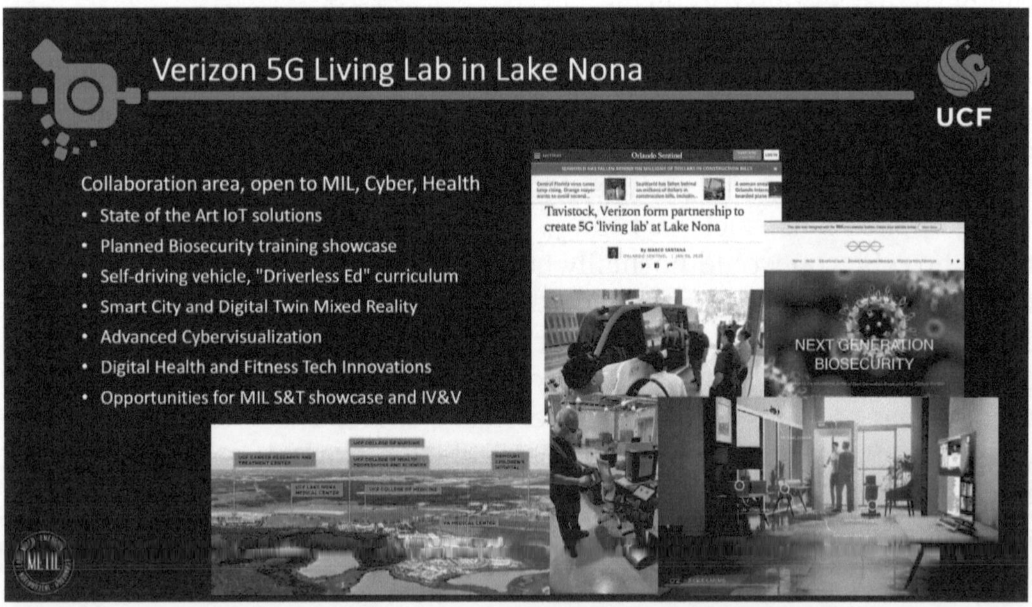


We're blessed to have the Lake Nona district of Orlando that is really a living lab and an innovator's dream. We get to test out the latest in self-driving vehicles, the latest in hospital technology, the latest in 5G technology with Verizon's 5G lab. Anything from robotics to the advances that you might have in health and wellness are part of this community. And the residents tend to get very involved in these studies and these study groups. It's been a pleasure to be able to see, at scale, smart cities technology and the digital twin of the whole community be able to put forward towards looking at health, environmental, and education over the course of time.

We're privileged to have our own College of Medicine there, UF's pharmacology school, the most visited VA in the nation, a freestanding Nemours Children's Hospital, and a number of other health related disciplines and areas within this one centralized community. It's been very collaborative and effective to be able to have this and to see these types of real-world solutions where the AI and the blockchain and the security of these are not screamed about front and center but are part of every single solution of these emerging technology disciplines that you think of having proper intelligent systems architecture below each of these different solutions.

One of the things we think about quite frequently in Florida is, of course, is hurricane season and natural disasters, which happen everywhere, but we tend to be able to have a few more hours, if not days to plan for them. We have these collaborative virtual command centers that can be secured, that can track this and use Artificial Intelligence over time to see how you can plan for predictive analytics, but also how you can plan recovery and logistics and supply. We're seeing groups like Mobility Insights and other groups using these tools and how they can do things even in places like the Gaza Strip right now to plan for those type of disasters.

We've had the privilege of working with places like Kant Consulting, who all the way since 9-11 have been designing solutions that can be low code / no code and able to be delivered very, very quickly. In just a matter of hours to a few days, you can have a full working portal that can keep track and secure all of your information for a one-stop location that also has some smart predictive analytics. Those are the types of things that we're getting to work on that are real-time, that are data-driven and that are looking at the next areas that we might see Artificial Intelligence really having an impact on. We can even have custom reports that are generated in seconds rather than with great effort over time using low code / no code solutions that Artificial Intelligence is going to be driving.

We're quite excited about the opportunities. And for those of you who both are here participating, as well as those that might think about how you can leverage some of this technology, some of these past projects and past work that's been done, your public universities, not just UCF, are really at that epicenter. We are in a good position to be able to bring industry, hospitals, health systems, nonprofits, and government entities together. It's sort of like being that neutral zone that can work on big societal problems. Doing that inside of a very diverse organization, like our university, which is a Minority Serving Institution, you can see for yourself firsthand what that might look like for these next generation technologies. At the same time, we are developing the next generation of leaders and technologists.

If you have opportunities or problems, that maybe need a lot of smart people pointed at it, or that you need a system that you can control to be able to have these AI-as-a-Service or Large Language Model-as-a-Service offerings that can be even within your secure systems and managed, those are the types of things that we're working on right now. This approach is leading to and informing the opportunities that we're taking with the Intelligent Health Association and the Intelligent Health series of books to build out a community. One of the best ways to do that is by having conferences like this, like the KPMG co-sponsored Health Data and Equity for Good conference that they recently did, as well as producing things like a book or an artifact after the fact. We really think that the ABCs for the next generation of intelligent systems architecture is going to drive our future across a number of different disciplines and areas and with particular emphasis in healthcare.

# Chapter 6:

# Trust as a Driver for Growth, Innovation, and Efficiency

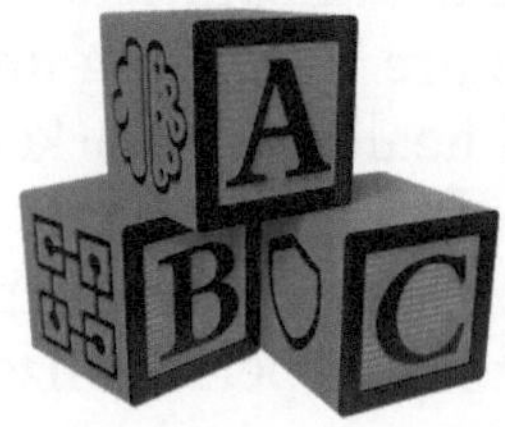



**Oita C. Coleman**
*Senior Advisor*

*Open Voice TrustMark Initiative*

*Linux Foundation AI & Data Foundation*


## *Editor's Note*

In this chapter, Oita Coleman furthers our discussion of standards, capabilities, and trust as they highlight efforts underway at the Linux Foundation around data security, voice, AI in the context of a TrustMark Standard. Having a good housekeeping seal of approval that confirms privacy, security, and trusted verification will enable next-generation solutions leveraging blockchain and cybersecurity practices. We'll continue to bolster the acceptance and adoption of these important technologies throughout the healthcare system.

The US health sector is crucial for the national and global economy, representing 18% of its GDP (gross domestic product).

Three technological domains will likely keep transforming the health sector: **AI, Blockchain, and Cybersecurity**. Looking ahead, we can see the relevance of the ABCs of this next-generation technology, which can pay dividends to the quadruple aim of improving, accelerating, and reducing the cost of health services while respecting and empowering the providers.

What if we combine these technologies? We could enhance applications that ensure privacy, trust, automation, and intelligence, which could have the positive impact on society that we aim to achieve. Yet, these new technologies bring ethical, legal, and technological issues. There are significant reasons why the need, adoption, and use of these technologies are increasing and why they are so important. First, there is a shortage of healthcare workers worldwide. This shortage is leading to disparity in healthcare delivery – especially for underserved populations. Additionally, there is a growing trend in the healthcare industry towards a more distributed and personalized care model – leading to the need for more complex systems, particularly AI, to manage healthcare tasks.

Trust is key to the relationship between healthcare professionals and their patients (Mechanic, D., & Schlesinger, M.,1996). According to the General Medical Council, doctors must earn and keep the trust of their patients by providing high-quality and ethical care (*Good Medical Practice 2024*, n.d.). This principle also applies to other healthcare professionals, such as nurses (The Nursing and Midwifery Council, n.d.) or psychotherapists (*British Psychological Society*, n.d.). Patients need to trust their healthcare professionals to act in their best interest and achieve the best possible outcomes (Hall et al., 2001). Therefore, trust in the healthcare professional is essential for effective treatments (Calnan & Rowe, 2006) and patient-centered care (Sakallaris et al., 2016).

## *The Speed of Trust*

Trust is a catalyst for positive change in health care. According to Stephen Covey's book "The Speed of Trust", trust is not merely a soft, social virtue but a hard-edged economic driver (Covey & Merrill, 2011). The "speed of trust" concept refers to the idea that things get done more quickly and efficiently when trust is high. When trust is present in a relationship, organization, or society, it can significantly accelerate achieving goals and resolving challenges. In a high trust relationship, it's like a dividend that pays off in terms of increased collaboration, innovation, and speed. Conversely, when trust is low, it acts as a hidden cost that slows down processes and hinders progress (Covey & Merrill, 2011).

Covey's statement that "trust is the one thing that changes everything" emphasizes trust's foundational and transformative role in various aspects of personal and professional life (Covey & Merrill, 2011). In the context of healthcare, trust is crucial for building strong relationships between healthcare providers, patients, and other stakeholders. Here's how trust can accelerate improvements in efficiency and patient outcomes in the healthcare sector:

Improved Patient Satisfaction and Engagement: Trust fosters open, honest communication between healthcare providers and patients. When there's a high level of trust, patients are more likely to share important information about their health, symptoms, and lifestyle, enabling healthcare professionals to make more informed decisions. Patients are more likely to follow treatment plans, adhere to medications, and adopt healthy behaviors (Coulter, 2002).

Collaboration and Teamwork: Trust is essential for effective cooperation between healthcare professionals. In a trusting environment, healthcare teams can collaborate seamlessly, share information, and leverage each other's expertise, ultimately leading to better patient care and outcomes (Wang et al, 2023).

Reduced Legal and Ethical Issues: Trust helps reduce legal and ethical challenges. When there is a high level of trust between healthcare providers and patients, misunderstandings and disputes are less likely to occur, contributing to a more positive and efficient healthcare system.

Adaptation to Change: Trust facilitates the acceptance of change. In an environment of trust, healthcare professionals are more likely to embrace new technologies, processes, and innovations, leading to continuous improvement and adaptability in the face of evolving healthcare practices.

Efficient Resource Allocation: Trust allows for more efficient use of resources. When there is trust among healthcare team members, there is smoother coordination of tasks, leading to optimal resource allocation and utilization.

# Guiding Beliefs

The **Open Voice TrustMark Initiative** upholds guiding beliefs that are essential for building trust between patients and providers to achieve positive impact in the use of advanced technology:

- **Do no harm** – an oath to protect the rights of patients and providers
- **Duty of care** – a legal and ethical duty to ensure the safety, well-being, and best interests of others
- **Worthy of trust** – an ethical commitment to ensuring that AI technologies promote benefits while minimizing harm

These guiding beliefs should not be considered obstacles to innovation or progress in next-generation AI, blockchain, or cybersecurity technology. Using these technologies requires careful consideration of legal and ethical issues to minimize risks while advancing patient outcomes. Trust is an accelerator to overcome these challenges. The Open Voice TrustMark Initiative provides guidance for risk mitigation.

# ABC4Health and the Need for Trust

Hospital triage has historically been essential to the healthcare system in helping to ensure that patients receive the prompt and efficient medical attention they need. A group of skilled medical professionals who are trained to evaluate and rank patients according to the severity of their conditions are at the core of the system.

Upon arrival at the hospital, patients undergo a prompt assessment by a triage nurse who records vital signs, medical history, and symptoms. Based on the severity of the patient's condition, the nurse then designates a priority level for them. Patients who are experiencing a life-threatening illness, like a heart attack or stroke, are given top priority and receive care right away.

Patients with less severe conditions are assigned lower priority levels and may have to wait longer to be seen by a doctor. Once a patient has been assigned a priority level, they are directed to the appropriate area of the hospital for treatment.

Overall, the hospital triage system plays a critical role in the healthcare system, helping to ensure that patients receive the medical attention they need promptly and efficiently. Thanks to the expertise of the medical professionals who operate the system, patients can rest assured that they will receive the highest level of care, no matter the severity of their condition.

In the hospital metaphor, we can explore how advanced technologies are continuing to reshape the landscape of the healthcare industry:

- **AI as a Diagnostic Tool:** AI-powered tools can analyze patient data, such as vital signs and medical history, to help identify patients who require urgent attention (EurthTech, 2023). One important way AI technology is being used in triage is through the development of chatbots and virtual assistants – called conversational AI. These tools can help patients navigate the triage process by answering questions about their symptoms and directing them to the appropriate level of care. Chatbots and virtual assistants can also help reduce wait times by providing patients with real-time updates about their status and estimated wait times. By analyzing patient data and identifying subtle changes in vital signs, conversational AI tools can help expedite patient care. The use of conversational AI technology in the triage process can greatly improve the efficiency and accuracy of the system. By analyzing patient data and identifying patterns and trends, AI-powered tools can help doctors and nurses make more informed decisions about patient care, ultimately leading to better patient outcomes (Bria, 2023).

- **Blockchain as a Secure Record-Keeping System:** Imagine the hospital's blockchain as a secure and transparent record-keeping system. Blockchain technology can provide a distributed ledger where all transactions and activities related to patient care are recorded. It can be used in the verification of the authenticity of AI algorithms, to securely store sensitive data, and to provide an auditable trail of activities. It helps build trust by providing a verifiable history of actions and ensuring the integrity of critical information (Song, Jien, et al, 2022).

- **Cybersecurity as Protective Measures:** Cybersecurity represents the protective measures to safeguard the hospital's network, systems, and patient data. Similar to how medical professionals prioritize patient safety, cybersecurity measures prioritize the security and confidentiality of data and systems. They use strategies like intrusion detection systems, encryption, access controls, and frequent security audits to guard against data breaches, illegal access, and other online dangers (Open Voice Network, 2020). Cybersecurity measures are crucial for ensuring trust in the AI and blockchain systems by proactively addressing vulnerabilities and mitigating risks.

The hospital triage example highlights the importance of assessing, prioritizing, allocating resources, and collaborating in the context of trust between **AI, blockchain, and cybersecurity**. The connection between trust, AI, blockchain, and cybersecurity lies in the cohesive functioning of these elements. Trust is built when AI algorithms demonstrate accuracy and reliability, blockchain provides a transparent and secure framework for recording and verifying data, and cybersecurity measures protect critical information.

**Figure 1**
AI "Jobs to Be Done" in Healthcare

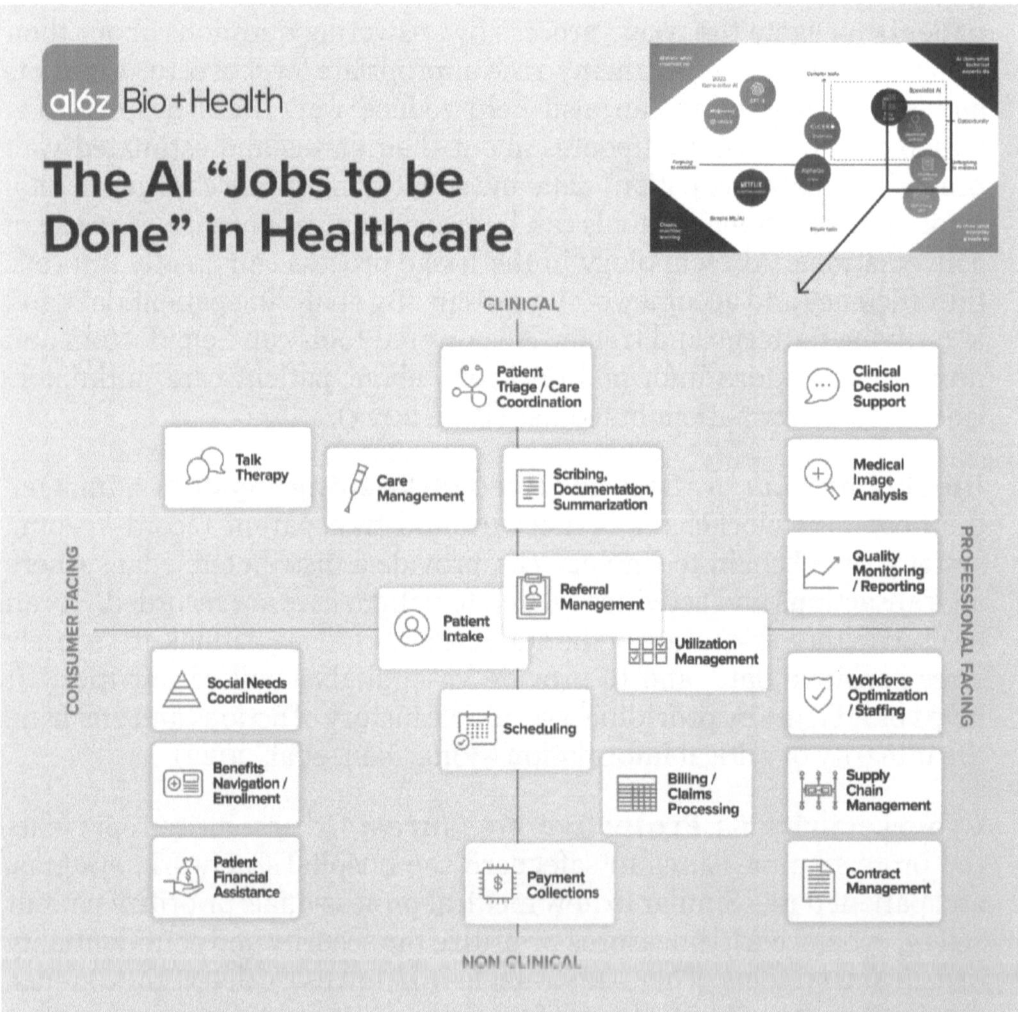


Note: Opportunities for AI within the healthcare tasks, are divided along two axes: clinical vs. non-clinical, and consumer- vs. professional-facing where there is the greatest opportunity for impact to manage complexity. https://a16z.com/commercializing-ai-in-healthcare-the-jobs-to-be-done/

An integrated ABC solution is an excellent fit to manage the complexity for three main reasons:

1. The tasks require processing large amounts of complex and specialized data quickly and accurately to support critical decisions or actions (Rughani et al., 2023).

2. The tasks are time-consuming, compounded by staffing shortages (Rughani et al., 2023).

3. The tasks are very challenging and demand high-quality results.

By working together, these components create a robust ecosystem where trust is established, enabling the effective and secure deployment of AI and blockchain technologies in various applications, such as:

- **Secure Patient Data Sharing:** Blockchain can create a secure and immutable ledger of patient health records. Conversational AI interfaces can then access this data securely to provide relevant information during patient consultations. Patients can control access to their health data and grant permissions to healthcare providers through conversational AI interfaces, ensuring privacy and data security.

- **Patient Identity Management:** Blockchain can serve as a decentralized and tamper-proof ledger for patient identities. Each patient would have a unique digital identity stored on the blockchain. Conversational AI interfaces can interact with the blockchain to verify patient identities during various interactions, such as appointment scheduling, telehealth consultations, or accessing personal health records.

- **Credential Verification for Healthcare Professionals:** Blockchain can be used to store and verify the credentials of healthcare professionals, reducing the risk of fraudulent claims (Walling & Walling, 2023). Conversational AI can assist in verifying the credentials of healthcare providers during recruitment processes or when patients seek information about their caregivers.

- **Decentralized Clinical Data Repositories:** Blockchain can support the creation of decentralized clinical data repositories, allowing patients to control their health data. Conversational AI interfaces can help patients securely manage and share their data, ensuring that healthcare providers receive accurate and up-to-date information.

- **Interoperability and Health Information Exchange:** Blockchain facilitates secure and interoperable health information exchange between healthcare entities. Conversational AI interfaces can assist in querying and exchanging health information seamlessly across various platforms while maintaining data integrity.

# Conversational AI in the Healthcare Enterprise

## *Working Definition of Conversational AI*

Conversational AI implements voice technology in audible and/or textual automated interchanges between a human and digital device that facilitates Interactive, automated patient engagement; inclusive engagement; accessible engagement; and biomarker precision medicine.

AI technologies are a revolutionary innovation for enhancing, speeding up and lowering the expense of health services, while respecting and empowering the providers. Conversational AI technologies enable this transformation by allowing natural and effective communication between humans and machines.

Broadly defined, voice technologies offer the following, through software that can reside on multiple types of devices (Open Voice Network, 2023):

- **natural language understanding and processing** – the ability of a computational device to "listen" to human utterances and translate spoken words into text, across dozens of languages and dialects
- **natural language generation** – the ability of a computational device to turn text into human-like speech across dozens of languages and dialects
- **voice assistance** – through which a computer can proactively interact with a human (e.g., providing reminders, a clinical interview, or entertainment) or respond to human inquiries with trustworthy information on a 24/7 basis. **This can enable interactive, automated patient engagement,** including
    - brief verbal diary entries
    - conversational apps with patient/caregiver instructions and virtual coaches

  - data-gathering/reporting tools that use voice technology to gather and report new data and interact with wearable devices that track fitness and health conditions through blood pressure, glucose, heart rate, and digital ECG/EKG monitors

- **a means for continuous care and evaluation of chronic conditions,** providing
  - Information on leading health indicators
  - automated reminders
  - instruction/education
  - caregiver coordination and decision support
  - companionship
  - A trustworthy source of 24/7 information

- **inclusive and accessible patient engagement** across multiple languages, dialects, speech differences, and underserved populations (Pew Research Center, 2021)

- **AI-based speech/voice analysis,** which can provide assessments of leading indicators of the speaker's mental and physical health, as well as identify (with increasing accuracy) the speaker's gender, geographic region, ethnicity, educational-income level, body mass index, upper body strength, and personality type, and emotion. The human voice is
  - a biometric identifier, similar to fingerprints in the ability to identify a unique individual
  - a biomarker (defined as a measurable substance in an organism whose presence is indicative of some phenomenon such as disease, infection, or environmental exposure), which, in voice, can provide increasingly precise indicators of mental and physical illness, ranging from schizophrenia to Parkinson's and respiratory conditions such as COVID-19 (Püntmann, 2009).

Generative AI chatbots can perform tasks such as reading patient records and summarizing their main points. They can also translate documents and conversations in different languages and use a synthetic voice to speak the results. Generative AI involves natural language processing, understanding, and generation, and the AI technologies that enable machines to comprehend the intent of a human question, and to produce relevant answers to that question. Conversational AI technologies increasingly incorporate generative AI and large language models. One of the most famous models is OpenAI's ChatGPT.

# Voice Data Analysis

The human voice is composed of distinctive sonic characteristics such as tone, speed, duration, volume, and pitch. These characteristics are unique to each individual.

**Figure 2**
Voice Data Analysis

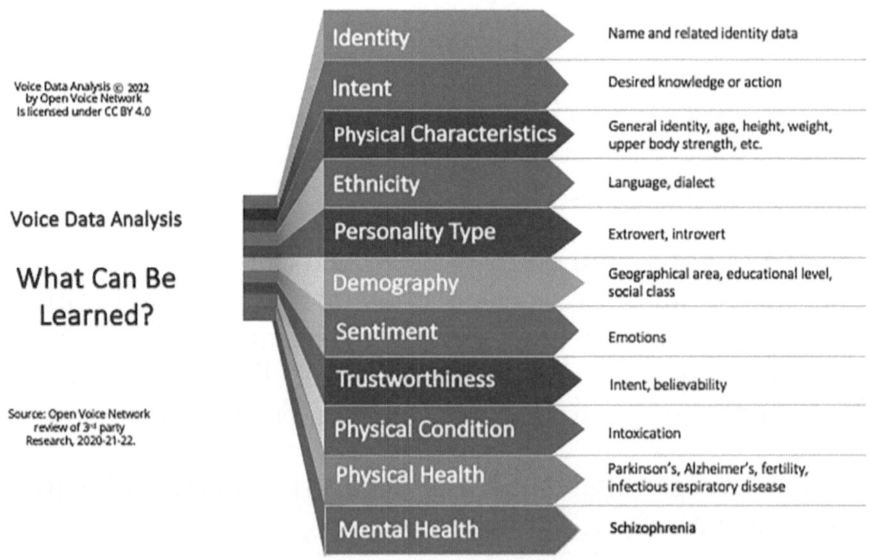


Voice technology can identify, analyze, and deduce sensitive and personal information about an individual from these distinctive characteristics in the sound of their voice and ambient noise. This can include information about an individual's identity, such as their name, location, socioeconomic status, physical characteristics, physical health, mental health, emotions, intent, and more.

These characteristics can be processed and analyzed for various purposes, including:

- Voice authentication can be used for purposes such as fraud detection, call center identification verification, contactless login, two-factor authentication, digital signatures, workforce management, and more (Maureen, 2023). Benefits include saving time and money, increasing security and accessibility, and ease of implementation.
- **Patient intent analysis and understanding,** a proven, increasingly accurate capability that enables automated communication with patients – reminders, intake interviews, patient requests, and search for medical information.
- Acoustic biomarker analysis of leading indicators of physical and mental conditions is a rapidly growing area of research and is increasing in use in clinical implementations. This promises significant value in service delivery and efficiency.

In all cases, clinicians and providers must review carefully: what data is collected; why the data is collected – the purpose and expected outcome; which specific data is analyzed and for what purpose; who is collecting the data; how the data is collected and stored; how long data will be stored; inherent biases within the data that may shape results; and how the analysis will be interpreted (Open Voice Network, 2023).

# Conversational AI Risks

**Figure 3**
Conversational AI Risks

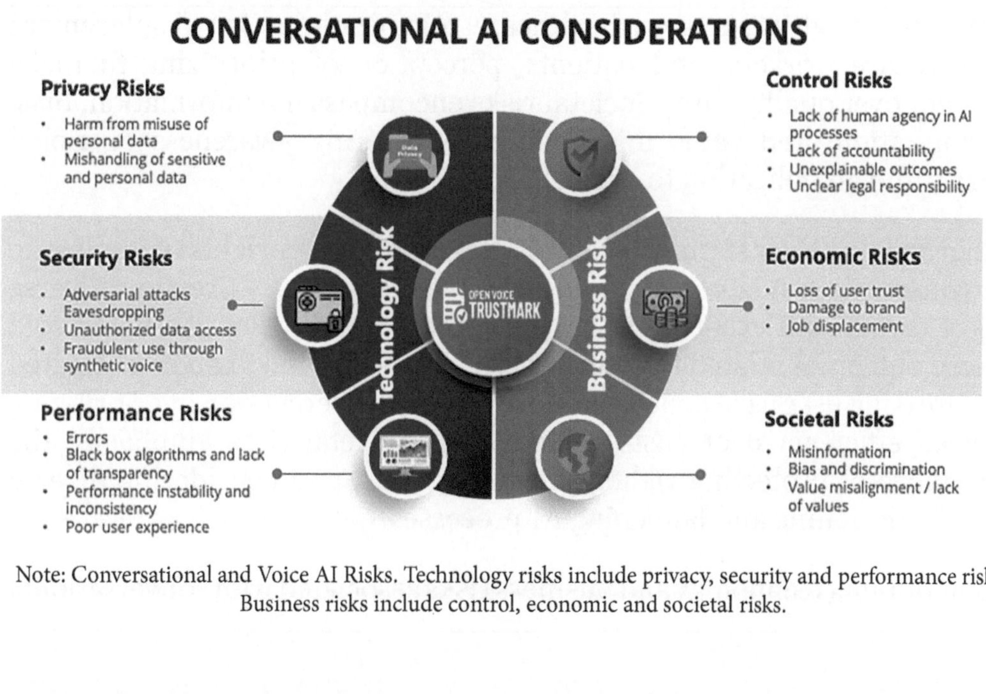


Note: Conversational and Voice AI Risks. Technology risks include privacy, security and performance risks. Business risks include control, economic and societal risks.

The risks in business related to conversational AI can be categorized into three groups: privacy, security, and performance. Privacy concerns emerge from inadequately secured storage and transmission of patient data, compromised systems becoming susceptible to unauthorized access by hackers and other malicious entities, dissemination of inaccurate medical information, and data theft. Establishing trust is particularly vital, especially in healthcare scenarios involving voice-only interfaces where privacy concerns are heightened. It becomes imperative to implement robust mechanisms to safeguard patient privacy when trust is compromised.

Security risks pertain to the vulnerability of digital information and systems, including applications like conversational AI, to attacks and malicious interference. In healthcare, voice technology may be exploited to impersonate public figures, introducing risks of spreading misinformation and manipulation. However, complications arise with the use of "black box" AI methods, particularly in healthcare applications, lacking transparency in decision-making. This opacity can result in potential inaccuracies and a lack of clear ownership of identifiable content. Performance risks include the expectation that the use of technology achieves shared goals, but challenges arise with the use of "black box" AI methods that lack transparency in decision-making, leading to potential inaccuracies and a lack of identifiable content ownership (Open Voice Network, 2023).

Business risks associated with conversational AI fall into three categories: control, economic, and societal. Control risks involve issues such as a lack of human agency, accountability, and unclear legal responsibility, which can erode trust and lead to negative reputation. Economic risks include financial impacts on healthcare organizations, job displacement of healthcare workers, and patients' perception of prioritizing financial efficiency over quality care. Societal risks encompass misinformation, bias, discrimination, and value misalignment, requiring awareness of global impacts and an obligation to protect rights.

Acknowledging their significance and safeguarding user rights of disclosure and consent is fundamental to address business risks. Creating diverse project teams with expertise in law, technology, and policy can help avoid adverse outcomes related to control risks. Economic risks can be mitigated by addressing user trust concerns and avoiding the perception of prioritizing financial efficiency over customer service. Societal risks emphasize the importance of protecting rights, preventing bias, and considering diverse values in designing and launching AI processes.

Understanding technology and business risks associated with conversational

AI enables the formulation of ethical principles to support voice technology. The Open Voice TrustMark Initiative is dedicated to addressing changes in risk factors and providing continuous education for all stakeholders.

# Open Voice TrustMark Initiative

**Figure 4**
Ethical Principles for Trustworthy Conversational AI

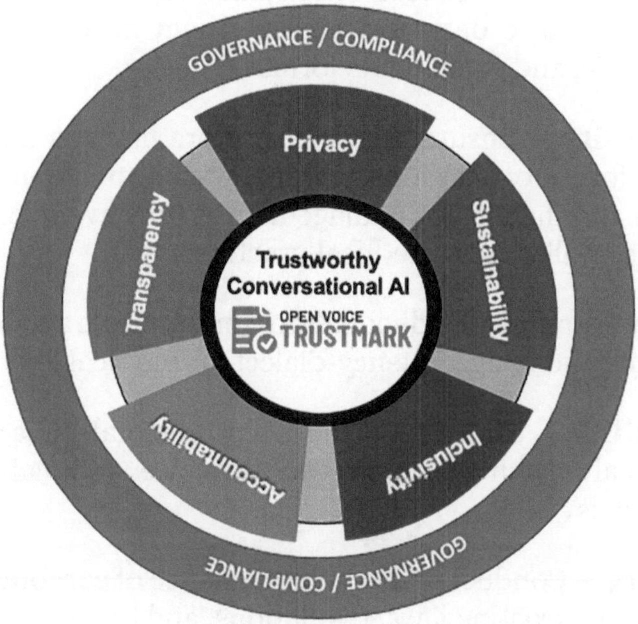


Note: At the core of this initiative is a public-facing pledge to uphold and promote the ethical principles of privacy, transparency, inclusivity, accountability, sustainability, and compliance in the development and deployment of conversational AI technology.

In March 2023, the Open Voice TrustMark Initiative, a project of the Linux AI & Data Foundation, published an important overview of the ethical principles essential to the use and practice in the use of conversational AI, which includes definitions and suggested mitigation strategies distilled from the extensive body of AI ethics research, global regulations and standards, and legislation. It translated the guiding beliefs – "do no harm," “duty to care,” and “worthy of trust” – into six ethical principles:

- **Privacy** – A fundamental human right. Collect voice data only for a specific purpose and duration. Users [e.g., patients] must understand how voice data is used, collected, and shared; must give explicit consent to how it is used, collected, and shared; and, must be able to easily access, rectify, suppress, limit, oppose, and transport voice data. Numerous government and industry-specific regulations govern the protection and use of information that can identify or be ascribed to an individual. Existing regulations that protect patient and user privacy include the Health Insurance Portability and Accountability Act (Health Insurance Portability and Accountability (HIPPA) Act of 1996, 1996), the General Data Protection Regulation (General Data Protection Regulation (GDPR) – Official Legal Text, 2022) of the European Union, and many national or state-based data privacy laws (Open Voice Network, 2023).

- **Transparency** – Disclose decisions regarding acquiring and using personal voice data and present them in an easily accessible, understandable, and explainable format.

- **Accountability** – Ensure that one or more humans are identified as responsible for every decision regarding data acquisition, analysis, use, and storage and that senior management is fully aware of the potential harm caused by illegal or unethical practices.

- **Inclusivity** – Enable all individuals to communicate and be understood, regardless of gender, age, fluency-dialect, or physical ability.

- **Sustainability** – Understand the environmental impact of the large computational resources demanded by voice and natural language training models

- **Compliance** – Conduct proactive governance of corporate practices in accordance with existing laws, regulations, and best ethical guidelines.

Ethical principles play a crucial role in shaping technology's ethical and responsible use. Organizations and developers need to consider these principles when designing, implementing, and managing healthcare solutions to ensure they align with societal values, legal requirements, and sustainability goals. Additionally, continuous efforts should be made to adapt systems to evolving ethical standards and regulatory landscapes.

**Figure 5**
TrustMark Tools

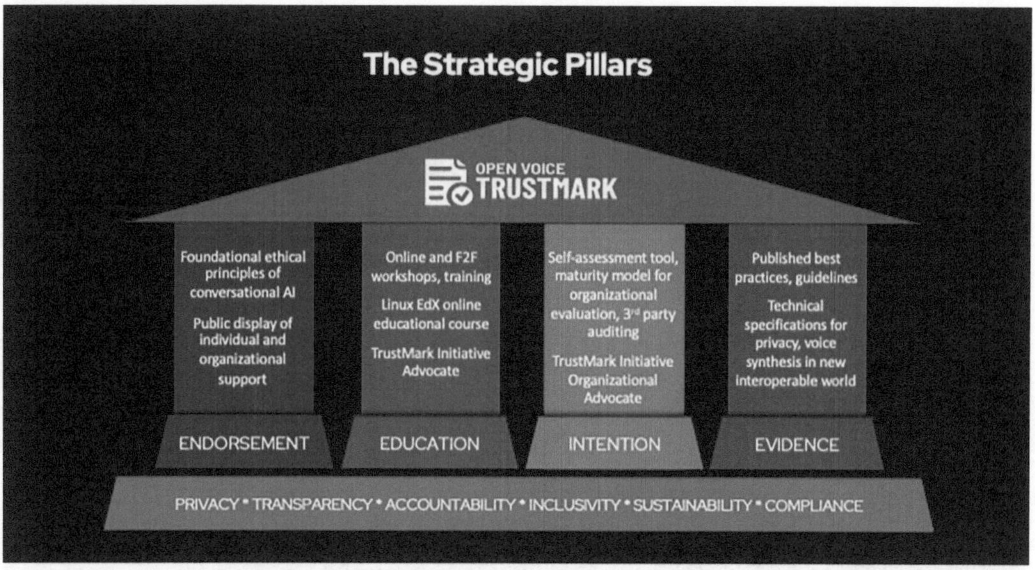


Note: The TrustMark Initiative works by establishing a set of criteria for trustworthy conversational AI products and services based on the foundational ethical principles.

The Open Voice TrustMark Initiative delivers comprehensive legal and ethical risk mitigation tools for all stakeholders who develop and use conversational AI. The tools include

- **EDUCATION:** Online and in-person training courses designed for all stakeholders of voice/conversational AI, from individuals to organizational employees/associates
- **INTENTION:** An online self-assessment/maturity model tool that will allow organizations of all sizes to evaluate policies, practices, and implementations against best practices
- **EVIDENCE:** Technical "building block" standards that will allow ethical practices to be "designed in"

The Open Voice Trust Mark Initiative establishes tangible steps to legal and ethical risk mitigation. Grounded in a study of extant AI ethics literature, regulations, and guidelines, its areas of work include privacy, security, voice synthesis, and ethical requirements for interoperability of conversational AI technologies. The initiative has also launched an online educational course via EdX and an organizational self-assessment tool. Although focused on conversational AI, the tools equally apply to blockchain and cybersecurity solutions (Open Voice Network, 2023).

**Figure 6**
TrustMark Stakeholders

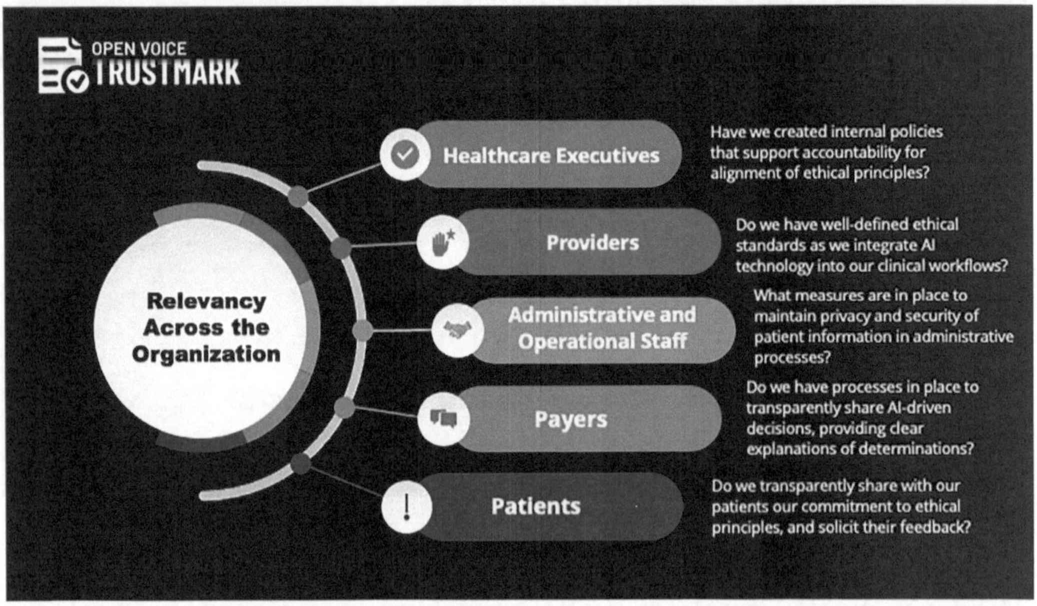


Note: Everyone who contributes to or benefits from these systems has a duty to ensure that they uphold established laws and human rights and avoid unjust negative repercussions to individuals and organizations.

The components of the program can bring significant benefits to all stakeholders in the healthcare ecosystem, including the C-suite executives, healthcare providers, support staff, supply chain participants, and payers. For example

- Training ensures that healthcare executives understand the ethical implications and align their conversational AI initiatives with the organization's values. Self-assessments can gauge the extent to which AI implementations adhere to ethical standards.
- Providers can benefit from training to understand the importance of responsible data stewardship and how to mitigate risks of bias in using the technology.
- Self-assessments can help all stakeholders identify potential risks associated with conversational AI adoption and use. Understanding these risks enables proactive measures to address ethical concerns in daily operations.

- Patients can be educated to make more informed decisions about data sharing and privacy considerations, thus increasing their trust in the secure use of conversational AI as part of their healthcare treatment.

- Training can guide payers in making fair and unbiased decisions and developing and using conversational AI models. Self-assessments can ensure decision-makers are aware of and adhere to ethical standards in coverage determinations and claims processing.

By investing in training and self-assessment programs, stakeholders across the healthcare spectrum can enhance their understanding of AI-related ethical, privacy, and security considerations. This, in turn, fosters a culture of responsible AI use, improves decision-making, and contributes to building trust among all stakeholders in the healthcare ecosystem.

# Conclusion

In conclusion, conversational AI is a powerful and promising technology that can enhance the delivery of healthcare services, especially remote patient monitoring. By leveraging natural language processing, data analysis, and generative AI, conversational AI can provide continuous care, improved outcomes, and operational efficiencies for patients, clinicians, and providers. Conversational AI can also detect and prevent various physical and mental health conditions through biomarker analysis. However, conversational AI also poses significant challenges regarding privacy, ethics, and trust.

Trust is a catalyst for positive change in health care. The Open Voice TrustMark Initiative provides a framework for building and maintaining trust, outlining specific behaviors and principles that overcome these changes. Following the guidelines and best practices outlined ensure the responsible and secure use of conversational AI technologies.

Integrating the use of conversational AI with blockchain and cybersecurity technologies within healthcare systems intentionally cultivates trust. The connection between trust, AI, blockchain, and cybersecurity lies in the cohesive functioning of these elements. Trust is built when AI algorithms demonstrate accuracy and reliability, blockchain provides a transparent and secure framework for recording and verifying data, and cybersecurity measures protect critical information. These promising technologies can allow organizations to operate at a higher speed, achieving their goals more rapidly and effectively.

# About the Open Voice TrustMark Initiative of the Linux AI & Data Foundation

The Open Voice TrustMark Initiative is an incubation project of the Linux AI & Data Foundation, dedicated to making conversational AI worthy of user trust, and formed in March 2023. The TrustMark Initiative

- translates an ethical code that respects the individual's privacy rights, regulations, and legislation for conversational applications into implementable actions that mitigate risk for developers, clients, and the public and promote values of transparency, accountability, inclusivity, and sustainability;
- provides public/industry education on critical ethical issues and best practices through training courses, published policies/guidelines, and a self-assessment and maturity model for organizations; and
- Enables public identification of individuals/organizations (through badges/certifications) who strive to implement best practices outlined by the TrustMark initiative.

For more information, visit https://openvoicenetwork.org/trustmark-initiative/.

# About the LF AI & Data Foundation

The LF AI & Data Foundation supports and sustains open-source projects within artificial intelligence (AI) and the data space. It is a greenhouse, growing and sustaining open-source AI and data projects from seed to fruition. We provide support to projects for open development among a diverse and thriving community, in addition to a number of enabling services that include membership and funding management, ecosystem development, legal support, PR/marketing/communication, events support, trademark management, export control filings, and compliance scans.

For more information, please visit https://lfaidata.foundation/.

# About The Linux Foundation

Founded in 2000, The Linux Foundation is supported by more than 1,000 members and is the world's leading home for collaboration on open-source software, open standards, open data, and open hardware. Linux Foundation's projects, including Linux, Kubernetes, Node.js, and more, are critical to the world's infrastructure. The Linux Foundation's methodology focuses on leveraging best practices and addressing the needs of contributors, users, and solution providers to create sustainable models for open collaboration. For more information, please visit linuxfoundation.org.

# About the Author

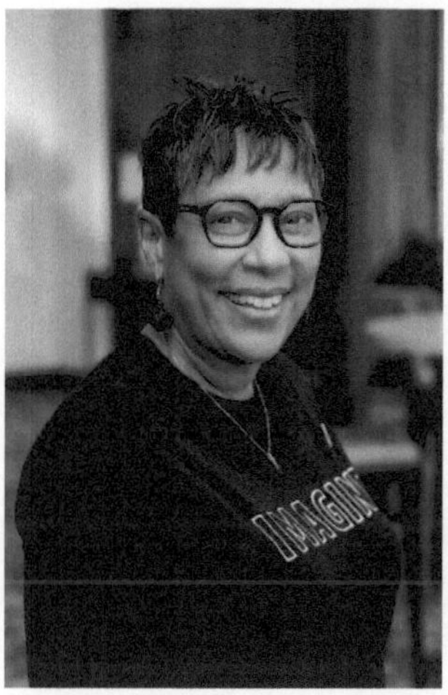

Oita Coleman is a performance-driven executive known for cultivating relationships and building exemplary global teams. As the head of the Open Voice TrustMark Initiative, she leads the global Linux Foundation project dedicated to establishing open standards and best practices for conversational AI technologies. In her role, she assumes the responsibility of formulating and implementing an ethical framework that safeguards individuals' privacy rights, adheres to relevant global laws and regulations, and minimizes risks for developers, clients, and the public. She has a strong background in software quality research and development, having previously worked as the Vice President of Research & Development for Software Quality at SAS Institute, where she provided oversight for global processes, standards, and policies, further emphasizing the importance of delivering exceptional products and experiences to customers.

# Chapter 7:

## The Elixir Effect of ChatGPT in Healthcare

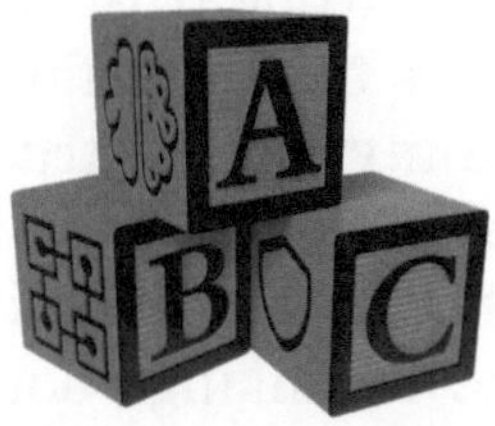



**Yaa Kumah-Crystal**
**MD, MPH, MS**
*Assistant Professor*
*Biomedical Informatics*

*Vanderbilt University*
*Medical Center*


### *Editor's Note*

Dr. Yaa has built an incredible reputation over the years as a doctor, who leverages the best of technology for the benefit of her patients. She has taught countless physicians and healthcare providers, how to best lives state of the art technologies to get the most out of digital health. This includes *ABC* technologies, with particular interest in the current state of artificial intelligence. In this chapter, she provides a pragmatic and easy to digest understanding and sets of examples that can be put into practice today.

I'm a pediatric endocrinologist here at Vanderbilt University Medical Center in Nashville, Tennessee and I'm going to be talking to you about considerations for these tools as it comes to healthcare. So, I rendered this picture using one of the tools called DALL-E, which is a text to image generator, and I put in there a robot doctor caring for a young child in the style of Norman Rockwell because you can just do that now. You can essentially transfer the contents of your mind into a visual representation and this is where we are with technology. The start of age is just pretty amazing. But after the picture came to being I had some feelings about it. I am a big tech enthusiast, and I was the one who instantiated this image, but it made me a little uncomfortable just seeing this picture of this kind of robot doctor giving some kind of medicine or elixir to a young child and it made you think and pause and wonder why would we, why would anyone trust the care of some of our most vulnerable treasures to machines to algorithms? Who knows what could go wrong there's so much uncertainty we can't trust these things can we and certainly humans are far better providers of care and our children and our colleagues ourselves are better in the hands of humans, right? Well, that's actually what we're going to be talking about today.

So, let's go to the concept of an elixir. So, in medicine the term elixir has evolved over time. It went from being just something that would enhance a medication, to make it easier to swallow something that would sweeten it add flavor, aroma, and then more over time into the concept of a panacea, cure-all that would just make everything better and you could buy them at the store. And with that the connotation of more negative implications of elixirs came into being as something that was more smoke and mirrors and maybe the term snake oil you'll hear because there's nothing that can fix everybody's problem and anything that proposed to do so was held with great skepticism. So where does that align with everything we're talking about today? Well let's talk about ChatGPT.

So, another image that I rendered with DALL-E. So, ChatGPT is kind of the marquee and flagship tool that people think about today when they hear the word AI (Artificial Intelligence). It's become synonymous with the generative era and these new tools and it's essentially about the Kleenex of large language models. So, I asked for you know ChatGPT Kleenex image, and this is what the tools came for me. So, I'm going to be using the term to describe a lot of the concept of these large language models but there are many other cousins of these tools like Bard and Llama and Gemini which we'll talk about shortly that do similar things but let's talk about what these things are that they do. So very high level not to get to the weeds here because I presume most of you who are attending this are here because you have a general understanding or interest but large language models very much as they attest to be are models based on a lot of information about language. They're trained on the Internet and just vast amounts of content and the magic under the hood is that they can predict logical words in a sequence. Twinkle twinkle little... star or boat, what have you, but it's trained on enough words to make concepts make sense to it so it knows that king is to queen like prince is to princess and then it's been finely tuned on instructions which means that you can now ask it to do things and it can, again, understand. I'm going to use a lot of these words that sound like I'm personifying the tools but it's the easiest way to communicate what it is these exchanges are but what's most important what I want to highlight is that they can eerily mimic human understanding and reasoning.

So, going back to ChatGPT, this Kleenex, this marquee model so ChatGPT very lately was considered the hallmark, the most capable model that we have, but last Wednesday on the 6th Google released something called Gemini and they had this amazing demonstration of this new model and it could follow along in real time and it could see someone doing rock paper scissors and guess what it was doing someone was drawing a picture of a blue duck and it was trying to figure out what the blue duck was and using silly phrases like what the crack and people were just astonished with this real-time interaction problem solving. Well, the very next day, and honestly just the same day several hours later, there were reports that Google's demo of the Gemini Pro was mostly staged. The video was largely edited to remove a lot of the latency, there were some additional prompts that were given that were not shown as part of the demonstration, and this exaggeration of its capability raised a lot of doubts about what Google could actually deliver. So, any of you that work in tech or tech adjacent fields understand the concept of over promising. Essentially you want to be careful about your own excitement enthusiasm about the tools you can see the vision of the future and everything it can do and all the things you want to be able to do but this rosy vision might not really match the reality of what it's capable of doing right now and that last mile to get to what your rosy vision is might be the hardest part of it all. And that might be the point where people might actually start believing you, but if you sell a vision versus what's capable of doing right now, you're gonna lose some trust and that's what's happened with Google just over the past couple of days.

So, we essentially have found that we have these two camps of folks when it comes to these new AI tools. You have the fanatics and the skeptics. And then there are people who are kind of temid in the middle they don't they haven't heard about these tools they haven't really used these tools yet but it's very divided. And I just found that was such an interesting way for these solutions to fall together especially in the age that we're in. And I'll let you guess which camp I'm in after this talk. And then it comes down to this concept of an elixir again this potential cure all, these magical tools that can solve all of our problems and the skeptics think that there's a good degree of smoke and mirrors based on the Google demo where it should be all these things but really when you pull back the curtains there was really a wizard behind the curtain. But then we have reports like this.

So, this happened in September just a few months ago where there was a very astute and diligent mom who had a child that was suffering. She had taken him over several several years to several doctors several consultants and could not get an answer for while her child was in pain and ChatGPT ultimately made the diagnosis. So, it was a very interesting story if you read the details starting with, they had gotten a bounce house, he was using the bounce house over to COVID, started to have some pain and teeth grinding, so first she went to a dentist, and then they thought he might have some breathing problems with his airway. So, they did some spacers, he went to an orthodontist, went to a neurologist, he went to a psychiatrist, and a counselor. No real explanation as to the symptoms he was having this pain, this discomfort, this behavior, he was having that was different and he even started to have some actual symptoms. And one of the more poignant things that mom mentioned, and she noticed that he wasn't even able to sit crisscross applesauce anymore which she just thought was striking. And again, she was on this diagnostic journey where she sought the advice of many consultants, and she was asking information. She had lots and lots and lots of tests done but no one could figure out what was going on with this child. And one of the things that struck me about her description of her experience is, no matter how many doctors the family saw the specialist would only address their individual area of expertise. No one was willing to solve for the greater problem. And as a specialist as a pediatric endocrinologist, I have to admit that that's true. You have your domain that you're expert in and if someone has other symptoms or concerns you say, well you should probably follow up with your pediatrician, or you might want to see neurology, or GI because that's just not where your expertise is and you want to stay in your lane to make sure you're doing the right thing for the patients. And there are even means that speak to some of this, like super specialization in medicine and how we are very focused on what we're trying to solve for, but there's nothing really bringing everything together.

So, this is just a meme of a gentleman trying to go to an ophthalmologist and he has to decide whether he needs to see a right eye specialist or a left eye specialist. This is another image that was generated by DALL-E and there are some inaccuracies in it. I'll see if you can figure out and draw to your attention later on whilst I am trying to make a point here. But the promise of AI in medicine is very much this, connecting the dots. Because in the previous example this mom saw lots of experts, lots of human experts, tried to get information, and they were both able to identify something about his symptoms and their specialty to address components of it. But it wasn't until she put all the symptoms together. She typed in all the relevant things and his clinical notes that she had access to, things from his imaging scans, MRI and among the information she got back in the differential diagnosis was something for consideration of condition called Tethered Gourd Syndrome. And she raised this with one of her doctors and they looked further into it and that was pretty much exactly what he had. He's since been treated for it and is doing much better.

So, again the promise of AI in medicine connecting the dots and bringing things together in a way that the way our health systems are currently structured right now we are not doing a great job of. So, for patients these tools can help us understand the decisions that are being made on their behalf. It can help them decipher complex medical jargon and information. And help them engage and understand their health and even what questions to ask when they go see their doctors. For providers it can help us forage through the mountains of information, because certainly I want to understand what's going on with the patient and see what their considerations are, but if there's a ton of information to go through there's just not the potential to be able to delve through it all. It could help surface patterns and help us derive insights about what's going on with these patients to pull these things together to say, hey, did you consider this test that was done by rheumatology three months ago that's positive, and these other tests that you've had, and putting those together? What could be going on with this patient? And it also helps communicate the complexities of the medical decision making.

So, this concept of bespoke information and what these tools, what these large language models allow, is for you to have an interaction with Artificial Intelligence with these large tools and get information that's curated to the question that you're asking. Information exists today. You can go to Google or Bing or what have you and search for something and what it will give you are these references, these sources of truth that you can go to and decipher and comb through and put together a piece of information yourself. These tools are able to now bring together the information for you, organize it for you, and disseminate it to you in the way that you understand best. And it's also able to do it on a reading level that makes sense to you. And you can dig more into particular areas that you have questions about and get a fuller sense of what is going on in a way that you just weren't ever able to before these tools become more mainstream.

But these tools have limitations going back to this picture that I put in the DALL-E image creator. I said, give me a picture of a right eye specialist and a left eye specialist. The word specialist here is spelled wrong. I promise you I typed that in correctly but these tools this one specifically is not trained on how to spell words. It's not skilled at how to do that. So, the information I'm going to get back is going to look funny. If I wasn't specifically looking for that, if I wasn't looking to validate that, I might have missed that. Very low stakes when this is just a talk that I'm giving and it's just a silly image that I want to include on there, but you can see how this could be higher stakes when we're considering information that people are going to make decisions based on.

So, this is the concept of hallucinations. And hallucinations are a function of these tools and how they work. Essentially, they predict the next word that makes sense in a sequence based on the information they have available. So, twinkle twinkle little... star. That makes sense. If I didn't have that in the training set, I didn't know about the song, I might say twinkle twinkle little... diamond. That's just as reasonable, but that's not right. So, when you have information that's considered truthful and valid and there's a source of truth and there's a right answer, but the data sets have never been trained on it, it's not going to pull up what's considered correct to you. But it's not trying to trick you, it's not being malicious, it's not lying. It's doing exactly what it's designed to do which is to pull up the most probable word that makes sense. So, twinkle twinkle little star. That could be a delightful song as well.

But the problem we find here is that humans are very easily led. I'll just give you a second to digest this slide. So, because humans are easily led, we are having to make decisions about how to consider the usage of these tools that can lead people awry. Going back to the concept of AI art, what I love about AI art is that it really allows you to see, like visually, it literally illustrates some of the shortcomings of Artificial Intelligence and Generative Artificial Intelligence. So, until very recently these tools were horrendous at rendering hands and fingers, like monstrosities really, like nightmare people. And you could see that right away. Like, anyone looking at these pictures would say, whoa what is going on here? That is not okay. Because, you know, we know what hands look like. We all have hands and it's very easy to know what's right and what's wrong and what's different and what's unusual. But with words, with text, with information, unless you know more than the source, unless you know more than what's pulling out, you won't be able to detect where the errors are.

So, computers can lead us astray. We know that now. We understand that now. But I don't know that we can say that humans are perfect either. In the 2000s there was a report by the Institute of Medicine that was essentially claiming almost a hundred thousand people died annually due to medical errors in hospitals and the set toll was higher than motor vehicle accidents, breast cancer, HIV, AIDS, but wasn't getting half the public attention that any of those were getting. Because to err is human. We understand that we are flawed we're not perfect, but we expect our tools to be.

So, going back to this concept, this, algorithmic aversion. Why is it that we will tolerate error in humans more so than in tools that could potentially help us accomplish things? This is a very interesting area of psychology that I think we need to better fully understand in order to figure out how to make these tools useful. And how to reasonably implement them in the work we do and the lives of our patients. We have a real-life trolley problem here. We know for a fact that humans miss things, humans make errors, and we know these tools, if they're not trained well enough, are going to potentially make errors also and these errors could also have really negative implications. So, what do we do? Do we just pack it up and say, well that's that. These are not good enough. We just need to continue on the way we're doing. Or is there more we need to do to ensure that we're being thoughtful about these tools and can leverage them in order to take better care of our patients?

I just want to give a quick demonstration of how these tools can really help to guide patients to get the information they need and give this kind of bespoke information to help people solve the problems that they have. So, this is just my ChatGPT, and I put it in, I just asked a question. I was like, oh I can't get my child to take the medicine. Do you have any recommendations for me? And then within minutes, it gave some really good recommendations about things to consider if you're trying to get a child to take medicine. Explaining the importance considering, making it a fun game, adding flavor into it. So, adding elixir, full circle. And I went on to give it some other examples. I'm like, well he took the medicine, but now he has a rash, because you know what, you can add images to this also. And I was like, what do I do? It went on to describe the rash and it gave recommendations about things to do. It says, call your healthcare provider, stop medication, and contact your healthcare provider. This could be an allergy. Make sure he's wearing loose clothing so that he doesn't get irritated. And I was like, okay look about that, that's a great suggestion and on and on. What kind of medications can I give to help with a rash? And then at the end I said, well my kid has had a really long day can you write them a bedtime story to help him feel better about everything he's been going through? And it wrote me a story about a brave little bear.

So, technology is there. This is something called a technology acceptance model that shows how people use these tools. And at the end we have this concept of actual system use. The things that provide system use or perceived ease of use and perceived usefulness and people's attitudes towards it, this has happened already. We have patients that are using these to diagnose their children when doctors have failed them. We have doctors that are using this to better understand medical cases, but we have gaps in the information. So, what we need to do is not understand whether we should but understand how we should incorporate these models safely in healthcare. How patients are using them right now. When they fall short, why they fall short, and how to improve the performance and the existing principle and techniques. Because the problems that we have are real. The problems the patients have are real. And we can't just keep ignoring them. This is not a cure-all, but it really can be something that can add some flavor and vitality and improve the way that we're taking care of our patients.

# Chapter 8:

## Navigating Challenges and Opportunities in Implementing AI in Disease Management: AI and the State of Rare Diseases in Healthcare

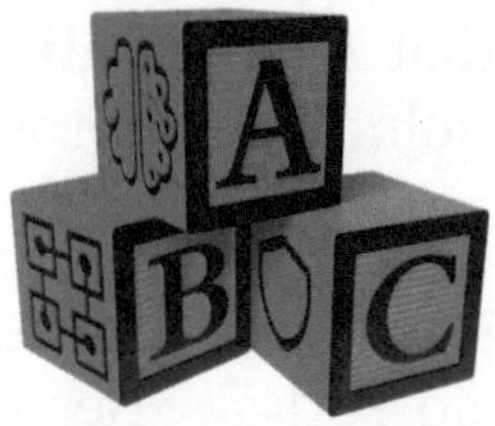


**Laura Elizabeth Hand, M.A.**
*Education Specialist and Associate Director*

*Spark Growth, LLC*

*Assistant Director of Career Services*

*Eugenio María de Hostos Community College of The City University of New York*

### *Editor's Note*

In this chapter, Laura Hand tackles the promising but daunting area of next-generation health research in the context of ABC. Her perspective combines the philosophical and ethical with the pragmatic and the promises for future generations' capabilities. The early examples that she provides will serve as a pointer for for future researchers and a blueprint for for addressing current and future issues and capabilities.

This chapter seeks to explore the transformative impact of Artificial Intelligence (AI) in the management of rare diseases within healthcare, examining both the potential benefits and the challenges posed by AI, blockchain, and cybersecurity technology in this rapidly evolving field.

In the healthcare sector, the advent of Artificial Intelligence (AI) heralds a new era of possibilities and challenges. While AI's potential in mainstream medicine has garnered significant attention, its impact on the management of rare diseases represents a paradigm shift yet to be fully realized. Rare diseases, often complex and poorly understood, require a nuanced approach to diagnosis, treatment, and patient management (Wotjara et al., 2023). AI offers novel tools for tackling these challenges, from refining diagnostic processes to personalizing patient care. This concept is further substantiated by Sharma, Rawal, and Shah (2023), who emphasize that AI integration in telemedicine offers opportunities to tailor healthcare solutions, improve patient experiences, and enhance healthcare outcomes.

This chapter delves into the multifaceted role of AI in rare disease management. Drawing insights from experts in the field and a series of participant interviews with rare disease sufferers and their immediate family members, the chapter explores how AI is reshaping healthcare dynamics. However, as Sharma, Rawal, and Shah (2023) point out, implementing AI in telemedicine presents challenges such as ensuring safety, regulatory compliance for patient privacy and data security, and financial constraints in integrating AI technology. The text examines challenges such as data analysis, patient privacy, and ethical considerations while highlighting AI's role in clinical trials, drug development, surveillance, and patient embodiment.

Within the framework of this chapter, the concept of kuru sorcery among the South Fore people of Papua New Guinea provides a striking parallel to contemporary challenges in healthcare, especially when viewed through the lens of AI integration. Kuru, a prion disease akin to Creutzfeldt-Jakob Disease, was once attributed to sorcery by the Fore people (Lindenbaum, 1979). This cultural interpretation of disease highlights the importance of understanding and integrating diverse cultural perspectives and historical contexts into AI-driven healthcare systems. AI, with its data-driven diagnosis and treatment recommendations, must navigate and respect these cultural nuances to be truly effective and accepted in global healthcare practices.

While the integration and acceptance of AI in rare disease management marks a significant advancement, it is also crucial to consider the role of emerging technologies like blockchain, which can further enhance data security and patient care.

# Blockchain's Role in the Implementation of AI in Healthcare

Exploring the intersection of AI and rare disease management also necessitates understanding the increasing role blockchain technology plays. Blockchain's decentralized ledger system ensures the integrity and provenance of medical records, as highlighted by Kumar et al. (2022). Integrating blockchain with AI could also facilitate more secure patient data exchange across different healthcare platforms, ensuring consistency and accuracy in patient care, especially for those with rare diseases for whom communication can facilitate treatment, given the rarity of information and specialists (See **Table 1**). As one participant with lived experience insightfully pointed out, "there are a lot of really bad experiences with doctors and physicians when patients go to them."

In many cases across the globe, practitioners and students cannot adequately define rare diseases, let alone support effective diagnosis and treatment practices. Participants' experiences reflected this global issue, as they narrated struggles with medical professionals who treated conditions as textbook cases, misdiagnosing conditions, excluding differential diagnoses, relying on inconsistent or insufficient protocols, and failing to recognize the participants and their family members as autonomous individuals.

In Poland, 85% of nurses and 75% of nursing students consider adding coursework on rare diseases necessary, and most doctors in Kazakhstan reported feeling inadequately prepared to care for patients with rare diseases, with only 9.9% rating their knowledge as sufficient for application in the field (Gómez-Díaz et al., 2023). These observations reinforced the necessity of integrating blockchain and AI to enhance the understanding and management of rare diseases among healthcare providers.

To better understand the current landscape of rare disease knowledge among healthcare professionals, **Table 1** presents a summary of various studies and their key findings.

## Table 1

### *Published Assessments of Rare Disease Knowledge among Students and Practictioners*

| Study | Survey Aims & # Items | Target Population & Participants | Findings |
|---|---|---|---|
| Iranian future healthcare professionals' knowledge and opinions about rare diseases: cross-sectional study | Knowledge, Awareness (26 items) | Medical students (40%), Nursing students (34.2%), Other students (25.8%), Total: 6838 | Gap in medical students' knowledge of RDs reported. No significant difference in knowledge and attitudes. Participants feel unready to care for patients with RDs. |
| Physicians' knowledge on specific rare diseases and its associated factors: a national cross-sectional study from China | Knowledge (102 items) | Physicians from ~200 hospitals across six Chinese provinces, Total: 3197 | Two-thirds of participants had average or good knowledge on specific RD. Higher knowledge scores are associated with certain genders, income ranges, and medical specialties. |
| Awareness of Rare Diseases Among Medical Students and Practicing Physicians in Kazakhstan | Knowledge, Perceptions, Awareness (28 items) | Students (67.2%), Physicians (32.8%), Total: 308 | Over 80% recognize RDs as a public health issue, but less than 13% feel knowledgeable enough. Lack of special training on RDs noted. |
| Awareness and Knowledge of Rare Diseases in German Dentists, Dental Specialists, and Oral and Maxillofacial Surgeons | Knowledge, Awareness (37 items) | Dental Specialists and Oral and Maxillofacial Surgeons, Total: 297 | Majority acknowledge the importance of RD knowledge in dental practice but admit to inadequate knowledge. |
| Knowledge level of medical students and physicians of Rare Diseases in Peru | Knowledge, Perceptions, Awareness (38 items) | Students (46.9%), Resident doctors & MDs without specialty (25.7%), Medical specialists (27.4%), Total: 720 | Preference to prioritize common diseases. Recognition of RDs as a public health issue but lack of preparedness to care for them. |
| Knowledge and Attitudes of Future Healthcare Professionals Toward Rare Diseases | Knowledge, Perceptions, Awareness (28 items) | Nursing students (17.3%), Physiotherapy students (26.5%), Medical students (56.2%), Total: 654 | 95% consider their RD knowledge insufficient. Highlights educational gap in future healthcare professionals. |
| Are rare diseases overlooked in medical education? Awareness among physicians in Poland | Knowledge, Perceptions, Awareness (28 items) | Physicians in specialization courses, Total: 165 | 94.6% perceive their RD knowledge as insufficient. Less than 5% feel prepared for caring for RD patients. |

| Study | Survey Aims & # Items | Target Population & Participants | Findings |
|---|---|---|---|
| Needs assessment study of rare diseases education for nurses and nursing students in Poland | Knowledge, Perceptions, Awareness (28 items) | Nurses (55.7%), Nursing students (44.3%), Total: 255 | High demand for RD education. Nurses and nursing students show insufficient RD knowledge. |
| Awareness of Rare Diseases in India | Knowledge, Awareness (26 items) | Nonmedical (67.7%), Medical (32.3%), Total: 599 | Low awareness across all categories. Over 70% lack basic RD knowledge. |
| Medical students' knowledge and opinions about rare diseases: A case study from Poland | Knowledge, Perceptions, Awareness (28 items) | Medical students, Total: 346 | High reliance on geneticists and pediatricians for RD education. Over 92% feel unprepared for RD patient care. |
| Information needs of physicians regarding the diagnosis of rare diseases: A study in Belgium | Knowledge, Perceptions, Awareness (25 items) | GPs (39%), Pediatricians (32%), Pediatric specialists (9%), Adult specialists (16%), Total: 295 | Most physicians encounter RD patients but have suboptimal awareness. Lack of RD knowledge in GPs. |
| Knowledge of rare diseases among health care students – Effect of targeted education | Knowledge (23 items) | Medical students (73.7%), Health Sciences students (14.4%), Pharmacy students (11.9%), Total: 270 | Initial poor RD knowledge among medical students, improved with targeted education. |
| Attitudes of medical students towards rare diseases: A cross-sectional study | Knowledge, Awareness (22 items) | 3rd-year medical students (59.2%), 6th-year students (40.8%), Total: 592 | 6th-year students have better RD knowledge than 3rd-year students; knowledge is still insufficient. |
| General knowledge and opinion on rare diseases among future health care and non-health care professionals | Knowledge, Perceptions, Awareness (20 items) | Resident doctors (17.1%), Nursing students (45.3%), Technical and vocational health education students (18.0%), Non-health-related university students (17.1%), Total: 234 | Resident doctors slightly more knowledgeable on RD. Overall, there is low RD knowledge among health and non-health professionals. |
| General knowledge and awareness of rare diseases among GPs in Bulgaria | Knowledge, Awareness (17 items) | GPs without specialty (19.36%), With one specialty (67.47%), With two or more specialties (13.17%), Total: 1002 | Low general knowledge and awareness among GPs. Indicates the need for increased RD awareness campaigns. |
| Assessing knowledge, perceptions, awareness and attitudes on rare diseases among health care providers and health students in Mexico | Knowledge, Perceptions, Awareness, Attitudes (15 items) | Health care professionals and students, Total: 944 | Satisfactory level of RD knowledge, except on orphan drugs. Significant differences in perceptions, awareness, and attitudes among groups. |

Note. Adapted from Gómez-Díaz et al., 2023.

As the parent of an adolescent rare disease sufferer pointed out, “Even when doctors are highly educated about a rare disease, they don’t see tons of it.” In the context of the discussion on the intersection of AI, blockchain technology, and rare disease management, the narrative of the parents of a rare disease sufferer offers a compelling case study (see **APPENDIX A**). This narrative exemplifies the challenges faced due to the lack of adequate knowledge and preparedness among healthcare practitioners in managing rare diseases.

The parents described a harrowing experience, which began with a startling phone call from an unfamiliar nurse announcing their newborn's diagnosis of galactosemia, a rare genetic disorder. The parent recalled, “This nurse called me... and she said, [your newborn’s] test is positive for galactosemia, which I'd never heard of. I couldn't even understand what she was saying. It's a weird word, right?” This experience underscores the initial shock and confusion faced by families when confronted with unfamiliar medical terminology, a common occurrence in rare disease diagnoses.

Instead of providing a detailed description of the condition, the risks, and the next steps, the nurse merely insisted that the child was dying and should seek care at the nearest Emergency Room. The narrative further illustrates the emotional and logistical turmoil experienced by the family. In interviews, one parent expressed, “[the nurse said] Your baby's dying... And I was like, ‘he doesn't look like it... But, of course, we'll go.’” However, upon arrival, the parents found a medical team with limited knowledge of the condition beyond an inconsistent protocol and a medical team that, eventually, directed the young parents to go home, try a mixture of breastmilk and formula, and see what happens. No treatment other than avoidance was suggested because of a lack of available knowledge and resources for treatment. This highlights the dissonance between the severity of the medical advice received and the observable condition of their child, a discrepancy that can often lead to confusion and distrust in the healthcare system.

Moreover, the narrative underscores the complexity and urgency in adhering to specific medical protocols, often characterized by a lack of clarity and support for rare disease sufferers. The parent detailed, “The blood test can only be sent to one lab... It's not going to get there. What are we supposed to do?” This statement reflects the logistical challenges and the sense of helplessness faced by families navigating the healthcare system for rare disease management.

The parents’ experience culminates in a profound observation about the healthcare system's approach to rare diseases. They stated, “People are treated as textbook, and no one is textbook." This encapsulates the core issue of the healthcare system's inability to fully accommodate the unique aspects of each rare disease case, often leading to a one-size-fits-all approach that neglects individual patient needs. The participant continued by recalling, "And you can observe, but obviously sometimes symptoms are not visible. [...] What do we do? But then people start acting like, well, we don't really know, it's just protocol."

These experiences align with global observations about the lack of preparedness among healthcare professionals in managing rare diseases. Studies such as those conducted in Poland and Kazakhstan, as cited in Gómez-Díaz et al. (2023), reveal a significant gap in knowledge and training among healthcare providers. This gap not only affects the quality of care but also impacts the emotional and psychological well-being of patients and their families.

The narrative of this parent, interwoven with global data, underscores the urgent need for integrating advanced technologies like AI and blockchain in healthcare education and practice. These technologies could significantly enhance the understanding, diagnosis, and management of rare diseases, leading to improved patient outcomes and experiences.

The participant later related the disconcerting feeling of calming down panicking nurses in epidemiology who recognized enough only to know that the condition, galactosemia, was rare and could be deadly. For the participant navigating the complexities of rare disease diagnosis for their children, this evoked the sense that "'Doctors aren't looking at a whole person. They're doing a protocol." This reflection and the participant's experience identifies a gap in care in which AI-driven healthcare systems, by incorporating a more patient-centric approach, can better address conditions such as rare diseases, which often present unique, non-textbook challenges.

The participant also recalled, on multiple occasions, watching providers "Google galactosemia" while waiting in the ER for their child to be served. The medical providers were taking the same steps the parent took when the nurse initially called, such that the experts had to rely on the accuracy of a websearch to serve as the foundation for their care plans.

The participant's experience underscores the urgency for blockchain and AI integration in healthcare to ensure accurate information dissemination and more personalized patient care. This integration may render rare disease and treatment knowledge more readily available to improve rare disease patient care and treatment, an idea the participant was enthused about:

"I mean, if I received a communication saying, hey, your child has been. Identified as having this there's a potential intervention, are you interested? I would follow up. [...] there're so little options. Anything that would show up as an option is is welcomed."

## Blockchain Values

In addition to the potential blockchain and AI offer for facilitating knowledge sharing, in "Blockchain Applications in Healthcare – A Review and Future Perspective," Narikimilli et al. (2020) propose that blockchain fosters a move from volume to value-based care in healthcare. Blockchain does so by enhancing the transparency, traceability, and protection of data, which are essential in the trust-based verification of AI applications, especially in the data-sensitive realm of AI-driven drug research for rare diseases (Kumar et al., 2022).

The inherent security of blockchain, where each block is securely linked to its predecessor, creates an incorruptible data chain crucial for maintaining the authenticity of complex medical data (Kumar et al., 2022). Moreover, the immutability of data recorded in blockchain, which, once recorded, "cannot be altered," underlies its capacity to enhance data security and reliability in the healthcare sector (Narikimilli et al., 2020). The transition Narikimilli et al. (2020) described, from volume- to value-based care, relies on blockchain's inherent transparency, traceability, and security to maintain error-free medical services and efficient drug supply chain management, which, as this chapter discusses, is essential to the growing field of orphan drug development and personalized pharmacological treatments.

Blockchain's application extends beyond data integrity; it introduces significant efficiency and reduces computational overhead in data management. Reducing computational overhead corresponds with the potential decrease in cost and, thus, launching process friction. Blockchain offers the integration of AI in healthcare through applications such as security and drug development (Kumar et al., 2022).

Kumar et al.'s (2022) proposed architecture, described in "A Novel Decentralized Blockchain Architecture for the Preservation of Privacy and Data Security against Cyberattacks in Healthcare," is able to speed up ledger updates by 63% and reduce network traffic tenfold when node numbers increase. In recent studies, researchers also took the opportunity to use blockchain as a ledger, storing patient care data, and suggested it could further "store various healthcare data like provider directories, care plans data, clinical trial data, precision medicine data, Pharmaceutical supply chain data, biomarker data;" this application suggests additional potential for blockchain in reducing administrative burdens and transaction costs for clinical research and healthcare providers (Narikimilli et al., 2020). These efficiencies, critical in handling large, complex datasets typical in rare disease research, extend blockchain's application beyond data integrity to operational enhancements in healthcare.

As a result, blockchain technology does not merely complement AI in rare disease management; it offers enhanced data security, reliability, and operational efficiency, thereby fostering an environment where AI can be applied more effectively and responsibly in the healthcare sector (Kumar et al., 2022).

Reflecting on the privacy concerns, a participant stated, "Having all of the information spread across all providers is crucial." However, the participant also highlighted the importance of treating patients as individuals, emphasizing the delicate balance between leveraging patient data for advancements and maintaining privacy.

A participant also expressed how documentation and data both helped and harmed. After a carefully monitored home birth for health and cultural reasons, the participant reported that documentation presented both a boon and a fear, an opportunity to validate decisions but also an easy platform by which to be misunderstood, stereotyped, or misrepresented. This was a shared concern among participants impacted by rare diseases, particularly those identifying as female, who reported significant challenges with disclosing and treating their conditions. Zhang et al. (2021) support this with research showing women's pain is likely to misinterpreted, ignored, or treated differently, a bias which has long been acknowledged in the healthcare system.

Therefore, integrating AI into healthcare systems necessitates a sensitivity to aspects of identity, including traditional beliefs and practices. The case of kuru among the Fore people exemplifies how deeply ingrained cultural beliefs can influence perceptions of disease and treatment. AI systems should be designed to recognize and respect these cultural nuances and communicate and operate in a manner that bridges traditional beliefs with modern medical practices. This integration ensures a more holistic approach to patient care, especially in communities with strong traditional beliefs.

# Surveillance and Monitoring in Healthcare

Surveillance, traditionally viewed as a means of control through self-regulation and knowledge manufacturing, has evolved with the advent of AI in healthcare. While AI-driven health monitoring and surveillance systems offer personalized care, they also introduce ethical dilemmas regarding patient privacy and autonomy, particularly in chronic and rare disease management. AI-driven technologies, while promising this personalized and efficient care, also extend surveillance into the daily lives of individuals, thereby reshaping notions of self and body.

Integrating robust cybersecurity measures is essential in protecting the sensitive patient data collected through AI-driven health surveillance systems. The security and privacy of this data are fundamental in maintaining patient trust and ensuring the ethical use of AI in healthcare, particularly in light of emerging post-quantum threats.

The evolving role of AI in the health industry– from information security to care– and AI's increasing presence in health care surveillance can first be marked in the movement toward the proliferation of health monitoring systems and telehealth platforms as early as the late 1950s when AI was conceptualized (Nesbitt, 2012). However, technological restraints limited the progress of AI in health care for the greater part of a century; the stalemate continued until, in the initial years of the 21st century, a significant advancement in overcoming prior limitations was achieved with the introduction of deep learning techniques.

Presently, artificial intelligence systems possess the capability to analyze intricate algorithms and engage in autonomous learning. This development heralds a new era in the field of medicine, characterized by the increasing application of AI in clinical practices (Kaul et al., 2020). Reflecting the increasing role of AI in healthcare, Hao Zhu, director of the Division of Pharmacometrics at the FDA, reported a drastic increase in drug applications incorporating AI/ML elements (Eglovitch, 2023; New drugs at FDA, 2023).

From just three submissions in 2018 to 170 in 2022, this trend underscores the growing reliance on AI technologies in drug development, particularly for rare diseases (New drugs at FDA, 2023). AI/ML tools were used for various purposes, including study design, patient selection, risk identification, dosing optimization, endpoint and biomarker assessment, drug toxicity prediction, and drug discovery or repurposing. Observations Kaul et al. (2020) made on the rise of these applications were rendered especially timely by the near-global institution of social distancing practices in response to the rise of the COVID-19 epidemic at the time Kaul and his contemporaries were writing (i.e., early in the COVID-19 Pandemic) and the subsequent need for rapid innovations in pathology, epidemiology, pharmaceuticals, and other fields.

**Figure 1.**

***Tracking Scholarly Works on AI in Healthcare January 1992 to January 2021***

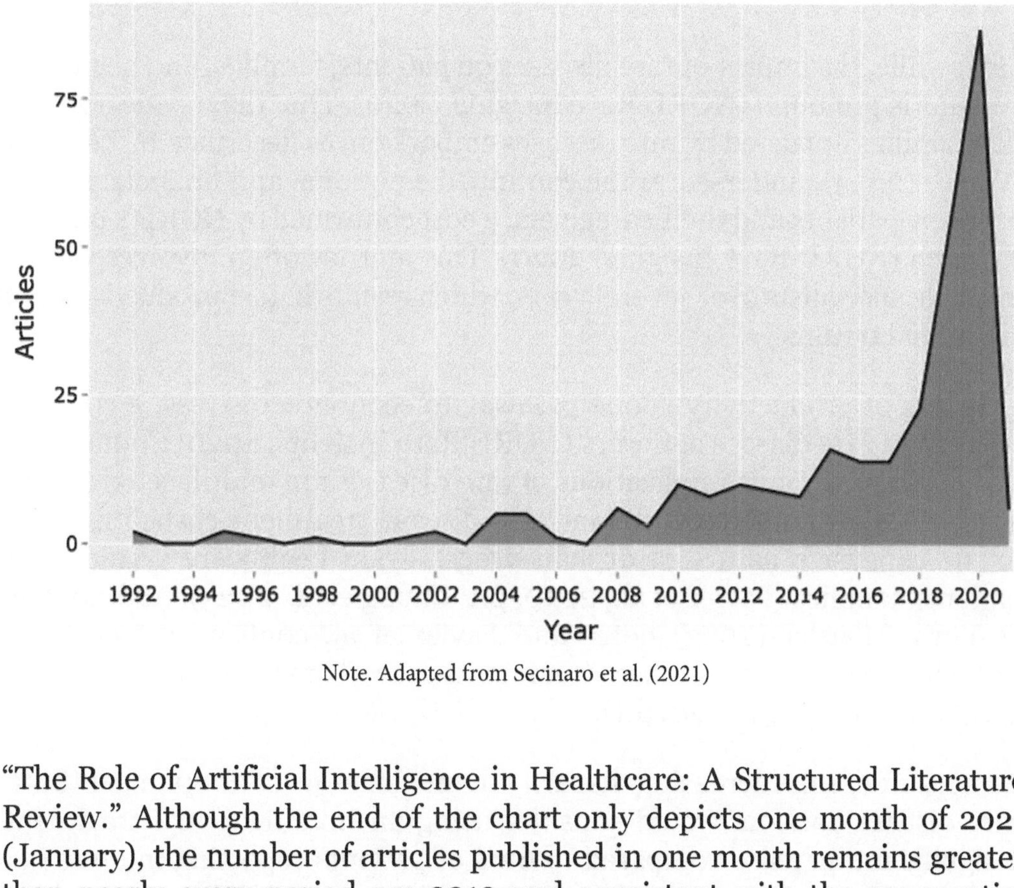


Note. Adapted from Secinaro et al. (2021)

"The Role of Artificial Intelligence in Healthcare: A Structured Literature Review." Although the end of the chart only depicts one month of 2021 (January), the number of articles published in one month remains greater than nearly every period pre-2010 and consistent with the exponential growth of the field.

The growing role AI plays in surveillance and monitoring in healthcare is multifaceted, offering both opportunities and challenges. Rare diseases offer both a field of prosperous research for medical AI and a promising lens for examining these facets of developments in artificial intelligence.

Rare diseases, characterized by their low prevalence but high complexity, pose significant challenges in the healthcare landscape (Hand et al.,

2023). These conditions, often genetic and life-threatening, affect a small percentage of the population. However, the total number of those impacted directly by rare diseases each year exceeds the number affected by cancer (Hand et al., 2023).

Therefore, clinical trials augmented by AI, as this chapter discusses, are necessary and essential, as approximately 90% of the 7,000 known rare diseases – and, as Michael Hund elaborates, the approximately 10,000 rare diseases estimated to be impacting the global population currently – do not yet have an FDA-approved treatment (NORD Rare Insights, 2020; Hand et al., 2023).

Meanwhile, the impact of rare diseases on patients, families, and healthcare systems is profound (NORD Rare Insights, 2020). The "diagnostic odyssey" that families impacted by rare diseases embark on, as described by Léon van Wouwe (2023), underscores the continued emotional and financial burden borne by patients and their caregivers, a cost confirmed by NORD's ongoing research (NORD Rare Insights, 2020). This journey often involves visiting multiple specialists over several years, which results in lost productivity and emotional trauma.

This loss of productivity is one pathway to economic distress, a common concern of rare disease sufferers (NORD Rare Insights, 2020; Chung et al., 2023). The economic implications of rare diseases are multifaceted (Faviez et al., 2020). Globally exorbitant rare disease treatment costs, often due to the expensive nature of orphan drugs, strain healthcare systems and patients' families (Faviez et al., 2020, p.1; Chung et al., 2023). Additionally, as Karin Hoezler (2023) notes and Faviez et al. confirm, the cost and distribution challenges of these treatments exacerbate the issue of equitable access (Faviez et al., 2020, p.1).

As a result of this increasing disparity in medicine, as of 2020, most (88%) rare disease patients would consider using an investigational treatment, a significant increase compared to 62% of patients reporting interest in a previous National Organization for Rare Diseases (NORD) survey thirty years ago (NORD Rare Insights, 2020). This rise is accompanied by an increase in telehealth services and a demand for these services, which AI can complement.

According to Bohr and Memarzedah (2020), AI applications are estimated to cut annual US healthcare costs by $150 billion in 2026. Meanwhile, the AI-associated healthcare market was projected to proliferate and reach over $6 billion by 2021, corresponding to a 40% compound annual growth rate;

more recently, the "Global Artificial Intelligence In Healthcare Market" was projected to grow at a CAGR of 45.5% from 2023 to 2030 (Verified Market Research, 2023). The market was valued at $6.48 billion in 2021 and is expected to reach $201.3 billion by 2030 (Verified Market Research, 2023).

## Limited Understanding and Misdiagnosis

Challenges in managing and treating rare diseases stem from several key factors (Wotjara et al., 2023). AI significantly reduces these challenges by enabling more precise diagnostic algorithms that recognize patterns and correlations in rare disease symptoms often missed in traditional approaches.

"Artificial intelligence in rare disease diagnosis and treatment" by Wotjara et al. (2023) notes that rare or orphan diseases are frequently misunderstood or misdiagnosed due to their rarity and unique symptomatology. Léon van Wouwe (2023) provides an example, noting that conditions like lipid dystrophy are often mistaken for more common diseases like diabetes. Similarly, participatants' narratives about rare diseases illustrated the consequences of misdiagnosis and limited understanding among healthcare professionals. One interview participant spent months on a birth control medication that significantly raised her risk of stroke due to her condition. Another experienced the panic of being told her child was dying by a provider who could not explain why they thought that or what the condition meant. Still others report having to wait while their providers Google and verify their condition. Misdiagnosis delays effective treatment and compounds patient suffering.

Additionally, research on rare diseases is often hampered by limited data availability: "The key challenge with RDs [Rare Diseases] is that there is often not enough data available to effectively train a model" (Wotjara et al., 2023). Small patient populations make it challenging to conduct extensive studies, leading to gaps in medical knowledge and treatment options. As forefronted by Erika Gebel Berg (2023), the lack of comprehensive natural history studies limits the current understanding of the progression and impact of these diseases.

# Clinical Trials and Drug Development Through AI

Data ownership and transparency are often core concerns in clinical trials and drug development (Committee on Strategies for Responsible Sharing of Clinical Trial Data et al., 2015). Therefore, these concerns likewise shift as AI is applied in clinical trials and drug development. The application of AI in clinical trials and drug development, particularly for rare diseases, presents a transformative approach to overcoming traditional barriers and raises new challenges (Faviez et al., 2020). AI can not only streamline the design of clinical trials for rare diseases but also aid in identifying potential patient populations, thus accelerating the path to innovative treatments.

The rise in FDA submissions with AI/ML components highlights the expanding role of AI in enriching the design of clinical studies. For instance, AI tools played a pivotal role in the emergency use authorization of Anakinra for COVID-19, where AI and machine-learning models were crucial for patient selection in clinical trials (New drugs at FDA, 2023). This example demonstrates the FDA's support and encouragement for the appropriate use of AI/ML in streamlining drug development, especially for rare diseases. In the following discussion, this chapter will consider the integration of AI into these processes and its implications.

In the realm of clinical trials and drug development, the incorporation of AI and blockchain technology, discussed throughout this chapter, offers a promising route for ensuring the integrity and traceability of data. Blockchain's unique capabilities in managing and securing clinical trial data can reinforce the authenticity and reliability of research findings, characteristics essential for the approval of AI-driven developments in treatments for rare diseases.

Additionally, AI's ability to identify potential patient populations for clinical trials, as discussed by Simon Alfano (2023), can revolutionize drug development. This application of AI can speed up the process of finding effective treatments, making clinical trials more cost-effective. For rare diseases, where the patient population size and the cost-to-profitability ratio of development previously served as inhibitors to research, this contribution of AI is monumental (Berdud et al., 2020). The research of Berdud et al. (2020) also indicates that these changes may signal a shift in factors correlating with the reasonability of orphan drug costs, thus reducing non-covered expenses for patients with rare diseases.

Additionally, AI tools enable researchers to design more effective clinical trials (Taylor et al., 2023; Vora et al., 2023). AI can optimize trial protocols by predicting patient responses and potential outcomes, making them more adaptive and responsive. Gebel Berg (2023) explains that this results in more efficient trials with a higher likelihood of success.

## Predictive Analytics and Targeting in Patient Management

Likewise, AI's ability to process and analyze vast datasets has revolutionized patient identification for clinical trials. The integration of AI in healthcare enables more accurate forecasting of disease progression in rare diseases, allowing for timely interventions and personalized care plans.

As highlighted previously in the chapter, the success of the recent work of Léon van Wouwe (2023) relies on the role of AI in pinpointing patient populations with rare diseases. This precise targeting makes clinical trials more efficient and opens the door to developing treatments for previously deemed too rare to study.

## Accelerating Drug Discovery, Repurposing, and Development

Using AI's advanced analytics for targeting can also significantly shorten the drug discovery timeline (Taylor et al., 2020). By rapidly analyzing biological data, AI aids in identifying potential drug candidates, as Simon Alfano (2023) noted. This capability is crucial for rare diseases, where time is often critical.

AI assists in identifying new uses for existing drugs, potentially accelerating treatment availability for rare diseases (Vora et al., 2023). As Léon van Wouwe (2023) notes, AI can play a pivotal role in narrowing down biological markers and focusing on specific disease states, thereby aiding in targeted drug development.

AI's ability to analyze complex biological data has already proven critical in identifying new drug targets; as previously observed, FDA data from 2022 shows a significant increase in drug and treatment approval for rare diseases, which correlates not with decreased rigor in regulation but with increased implementation of AI (New drugs at FDA, 2023). As Léon van Wouwe (2023) further observes, AI can analyze patterns in large-scale health datasets faster than traditional methods, leading to the discovery of potential drug candidates.

In AI-assisted drug discovery and development, the imperative of advanced cybersecurity cannot be overstated. Protecting the intellectual property and confidential information in this field is crucial, especially considering the risks posed by sophisticated cyber threats, including those beyond the scope of current quantum computing technologies.

In addition to impacting the global economy, this integration of AI in drug discovery and development marks a significant shift in the approach to rare diseases (Taylor et al., 2023). This technology is enhancing the efficiency and efficacy of the drug development process in several ways. https://deloitte.com/insights

AI's ability to analyze existing medical data has been used to uncover new uses for approved drugs, a process known as drug repurposing (Vora et al., 2023). The potential of AI in drug repurposing has been highlighted by several researchers and practitioners. By analyzing existing databases of drugs, AI can identify new therapeutic uses for medications initially developed for other conditions, offering a quicker route to treatment for rare disease patients (Vora et al., 2023).

## Enhanced Diagnostic Accuracy

AI algorithms have the potential to improve diagnostic accuracy significantly. AI algorithms, with their advanced pattern recognition capabilities, can offer a significant boost in diagnosing rare diseases, reducing the time and emotional burden associated with the diagnostic odyssey. Recently, AI has been harnessed for the early detection and diagnosis of COVID-19 by monitoring patients' demographic, clinical, and epidemiological characteristics (Abdallah et al., 2023). Similarly, by analyzing large-scale health datasets, AI can identify rare disease markers, reducing misdiagnosis rates and shortening the diagnostic journey (Kafkas et al., 2023).

KAUST's STARVar tool was designed and trained to have this capacity to improve diagnostic accuracy by interpreting symptom data in standardized and naettural language formats, demonstrating how AI can lead to significant advancements in diagnosing rare diseases, which are often misdiagnosed or misunderstood due to their complexity and unique symptomatology (Kafkas et al., 2023). The potential of AI for assisting in early diagnosis and pathological application is also exemplified in Léon van Wouwe's (2023) account of using AI to differentiate between lipid dystrophy and diabetes.

Léon van Wouwe (2023) also discusses how AI can reveal potential treatments for rare diseases hidden within existing medication portfolios, offering a quicker route to treatment. Van Wouwe (2023), a researcher with Volv, notes that Volv works: "with clients in the pharmaceutical industry specifically on these challenges. The company was formed around the true business problem, where the client has a drug in markets they know is a four-in-a-million disease and can only ever find one. So, where are the other three?" [...] Volv's research on making data science applicable and meaningful in the clinical setting for patients, healthcare communities, and drug development research settings focused on finding patients earlier (van Wouwe et al., 2023).

As van Wouwe (2023) reports, using AI tools, "most of our projects indicate that we can find the patients in the first instance." He later confirmed:

> We have data on file now [...] for one cardiovascular indication that, if you leave it be, can probably lead [...] to sudden cardiac death. We can potentially find these patients two to four years earlier. We need to look into this in more detail, but this may even be before the physical change to the heart is measurable to the point that they would qualify as having the disease.

Other projects addressing rare diseases, like the work of Michael Hund of EB Research Partnership, have found similar success through a commitment to applying evolving technologies (Hand et al., 2023). Many of these projects, researchers find, show that studies can locate two to three times more patients than are already diagnosed through AI-enabled processes analyzing potential patient data (van Wouwe et al., 2023).

In addition to finding three in four million, AI technologies enable predictive analytics to foresee disease progression and optimize patient management. AI streamlines the drug development process by predicting outcomes and patient responses, thereby reducing the time and cost associated with bringing a new drug to market. This streamlining is particularly beneficial for rare diseases, where the small patient populations often make traditional drug development processes impractical and economically unviable (Faviez et al., 2020). With over 10% of the global population affected by rare diseases yet only a small fraction possessing treatments, AI offers unique potential to revolutionize the status of rare diseases in investment and the global economy (Hand et al., 2023). Sharma, Rawal, and Shah (2023) argue for the importance of physician-guided implementation of AI in telemedicine to fully realize this potential, as it assists physicians in decision-making and healthcare delivery without replacing their comprehensive role. This proactive approach can lead to better patient outcomes and more efficient use of healthcare resources (Sharma et al., 2023).

These approaches rely on the use of AI to sift through large-scale healthcare data, enabling early detection of rare diseases, a process that often outpaces traditional diagnostic methods. In the case of Volv, AI algorithms have been effectively employed to identify patients with rare diseases. Likewise, their recent research has also shown that AI processing of big data and predictive tools can potentially predict the occurrence of a rare heart condition two to four years before the manifestation of physical signs. These algorithms have the capacity to detect diseases even before significant physical manifestations occur, enabling early intervention and potentially altering the course of the disease.

This scenario underscores a fundamental shift in the concept of embodiment within the medical field. AI redefines the patient's identity from a current state of health to a predictive model based on data analytics. This shift prompts a reevaluation of the patient's embodied experience, where the line between actual and predicted health conditions becomes blurred, challenging conventional perceptions of disease progression and patient identity.

## Patient Data and Privacy: A Balancing Act

Integrating AI in healthcare also brings heightened concerns about cybersecurity (Radanliev & De Roure, 2022, p. 924). Ensuring data privacy in AI-driven healthcare systems necessitates strong cybersecurity measures to protect sensitive patient information, especially in rare disease treatment and research personal health data.

In addressing the cybersecurity challenges associated with AI in healthcare, the insights from Anthony Ugochukwu Nwosu, S. B. Goyal, and Pradeep

Bedi (2021) underscore the urgency of adopting blockchain technology in the healthcare sector to combat the rising threat of cyber-attacks, which have become increasingly sophisticated, targeting sensitive electronic healthcare records and disrupting services. Safeguarding sensitive patient data against breaches is paramount, as this data is invaluable not just in a medical sense but also in a personal context for patients and families. As the chapter will explore, this data is often, while external to the body, fundamentally linked to the patient's understanding of identity and embodiment.

The research by Nwosu, Goyal, and Bedi (2021) highlights the vulnerability of current cybersecurity platforms in healthcare to various cyber-attacks. By incorporating blockchain technology, Kumar et al. (2022) and Nwosu et al. (2021) suggest, innovators on the intersection of the ABCs of Healthcare can create a more resilient framework for AI applications in healthcare, safeguarding against data breaches, identity theft, and unauthorized data manipulation. As this chapter explores the integration of AI in disease management, it is essential to consider the potential of blockchain technology– as well as the challenges. According to Nwosu, Goyal, and Bedi (2021), blockchain not only fortifies cybersecurity but also facilitates the safe and efficient sharing of medical data, thereby enhancing the development and deployment of AI solutions in healthcare. However, as data sharing becomes more secure and easier, however, some questions remain.

The use of AI in healthcare by researchers and corporations like Volv, particularly in rare diseases, necessitates a careful balancing act between leveraging patient data for medical advancements and safeguarding privacy (Wang et al., 2022). The growing trend of patient-led data collection and management brings this issue to the forefront.

Continuous data collection and analysis through AI provide healthcare providers in-depth insights into patient health trends and disease progression. This surveillance, as discussed by Léon van Wouwe (2023), is invaluable in understanding and managing rare diseases. AI enables personalized monitoring of patients, particularly those with rare diseases. This approach allows for real-time tracking of patient health and swift responses to any changes in condition. Simon Alfano (2023) notes the potential of AI in managing conditions like hemophilia, where apps can predict critical health thresholds.

The evolving utilization of AI in risk assessment models has also been instrumental in enhancing the accuracy of diagnoses and optimizing the efficiency of medical workflows (Kaul et al., 2020). These technologies, as highlighted in "Intelligent Telehealth in Pharmacovigilance: A Future

Perspective" by Edrees et al. (2023) and "Artificial intelligence in medicine: A comprehensive survey of medical doctor's perspectives in Portugal" by Pedro et al. (2023), not only facilitate predictive health care but also raise substantial concerns regarding data privacy and patient autonomy.

As healthcare moves towards more open data-sharing models, finding a balance between data accessibility for research purposes and protecting patient privacy is critical. The experience of one participant, interviewed for this chapter about their experience and their children's medical journey, sheds light on this critical balance. The participant's willingness to share personal experiences for the betterment of rare disease research while emphasizing the need for data privacy and security demonstrated the delicate interplay between data sharing and patient privacy in AI-driven healthcare, as did the participant's insistence on care in dissemination of information.

The participant, who is raising two medically fragile children with rare diseases, emphasized their fear that information sharing, especially if executed poorly, can result in issues such as medical kidnappings. Recently prominently featured in the news, media, and a Netflix documentary, the Take Care of Maya case resulted in the Kowalski family being awarded 261 million dollars after the Johns Hopkins All Childrens Hospital reportedly medically kidnapped Maya, a child with a rare complex regional pain syndrome (CRPS) diagnosis, and battered her while in its care, in part due to misunderstanding and suspicion of her diagnosis. The jury also ruled that the hospital's choices resulted in the wrongful death of Maya's mother, Beata. A significant part of the ruled medical negligence in this case was related to concerns of: misunderstandings of diagnosis, miscommunication between providers, provider's lack of knowledge of a rare condition, and disagreement regarding the limited options for treatment (Bruce, 2023). Maya's case is just one of many cases recently contested. An interview participant for this chapter experienced similar concerns as a parent after a Child Protective Services (CPS) worker was sent to their household. The household had been reported as medically negligent due to issues with data sharing and documentation regarding next steps for a medically fragile child with a rare disease. The case was later dismissed as unfounded, though the family now faces anxiety regarding information sharing, autonomy, and transparency.

These frequent challenges are well-articulated by Gebel Berg (2023), who discusses the need for equitable data access while ensuring patient data ownership and transparency. As the field progresses, evolutions in AI have given rise to needs in Cybersecurity and informed advancements in research.

## Ethical Considerations and Privacy Issues

While AI-driven surveillance offers significant benefits, it raises ethical concerns regarding patient privacy and consent (Wang et al., 2022). The constant collection of health data must be balanced against the need to protect individual privacy, as highlighted by experts' discussions in medical AI innovation and drug discovery (van Wouwe et al., 2023).

According to Wang et al. (2022), "The healthcare sector in the U.S. perennially experiences the highest costs incurred for data leaks compared to all other commercial sectors, with hospitals experiencing 30 percent of all large data breaches. Within the U.S., the average overall cost to an organization with a medical data leak was 10.1 million USD from March 2021 to March 2022" (p. 5). Correspondingly, Johns Hopkins University and Health System, subject to scrutiny in May 2023 as the result of a major data attack breaching thousands of employee and health records, has also come under fire for their Henry A. Kissinger Center for Global Affairs, named after a prominent and highly-contested former Secretary of State (Hayes, 2022; Johns Hopkins University, 2023). Among the Center's post-attack publications was a paper by Justin Lynch and Emma Morrison (2023), the Johns Hopkins Senior Director of Defense Special Projects and a national security professional who served at the House Armed Services Committee, respectively. The paper justifies "Deterrence Through AI-Enabled Detection and Attribution" (Lynch & Morrison, 2023).

This response is part of a movement validating AI as necessary and valuable in Cybersecurity responses to national security breaches, medical records, and FERPA- and HIPAA-protected personal identifying data (PID; Radanliev & De Roure, 2022). Likewise, in a National Academy of Medicine report covering the current and future state of AI implementation in health care, "the authors noted 'unprecedented opportunities' to augment the care of specialists and the assistance that AI provides in combating the realities of being human (including fatigue and inattention) and the risks of machine error" (Johnson et al., 2021, p.86). Understanding the impact of this movement toward integrating AI into health record-keeping and practice requires essential knowledge of the status and challenges of surveillance and embodiment in (tele)care.

Recalling the Panopticon, this chapter suggests that the constant collection of health data through wearable devices and other forms of telecare exemplifies a new form of medical gaze, wherein the patient's lifestyle and bodily functions are continuously monitored, echoing Foucauldian themes of disciplinary power, security, and enforcement; this schema recontextualizes the patient's body and reshapes the medical imaginary, informing not just the relationship of Cybersecurity and AI to the patient but also the relationship of the patient to the embodied self (Pols, 2012; Rice, 2003).

To better understand this relationship, understanding the Panopticonic concept is necessary. The Panopticon, conceptualized by English philosopher Jeremy Bentham in the late 18th century, represents an architectural design primarily used for prisons (Foucault, 1995, p. 195). Michel Foucault (1995) elaborated on the concept in Discipline and Punish, further defining and exploring the Panopticon and its mechanisms as figures in metaphor and reality. Characterized by its circular structure, the Panopticon features a central observation tower encircled by a ring of cells. This arrangement allows a single watcher to observe all inmates without the Panopticon's residents being able to tell if they are under surveillance. This design ingeniously merges architecture with social theory, aiming to induce a sense of perpetual visibility or the perception of observation as a form of control, thus altering inmate behavior. The Panopticon symbolizes the power of observation and has influenced discussions on surveillance, power dynamics, and social control (Foucault, 1995, pp. 195-228).

That the surveilled body responds to the evolving medical gaze and experience in a manner informed by the Foucauldian dynamic was substantiated by Tom Rice, who found that aural perception of a hospital environment invoked the possibility of surveillance, thus fundamentally impacting patient outcomes, self-perception, and behaviors (Rice, 2003). Additionally, an earlier study on pain perception lent credence to the idea that the patient's lived concept of the boundaries of their embodied self, and therefore their sensory experience, was impacted by their understanding of the non-dualistic body as existing in a tension between subject and object – a space now occupied by AI (Jackson, 1994).

Interestingly, the tech field and AI, in particular, are increasingly co-opting the Panopticon's theoretical framework, often without acknowledging its underlying theory. In 2022, Amazon Web Services (AWS), already widely associated with Panopticonic applications of AI, opened an office space in the prison Koepelgevangenis, designed after a Panopticon (Clark, 2023). Haarlem, Netherlands, the home of the Koepelgevangenis, converted the space into an area for tech companies, perhaps inherently understanding the connection between the surveillance age and the Panopticonic concept (Paul, 2021; Clark, 2023).

# The Impact of the Healthcare Environment on Patient Experience

Healthcare environments, encompassing architectural design, routines, institutional practices, and increasingly artificial intelligence (AI) technologies, profoundly impact patient well-being. These elements, integral to the healthcare experience, are crucial in shaping patient outcomes, experiences, and satisfaction.

## *Architectural Design Enhanced by AI*

AI-driven data analytics can inform the design of healthcare facilities, making them more patient-friendly and conducive to healing. For example, AI can analyze patient flow through a facility to optimize layouts, reducing stress and enhancing efficiency. AI can also contribute to creating healing environments by predicting the effects of natural light, green spaces, and room views on patient recovery rates, as suggested by studies like Ulrich (1984).

AI can also help mitigate environmental stressors in healthcare settings. For example, AI-powered sound management systems can reduce noise levels, while AI-driven monitoring can optimize patient flow and reduce overcrowding (Frąckiewicz, 2023; Alowais et al., 2023, p. 4). As healthcare evolves, AI is becoming an indispensable tool in designing patient-centered care and may be increasingly used to adapt environments for patient use (Taylor et al., 2020). AI's ability to process vast amounts of data can lead to environments that support both physical and psychological well-being, tailoring experiences to individual patient needs.

## *Soundselves: Sensory Experience and Surveillance in Healthcare*

Building on the theme of healthcare environments shaping patient experiences, Tom Rice's study in "Soundselves: An Acoustemology of Sound and Self in the Edinburgh Royal Infirmary" (2003) delves into how hospital soundscapes contribute to a Panoptic environment, influencing patient identity and behavior. Rice's work emphasizes the role of auditory and sensory experiences in the hospital setting, shaping the patient's perception of self and illness.

In the unit Rice studied, patients experienced a profound transformation in their sensory interaction with the environment. The use of "jammies," pajama suits designed to cover skin disorders and administer medication, served as a physical manifestation of the hospital's surveillance and control mechanisms (Rice, 2003, p. 6). These garments signified the patient's role within the hospital and altered their sensory experiences, such as touch, creating a barrier between the patient and their surroundings.

This sensory deprivation and the consequent redefinition of the body's boundaries realized the profound impact of the medical environment on the patient's sense of self. Rice's observations connect to broader themes of surveillance and embodiment in healthcare, showing how institutional practices physically and psychologically reshaped the patient experience.

Correspondingly, in 2019, Shivers, Llanes, and Sherman literalized an existing metaphorical relationship between the medical conception of the body, space, and technological – specifically Cybersecurity – innovations with their work on the implementation of artificial immune systems "to mitigate cybersecurity threats in unmanned aerial systems," the product of NSF-funded research at Embry-Riddle Aeronautical University (2018-2021).

Therefore, as this chapter explores the role of AI and Cybersecurity in healthcare and health education, this chapter suggests a complementary line of future study into the topology of a space in which the perspective of Chronic Pain sufferers, patients impacted by rare diseases, and other individuals with afflictions that evade traditional treatment offers insight into embodiment, thereby potentially augmenting the diagnosis and understanding of challenges and opportunities presented by innovations in AI and Cybersecurity.

## Telehealth and Remote Care: Lessons from the Pandemic

Treatment accessibility has always been a concern, but it is one that has grown substantially since 2020 and involved an increasing implementation of technological measures to sustain (Bohr & Memarzadeh, 2020). After the

Affordable Care Act was instituted and with recent increases in the demand for care for chronic conditions, partially due to Long COVID and the aging of the population, the overall demand for accessible care has risen in the US and globally (SAMHSA, 2023, p. 15). This effect is particularly remarkable in populations with rare diseases and made more evident by a shortage of physicians and allied health care providers (Vora et al., 2023; Bohr & Memarzadeh, 2020). Advancements in the application of AI in clinical and diagnostic tools, as well as conversational AI and AI-managed IoT systems, have begun to assist in addressing the care crisis.

As Erika Gebel Berg (2023) points out, the pandemic has transformed care delivery, making telehealth and remote monitoring more accessible. The COVID-19 pandemic has accelerated the adoption of telehealth and remote care, with AI playing a crucial role (El-Sherif et al., 2022). This shift has been particularly beneficial for patients with rare diseases, who often face challenges in accessing specialized care.

AI technologies have enabled remote diagnostic capabilities, allowing for earlier and more accurate disease identification. This advancement is crucial for managing rare diseases, where early intervention can significantly impact patient outcomes.

The integration of AI in telehealth services has also helped overcome geographical barriers, making specialized care accessible to patients regardless of their location (El-Sherif et al., 2022). Sharma, Rawal, and Shah (2023) further illustrate that AI in telemedicine can significantly enhance patient monitoring and disease management, especially in managing chronic diseases, by facilitating improved communication across healthcare delivery elements.

A 2020 report by NORD highlighted telehealth's impact on rare disease consultations. NORD reports, “Out of all patients who reported having had a telehealth visit, 92% described it as a positive experience, and 70% of respondents would like the option of telehealth for future medical appointments” (NORD, 2023). AI-enabled telehealth platforms have increased access to consultations in remote and underserved regions (El-sherif et al., 2022). This democratization of healthcare is vital for rare disease patients, often dispersed and unable to travel for specialized care.

## *Building Comprehensive Genomic Libraries*

Global access, as an advantage to telehealth and AI-driven medical innovation, is intrinsically linked to the concept of "Big Data," which Hoezler (2023) equates to DNA, our own Big Data that governs human functions and is largely still being interpreted.

Advancements in genomics, combined with AI, are paving the way for comprehensive genomic libraries that can enhance our understanding of rare diseases. Karin Hoezler (2023) discusses initiatives like the All of US research program, which exemplifies the potential of integrating global datasets for advanced research.

## *Global Collaboration and Data Sharing*

As Hoezler (2023) asserts, the ability to connect data sets globally is a crucial step towards a more inclusive healthcare landscape. Federated data models, in which data remains at its source but is accessible through shared algorithms, could revolutionize how we approach healthcare research and delivery. Dataset sharing has also been fundamental to the training of AI, though rife with controversy now extended to genetic profiles, where it has invoked ethical concerns and issues of patient trust (Alrefaei et al., 2022).

## *Overcoming Geographic and Economic Barriers*

AI has the potential to level the playing field in healthcare, making rare disease diagnosis and treatment accessible regardless of location or economic constraints. As healthcare data becomes more interconnected globally, the opportunity to address disparities in care becomes increasingly feasible.

However, as discussed in "Precision Medicine, AI, and the Future of Personalized Health Care" by Johnson et al. (2021), AI's impact on personalized medicine illustrates a shift in medical practice. AI algorithms tailor treatments to data such as individual genetic profiles, thereby redefining patient identity in terms of datasets. While beneficial, this revolution in treatment plans brings forth ethical dilemmas concerning data security and the potential for genetic and other discrimination.

Despite these developments, challenges remain, including ensuring equitable access to technology and maintaining the quality of care (Sharma et al., 2023). As AI continues to evolve, its role in shaping the future of telehealth and remote care will be critical, especially for rare disease management. In this context, Sharma, Rawal, and Shah (2023) highlight the essential role of education and training in AI-enabled telemedicine for healthcare providers, focusing on understanding AI capabilities, limitations, and ethical considerations.

As the American Psychological Association (APA) noted in 2021, "Psychologists are playing a larger role in the development and use of artificial intelligence, including how it can be used to improve mental health" (Abrams, 2021, p. 62). Using AI in mental health care through tools like AI-driven chatbots and mental health apps presents a dual-edged sword (Onisemo, 2023). As explored in "AI and Mental Health the Promise and Challenges of AI-Driven Mental Health Interventions" by Onisemo (2023), while AI-powered applications and tools may offer accessible and immediate care, these applications also involve continuous data collection– or the perception thereof– thus impacting how individuals perceive their mental health and further blurring the lines between care and surveillance.

In addressing the ethical implications of AI in healthcare, "Ethical and legal challenges of artificial intelligence-driven healthcare" by Sara Gerke, Timo Minssen, and Glenn Cohen (2023) delves into how AI-driven healthcare solutions must navigate the delicate balance between beneficial surveillance and infringement on personal freedom. Similarly, this chapter explores how AI, while offering unprecedented insights into health, raises concerns about the commodification of personal health data and the erosion of patient autonomy through Panopticonic practices.

## Navigating Global Disparities with AI-Enabled Healthcare Accessibility

The global challenge of disseminating AI-driven medical technologies to individuals with rare diseases highlights the Foucauldian principle of surveillance and power dynamics, reflecting broader social and economic disparities (See Kuiler & McNeely, 2023; Foucault, 1995; Wang et al., 2023;

Chung et al., 2023). Research on AI technology implemented in healthcare supports that the technology must also focus on bridging global disparities and social determinants of health, ensuring that innovations in rare disease management are accessible and beneficial to diverse populations worldwide to address the needs of the market and remain a viable solution (Chung et al., 2023; Berdud et al., 2020).

The conversation around making cutting-edge AI applications globally accessible demonstrates the uneven distribution of healthcare technology. AI's potential to revolutionize patient care is counterbalanced by disparities in access due to economic and infrastructural constraints in various regions. This situation is particularly acute in developing countries, where digital healthcare data is less available, necessitating the simplification of complex AI models for broader applications ("WHO issues first global report on artificial intelligence (AI) in health and six guiding principles for its design and use," 2021). The World Health Organization's 2021 report on AI in healthcare emphasizes the need to create adaptable AI systems that can function with limited data sets, particularly in low-resource settings (Ethics and governance of artificial intelligence for health: WHO guidance, 2021). This challenge is further complicated by bias in training sets ("WHO issues first global report on artificial intelligence (AI) in health and six guiding principles for its design and use," 2021).

In this scenario, the embodied experience of patients is significantly influenced by their geographical and socio-economic context. These disparities in access to AI technologies create varied healthcare realities across the globe, raising ethical questions about equitable distribution and the universal right to advanced medical care (Chung et al., 2023). This global disparity necessitates a reevaluation of the role of AI in healthcare, focusing on inclusive and equitable access. Alongside this, Sharma, Rawal, and Shah (2023) emphasize that AI in telemedicine must consider technical factors like trustworthiness, reproducibility, usability, and cost, as well as ethical considerations and governance for protecting healthcare data and ensuring responsible AI use.

Understanding this mechanism by which persons subject to surveillance develop alternate concepts of their boundaries and bodies through the language and values of their observers makes it possible to better understand the conflicts of suffering bodies with imaginaries altered by the threat of surveillance and control.

# The White Box: A Study in Surveillance and Self-Regulation

In Jeanette Pols' "Care at a Distance: On the Closeness of Technology" (2012), the "white box" telecare device is a pivotal example of the complexities of technology and healthcare. Pols challenges the traditional division of care into "warm" (human) and "cold" (technological) categories, demonstrating how surveillance and control dynamics manifest in patient interactions with the white box (Pols, 2012, p. 15).

Patients in palliative care, much like, as this chapter shall explore, the South Fore people, under the threat of kuru sorcery, experience a radical transformation in their social and individual contexts upon receiving a terminal diagnosis. Pols illustrates this shift, noting that the diagnosis not only affects the patient but also their wider social circle, including family and friends (Pols, 2012, pp. 29-30). This diagnosis creates a new dynamic wherein the patient, now under medical surveillance, must navigate their condition within the framework provided by the healthcare system.

As a telecare device, the white box becomes an extension or intermediary of this surveillance, asking patients to observe and report on their own practices. This self-surveillance blurs the lines between patient and caregiver, leading to a redefinition of the patient's identity and experience of illness (Pols, 2012, pp. 17, 28, 32, 41). Pols' observations highlight the transformative effect of technology in patient care, where devices like the white box assist in monitoring health and influence the patient's perception and understanding of their illness. The role of these devices is only increasing with the integration of AI tools.

# Patient-Centric AI Approaches in Healthcare

Still, the shift toward patient-centric healthcare, supported by AI, is a significant advancement, especially for those with rare diseases. This approach emphasizes the active involvement of patients in their health management.

AI-driven tools, as illustrated by Simon Alfano (2023), are enabling patients to take a more active role in managing their conditions. For instance, applications that help hemophilia patients monitor their factor levels show how AI can empower patients with real-time data and control over their health management.

AI is not only anticipated to assist in the development of solutions but also in the delivery.

## Supply Chain Challenges and AI Innovations in Healthcare

*Digital Innovations Reshaping Supply Chain Management*

In the healthcare sector, particularly in the context of rare diseases, the challenges of supply chain management have become increasingly prominent. The Deloitte Life Sciences Outlook 2022 highlights that global ocean freight rates and trucking spot rates saw substantial increases in 2021. This trend was further compounded by a rise in air freight rates in January 2022, indicating a significant strain on the logistics of healthcare supply chains (Deloitte, 2022, p. 63).

These challenges are not just logistical but are also closely linked to broader economic factors. As Abbott CFO Bob Funck explains, inflation and supply chain issues are intricately connected, impacting the cost and availability of raw materials crucial for healthcare provision (Deloitte, 2022, p. 63–64).

## AI as a Strategic Response to Supply Chain Disruptions

The complexities of these supply chain disruptions, especially in the realm of rare diseases, necessitate innovative solutions. AI stands out as a key technology in this regard. As described in the Deloitte Life Sciences Outlook 2022 report, various AI-driven digital innovations are being employed to mitigate these challenges:

1. **Control Towers and Data Lakes:** These digital platforms enable healthcare organizations to merge internal data with information from intermediaries and partners, providing real-time visibility into material

and product flow. This approach is particularly beneficial in managing the intricate supply chains of rare disease treatments.

2. **Machine-assisted Business Response using AI:** AI's capability to analyze supply chain, manufacturing, and market data helps in identifying potential issues such as stockouts of essential raw materials. These tools can suggest alternative suppliers or adjustments in production schedules, ensuring the uninterrupted supply of critical healthcare products.

3. **Machine-driven Resilience Management:** AI's predictive capabilities are crucial in forecasting events like logistics challenges and supply disruptions, enabling proactive responses to long-term risks.

4. **Market and Product Tracking with AI, IoT, and Blockchain:** These technologies are increasingly used to track and analyze various data types, including consumer sentiment and order patterns. This is particularly relevant for next-generation therapies in rare diseases, where tracking product movement and ensuring timely delivery are critical.

Deloitte then suggests that the integration of AI in addressing supply chain challenges presents a promising avenue for enhancing the efficiency and reliability of healthcare services, especially in the context of rare diseases (Deloitte, 2022). This approach mitigates logistical challenges and contributes to a more resilient and responsive healthcare system.

Integrating AI in healthcare has also opened new avenues for patient involvement in research. Erika Gebel Berg (2023) discusses how patient groups, through AI-enabled platforms, are now running their own registries and natural history studies. This active engagement enriches research data and ensures that the patient's voice is central to healthcare developments.

However, the changing role of healthcare professionals in an AI-dominated landscape is considerable. With the shift of focus to the patient, the practitioner has been recontextualized within the medical narrative. "The Changing Landscape of Healthcare: AI's Impact on the Role of Physicians" by Greenberg (2022) provides insights into this transformation. Among other changes, healthcare professionals are increasingly required to manage and interpret AI-generated data, shifting their traditional caregiving roles and influencing their perceptions of patients.

# Navigating the Diagnostic Odyssey

AI can significantly reduce rare disease patients' lengthy and often frustrating diagnostic journey. By analyzing complex health data, AI can provide early and accurate diagnoses, as indicated by Léon van Wouwe's (2023) experiences. This not only alleviates patient suffering but also streamlines their path to appropriate treatment. However, while innovative, the incorporation of AI in healthcare brings with it a host of ethical and social implications that must be carefully considered.

Surveillance (or the threat of surveillance) is often portrayed as a method of establishing control of the individual or social body through the instigation of self-regulation and the manufacture of knowledge.[1] By close reading depictions of imaginaries altered by the threat of surveillance and control, this chapter shows that subjects of surveillance internalize the conflict between the self and the observer-of-self by coming to understand their own boundaries and bodies through the language and values of their perceived observers; in doing so, this chapter also invites further contemplation of the regulatory and binding power of AI.[2] If medical knowledge can be conceived as a form of discipline or surveillance, as Foucauldian scholars have suggested, then demonstrating the mechanics of the relationship between the narrative subjects of medicine and their perceived observers is essential. This dynamic can offer insight into the internal conflict faced by other suffering bodies reimagined by the developing interdependence between medicine, AI, and cybersecurity as disease drives technology advances (AAAS, 2023).[3]

# Kuru Sorcery

Disease as a technological driver– and technology as a means of reconstituting the medical field is not a new concept. To illustrate the impact of cultural and historical contexts on healthcare, consider the example of the South Fore people of Papua New Guinea, whose experience with kuru disease offers valuable insights.

The ethnography Kuru Sorcery: Disease and Danger in the New Guinea Highlands surveys the South Fore people of New Guinea, particularly their response to disease and "intrusive phenomena" in a changing social landscape (Lindenbaum, 2013, p. 78). This case study offers insights into the dynamics of epidemic, care, and surveillance and how these intersect with technological advancements and disease management. The South Fore's experiences provide a foundational comparison for understanding similar dynamics in the context of the COVID-19 pandemic, AI, and cybersecurity.

Kuru, a notable epidemic among the South Fore, emerged around the same time as the early developments in AI. Prior to the kuru crisis, the South Fore peoples' concept of self and body extended beyond the individual to encompass their social relationships and environment (Lindenbaum, 2013, p. 52). Illness and death were attributed to external influences such as nature spirits, recently deceased ghosts, and sorcerers (Lindenbaum, 2013, p. 56). The unseen presence of these sorcerers, akin to the Foucauldian concept of a Panopticonic watcher, reshaped the Fore's perception of their bodily boundaries, internalizing the conflict between sorcerer and self (Lindenbaum, 2013, pp. 56–67). The sorcerers differed from ghosts and nature spirits in that neither a cure nor visible source could be located for sorcery-caused illnesses. However, by observing and collecting feces, hair clippings, and nail clippings, sorcerers were believed to be able to impact the body's internal processes. The sorcery practices, involving the use of bodily remnants like feces to exert control, mirrored contemporary concerns in AI and cybersecurity, where personal data, DNA, and digital traces become tools of influence and control (Lindenbaum, 2013, p. 61). Lindenbaum (2013) suggests that these practices and beliefs formed a kind of "social quarantine," prefiguring the social distancing measures of the 2020s (p. 68).

Kuru and other diseases proliferated in the early 1960s; amid the resultant political and agricultural upheavals, the number of (un)perceived sorcerers increased, intensifying the sense of Panoptic surveillance within the community (Lindenbaum, 2013, p. 7).[4]

Eventually, the decline of the kuru epidemic saw a corresponding decrease in the prominence of sorcerers. However, anthropologists and researchers replaced them as the new observers. Jeanette Pols, in her work Care at a Distance: On the Closeness of Technology (2012), describes a similar role for researchers in telecare, combining observation and interview techniques to understand the subject's experience (Pols, 2012, p. 15). This approach, paralleling Lindenbaum's, constructs knowledge that influences how communities like the South Fore perceive and interact with their environment and threats.

The South Fore's experience with kuru sorcery, as chronicled by Lindenbaum (2013), provides a compelling parallel to the modern challenges of AI and cybersecurity. The interplay of surveillance, belief, and the redefinition of self and community in the face of invisible observers mirrors the impacts of technological advancements in our era on the patient, likening the invisible observer to the invisible illness in its impact on the patient's lived reality (See Conrad & Barker, 2010).

Patients and their families play a crucial role in the AI-driven healthcare ecosystem, especially in the context of rare diseases. Recent research shows that patient groups are increasingly involved in data collection and management. Erika Gebel Berg (2023) emphasizes the growing trend of patient-led registries and natural history studies, which contribute valuable data for AI analysis and subsequent healthcare improvements.

Therefore, patients and their families are not just passive recipients of care; they are active advocates and partners in the treatment process. Their involvement is critical in shaping healthcare policies and practices more responsive to patient needs.

## Biological Citizenship

In "Biological Citizenship: The Science and Politics of Chernobyl-Exposed Populations" by Adriana Petryna (2004), the altered imaginaries of a suffering population redefine bodies, populations, and categories of citizenship in terms of surveillance as the collection and reconstitution of data by government groups and medical "experts."

Like the bodies in Rice's infirmary that were reconstituted by surveillance as "patients," the suffering bodies of Ukrainians post-Chernobyl recomposed themselves in an altered imaginary by identifying with the government surveillance's image of Ukrainians as constituted by dosimetrics. In the case of one Zone of Exclusion worker, Petryna recalls, "The new institutions, procedures, and actors that were at work at the state level, at the research clinic, and at the level of civic organizations were making their way into the couple's kvartyra (apartment). Anton's identity as a worker, his sense of masculinity, and his role as a father and breadwinner were being violently dislocated and altered in the process" (Petryna, 2004, p.263). The biomedical language of dislocation draws upon the physical transformation inherent in becoming a Zone of Exclusion worker and receiving a calculable "dose" of Chernobyl radiation. Anton's body received a "psycho-social" damages diagnosis (Petryna, 2004, p.263).

He was outwardly intact, but, like a dislocated limb, Anton was unable to function to his previous capacity, experiencing seizures, mood changes, and other side effects of radiation. Petryna relates Anton's condition further: "He found himself confronting the shameful option of breadwinning with his illness in the Chernobyl compensation system or facing poverty... The couple hoped this individual [the neurologist] would provide official support for Anton's claim of Cherobyl-related disability" (Petryna, 2004, p.264).

Anton is internalizing his dosage and his impairment as his desired self, a decision with which Petryna cannot empathize (Petryna, 2004, p.264). The values determining his understanding of his body have been reversed as a consequence of "dosimetric surveillance" and control (Petryna, 2004, p.258). His suffering was invisible and uncompensated until he could express his condition in the language and values of the observer, dosimetrics, and disability. To do so, he had to accept physical boundaries and limitations fundamentally conflicting with his self-image as a breadwinner and father, virile and capable. Anton's circumstances model a potential challenge whereby patients conceived of by AI in terms of datasets may find their physical boundaries and self-concepts evolving in the face of technological advancements in care.[5]

## From Kuru to Today's Biological Citizens: Global Data Integration and AI

The future of AI integration with healthcare appears promising (Deloitte, 2022). The current state of the medical research and development field is marked by a significant surge in drug discovery, especially in rare diseases. This assertion is substantiated by data from a 2023 report, which indicated that over fifty percent of the new drugs sanctioned by the United States Food and Drug Administration (FDA) in 2022 were targeted at rare disease therapies (New drugs at FDA, 2023).

**Table 2**

***2022 FDA CDER Novel Drug Approvals for Rare or "Orphan" Diseases***

| Total Novel Drug Approvals | Number Approved for Rare Diseases | Percentage |
|---|---|---|
| 37 | 20 | 54% |

Note. Refer to New drugs at FDA: CDER's new molecular entities and new therapeutic biological products, 2023.

**Table 3**
***Examples of 2022 FDA CDER Novel Approvals for Rare Diseases***

| Approval Date | Drug Name | Generic Name | Indication and Usage | Dosage Form |
|---|---|---|---|---|
| 6/13/2022 | Amvuttra | vutrisiran | Polyneuropathy in adults with hereditary transthyretin-mediated amyloidosis | Injection |
| 11/14/2022 | Elahere | mirvetuximab soravtansine-gynx | Recurrent ovarian cancer resistant to platinum therapy | Injection |
| 2/4/2022 | Enjaymo | sutimlimab-jome | Decreasing the need for red blood cell transfusion in adults with cold agglutinin disease | Injection |
| 10/21/2022 | Imjudo | tremelimumab-actl | Unresectable hepatocellular carcinoma | Injection |
| 1/25/2022 | Kimmtrak | tebentafusp-tebn | Metastatic or unresectable uveal melanoma | Injection |
| 12/22/2022 | Lunsumio | mosunetuzumab-axgb | Relapsed or refractory follicular lymphoma | Injection |
| 3/18/2022 | Opdualag | nivolumab and relatlimab-rmbw | Metastatic or unresectable melanoma in patients aged 12 years or older | Injection |
| 2/17/2022 | Pyrukynd | mitapivat | Hemolytic anemia in adults with pyruvate kinase deficiency | Tablet |
| 9/29/2022 | Relyvrio | sodium phenylbutyrate, taurursodiol | Amyotrophic lateral sclerosis (ALS) | Powder for Oral Suspension |
| 9/1/2022 | Spevigo | spesolimab-sbzo | Generalized pustular psoriasis flares | Injection |
| 10/25/2022 | Tecvayli | teclistamab-cqyv | Relapsed and refractory multiple myeloma after at least four prior therapies | Injection |
| 9/14/2022 | Terlivaz | terlipressin | Improved kidney function in adults with hepatorenal syndrome | Injection |
| 2/28/2022 | Vonjo | pacritinib | Intermediate or high-risk primary or secondary myelofibrosis with low platelet levels | Capsule |
| 8/31/2022 | Xenpozyme | olipudase alfa-rpcp | Non-central nervous system manifestations of acid sphingomyelinase deficiency (Niemann-Pick disease type A, B, A/B) | Injection |
| 3/18/2022 | Ztalmy | ganaxolone | Seizures associated with cyclin-dependent kinase-like 5 deficiency disorder (CDD) in patients aged two years and older | Oral Suspension |

Note. This table is a summary and may not include all drugs or their complete indications and information. Adapted from New drugs at FDA: CDER's new molecular entities and new therapeutic biological products, 2023.

These therapeutic innovations are at the vanguard of medical science, encompassing advanced modalities that leverage the latest genomics and artificial intelligence (AI) developments. The integration of AI in pharmaceutical research, as outlined by Léon van Wouwe of Volv Global, Heidi L. Rehm of Massachusetts General Hospital, Simon Alfano of McKinsey & Company, and Karin Hoezler of the National Organization for Rare Disorders, is revolutionizing the approach towards drug discovery, making it more efficient and targeted (van Wouwe et al., 2023). Similarly, advancements in genomics are instrumental in the progression toward personalized medicine, offering new avenues for treating rare diseases (Doe & Lee, 2023).

In the wake of these advancements, the STARVar tool presents a compelling case for continuing the exploration of AI as a solution in rare disease management (Kafkas et al., 2023). Developed by KAUST researchers, STARVar is able to analyze and interpret symptoms recorded in diverse formats, including both standardized medical language and free-form text. In doing so, STARVar accurately identified a solitary mutation in a young Saudi girl from a pool of nearly 800 gene variants. This mutation in the MMP2 gene was already known to be pathogenic and, therefore, offered a likely pathology for the girl's lumps, bone damage, and joint stiffness. STARVar successfully integrates data from various sources, such as genomic datasets, clinical symptoms, and scientific literature, suggesting that such an approach to tackling the complexities of rare diseases and unattributed symptoms is possible and productive (Kafkas et al., 2023).

Moreover, STARVar's approach addresses several critical challenges discussed in this chapter. It showcases the power of AI in enhancing diagnostic accuracy, especially in conditions where traditional methods fall short due to the rarity and uniqueness of symptoms. Furthermore, the tool's ability to interpret non-standardized symptom descriptions resonates with the ongoing conversation about patient data utilization and privacy (Kafkas et al., 2023).

## *From Sorcery to Science: The Evolution of Disease Understanding*

The integration of AI into healthcare signals a turning point in addressing the challenges posed by rare diseases. AI's capacity to process vast datasets and identify patterns undetectable to the human eye offers new hope in several key areas.

The transition from attributing diseases like kuru to sorcery to understanding them through scientific research mirrors the current shift towards AI in healthcare. Just as the South Fore's understanding of kuru evolved with scientific intervention, so too does the modern approach to rare disease management evolve with AI. By analyzing large datasets, AI can uncover patterns and connections in disease progression and treatment efficacy that were previously unseen, much like how anthropological and medical research unraveled the mysteries of kuru. This evolution from mystical interpretations to data-driven understanding underscores the transformative potential of AI in healthcare. As AI redefines the healthcare landscape, STARVar suggests a way toward more personalized, accurate, and efficient management of rare diseases through applications of AI for big data analysis and improved disease understanding (Kafkas et al., 2023).

Despite these advancements, the treatment landscape for rare diseases must be more comprehensive to address ongoing challenges (Faviez et al., 2020). Most rare conditions still lack effective diagnostic and therapeutic options, as Patel and Singh (2023) highlighted in their review of current treatment gaps. This situation underscores the continued need for technological innovation in this field and persistent advocacy for research and development of new therapies.

Another crucial aspect of this golden age of drug discovery is the challenge of ensuring equitable access to these novel treatments globally. Zhao et al. (2022) reported that disparities in access to healthcare resources and advanced treatments are prevalent, necessitating a global effort to bridge these gaps. This challenge points to the need for a more inclusive approach to the distribution and accessibility of advanced medical treatments, especially in underserved regions.

While this era represents a significant leap forward in the treatment of rare diseases, it also brings to the forefront the challenges of ensuring equitable access and addressing the unmet needs of disease therapy. The advancements in drug discovery for rare diseases not only bring about significant medical benefits but also profoundly impact the embodiment and self-perception of patients.

As Feldstein Ewing et al. (2012) explained, the advent of tailored therapies has led to a transformative experience for many patients, enabling them to redefine their identities beyond their conditions. The development of treatments such as tailored pharmaceuticals often means a shift from a life dominated by the constraints of a rare disease to one with greater autonomy and possibilities, which in turn can significantly alter a patient's perception of self, body, and cultural belonging (Prainsack, 2017).

Furthermore, the role of patient advocacy, engagement, and the evolving patient-physician relationship in the era of personalized medicine are crucial. Bombard et al. (2018) observed that patient engagement and advocacy groups have become instrumental in shaping research priorities and therapy development, leading to a more patient-centric approach in healthcare. This is reflected in the FDA's call for input on the integration of AI into pharmaceutic approval processes in recent reports. This evolving dynamic enhances patients' agency and involvement in their healthcare journey, further influencing their perception of self and disease (Bombard et al., 2018).

As highlighted by NORD (2020) in qualitative studies on patient experiences, the availability of effective treatments can result in a newfound sense of hope and empowerment among patients. This shift is particularly significant in the context of rare diseases, where patients often face isolation and a lack of understanding from the broader community (Chung et al., 2023). The psychological impact of these advances cannot be understated, as they not only address the physical symptoms of the disease but also foster a more positive self-image and a sense of belonging in society.

The significant increase in FDA submissions with AI/ML components is a testament to AI's transformative impact on healthcare. As Hao Zhu, director of the Division of Pharmacometrics in the US Food and Drug Administration's (FDA) Center for Drug Evaluation and Research (CDER) highlights, the agency is keen on understanding public opinion on AI/ML usage in drug development and manufacturing (Eglovitch, 2023; New drugs at FDA, 2023). This trend demonstrates AI's growing importance in healthcare and signals a future where AI-driven methodologies become central in managing and treating diseases, including rare conditions.

Looking forward, the convergence of AI and blockchain technology in healthcare, as explored by Nwosu, Goyal, and Bedi (2021), offers exciting possibilities. This synergy could lead to innovative solutions in disease management, particularly for rare diseases, where data security and integrity are paramount. The integration of blockchain technology is not just a security measure; as Nwosu, Goyal, and Bedi (2021) point out, it is a crucial enabler of AI in healthcare. By ensuring the security and reliability of data, blockchain paves the way for advanced AI applications in disease diagnosis, treatment, and patient data management.

## Table 4

***Use Cases: Blockchain Transforming Cyber-Attacks in the Healthcare Industry***

| S.No. | Use Case | Description |
|---|---|---|
| 1. | Stopping Security Breaches on Automated Systems | Blockchain technology recognizes and rejects corrupt commands in automated systems, enhancing security. |
| 2. | Verification of Software Updates or Downloads | Blockchain assists in verifying the legitimacy and security of software updates or downloads, ensuring they are virus-free. |
| 3. | Distribution of Public Key | Distributing public keys (e.g., passwords, usernames) via blockchain prevents hacker access. |
| 4. | More Secure DNS | Providing a decentralized Domain Name System (DNS) through blockchain enables stronger resistance against cyber-attacks. |
| 5. | Stopping Distributed Denial-of-Service (DDoS) Attacks | Using blockchain enables organizations to acquire additional bandwidth to counteract DDoS attacks. |
| 6. | Decentralized Data Storage | Blockchain's decentralized nature eliminates single points of entry, securing data more effectively. |
| 7. | Offering Digital or Biometric Identities | Implementing digital or biometric identities with blockchain provides a more secure alternative to traditional passwords. |
| 8. | Identity Authentication for Edge Devices | Enhancing the security of edge devices through a multi-step authentication process is facilitated by blockchain. |
| 9. | Device Hardware Provenance | Ensuring the authenticity of hardware components through blockchain prevents breaches by malicious viruses hidden in counterfeit hardware. |

Note. Adapted from Nwosu et al. (2021). This table summarizes the impact of blockchain technology on cybersecurity in the healthcare industry, particularly in preventing and mitigating various types of cyber-attacks.

In conclusion, integrating AI, health care, and cybersecurity signifies a paradigm shift in medical surveillance and practice. The integration of AI in healthcare, particularly in the management and treatment of rare diseases, represents a significant advancement in medical science. This technology has the potential to revolutionize patient care, from improving diagnostic accuracy to streamlining drug development and empowering patients and families. While offering personalized and efficient care, these technologies raise crucial questions about privacy, autonomy, and the redefinition of patient and professional identities in the healthcare domain.

In conclusion, this chapter has navigated the complex interplay of AI, blockchain, and cybersecurity technologies (ABCs) in healthcare, specifically in managing rare diseases. The chapter has examined the role of blockchain technology, the ethical considerations of data privacy, and the evolving patient-physician relationship, underscoring the importance of these advancements for future research and clinical practice. The involvement of AI in advancements in drug discovery and treatment for rare diseases may profoundly influence patients' embodiment, self-perception, and psychological well-being and offer cases on which to apply the lenses provided by Lindenbaum, Pols, Rice, and Petryna. As research into the ABCs of Healthcare moves forward, it is clear that AI will continue to shape the healthcare landscape. Its integration into various aspects of healthcare suggests a future where rare diseases are no longer insurmountable challenges but manageable conditions with effective treatments and improved patient outcomes.

# End Notes

1. The idea of surveillance as a method of instigating self-regulation is most often attributed to Foucault's Discipline and Punish. The choice of the word "manufacture" is justified by the forms of knowledge gained through surveillance, including "data," which is a mathematical image of observations that do not exist prior to surveillance and recording, "theories," which are constructed by observers and can be challenged and often disproven, and "nonknowledge," which is the recognized unknown, as in "Biological Citizenship: The Science and Politics of Chernobyl-Exposed Populations" (Petryna, 2004, p.258).

2. "Perceived" refers to surveillance as an unrealized threat (as is possible in the Panopticon), the subject of surveillance's image of the surveyor, and the subject's reassertion of control by adapting to and becoming a

part of the system of surveillance. Likewise, "observers" takes on the scientific definition, not limiting observations to visual sensory input. The "imaginary" (or social imaginary) is the set of values, institutions, regulations, and symbols shared by a particular social group and the related society through which individuals imagine their social whole (according to the definition by Charles Taylor).

3. "David Armstrong (1983), for instance, interprets Foucault's analyses as conceiving all medical knowledge as a form of discipline or surveillance. People start regarding themselves and others with a monolithic, totalitarian medical gaze. For these Foucault interpreters, subjectivity is not merely oppressed but is invaded and shaped by a medical logic that disciplines the ways individuals behave and perceive themselves. Without being aware of it, people reshape themselves according to medical norms" (Pols, 2012, p. 25; emphasis added).

4. "When the incidence of kuru reached its peak, in the 1960's, the South Fore believed their society was coming to an end" (Lindenbaum, 2013, p. 6). Note that kuru serves as the threat of punishment exercised by the panoptic observer.

5. Other interviewees share these traits. Negimba also insists on the power of Western pharmacology over the body, and Obeta employs "biomedical ideas about disease transmission" in his language (Lindenbaum, 2013, pp. 181-183).

# APPENDIX A

## Galactosemia Case Study

In the interview, the participant recalled the diagnosis process:

"This nurse called me. I've never met her. It wasn't his nurse. And she said, [your newborn's] test is positive for galactosemia, which I'd never heard of. I couldn't even understand what she was saying. It's a weird word, right? And she said, 'it's, it's fatal. He's gonna die. He's dying. You have to go to the emergency room right now. He's dying.' And I was like, 'I. Okay,' and it's like, 'hold on like I can't think. I can't process what you're saying. I'm gonna give the phone to my husband.'

"That came on really strong, right? Your baby's dying. And I was, and 'I'm holding him.' I was like, 'he doesn't look like it. He looks an A, but okay.

I mean, whatever you say. I will be right in.' And I gave the phone to my husband, and a friend of ours was there, and I was like, 'she's saying this, and so she's saying this.' So, [the friend's] Googling it, and we're trying to orient ourselves like, 'what is this? What are the symptoms? What is the science? What are these things?'

"They've got this baby right here. And this is like in minutes, right? This information is at your fingertips.

"You know, so [my husband's] on the phone, and they're telling him, and he's like, 'okay, okay, we gotta go to hospital. And you have to stop breastfeeding immediately. It's killing him. He's dying.' And, sure, that is true if a baby has classic galactosemia. But if a baby had classic, there's different variance, right? So, classic is the most life endangering. If a baby has classic galactosemia, you would know. They would be literally dying. They'd be lethargic. Yellow. Unresponsive? Dying, right.

"Our baby was still a 10 out of 10. We're like, 'this doesn't make sense. But we'll go.' And so we're freaking out. I mean, you can't even think straight, right? But at the same time, we're thinking, but. It looks fine. And it's not like it's our first baby, right? We had two more. They all seem fine, but of course we'll go. And so we went in, and they were like, 'we got to do all these blood tests and get them sent away right away. You have to stop breastfeeding.'

"Well, I'm holding my baby who's hungry, and I don't have formula.

"You know what I mean? I'm like, 'what am I supposed to do? He looks okay? It's killing him? I don't know.' And, they were like, 'okay, we've got it.'

"The blood test can only be sent to one lab. In the world. And it's in California, and the sample has to be kept under strict conditions, and it has to get there between Monday and Wednesday because then it has to process.

"There are all these stipulations, and I was like, 'but it's Friday. At like 5. It's not going to get there. What are we supposed to do?'

And they were like, 'well, we don't know.'

"And so I was like, 'this doesn't seem imminent to you? And our baby seems fine, but the nurse said I'm killing him.' You're trying to discern. Right? Amid very little information. Looking at your baby.

"And you can observe, but obviously sometimes symptoms are not visible. So knowing that too. Right? I believe that there could be something very wrong that we can't see, so we're here, right? What do we do? But then people start acting like, well, we don't really know, it's just protocol."

## References

Abdallah, S., Sharifa, M., I Kh Almadhoun, M. K., Khawar, M. M., Sr, Shaikh, U., Balabel, K.

M., Saleh, I., Manzoor, A., Mandal, A. K., Ekomwereren, O., Khine, W. M., & Oyelaja, O. T. (2023). The Impact of Artificial Intelligence on Optimizing Diagnosis and Treatment Plans for Rare Genetic Disorders. Cureus, 15(10), e46860. https://doi.org/10.7759/cureus.46860

Alowais, S. A., Alghamdi, S. S., Alsuhebany, N., Alqahtani, T., Alshaya, A. I., Almohareb, S.

N., Aldairem, A., Alrashed, M., Bin Saleh, K., Badreldin, H. A., Al Yami, M. S., Al Harbi, S., & Albekairy, A. M. (2023). Revolutionizing healthcare: the role of artificial intelligence in clinical practice. BMC Medical Education, 23(1), 689. https://doi.org/10.1186/s12909-023-04698-z

Alrefaei, A. F., Hawsawi, Y. M., Almaleki, D., Alafif, T., Alzahrani, F. A., & Bakhrebah, M.A. (2022). Genetic data sharing and artificial intelligence in the era of personalized medicine based on a cross-sectional analysis of the Saudi human genome program. Scientific Reports, 12(1). https://doi.org/10.1038/s41598-022-05296-7

Berdud, M., Drummond, M., & Towse, A. (2020). Establishing a reasonable price for an orphan drug. Cost Effectiveness and Resource Allocation, 18(1). https://doi.org/10.1186/s12962-020-00223-x

Board on Health Care Services; Institute of Medicine. (2012). The role of telehealth in an evolving health care environment: Workshop summary. Washington (DC): National Academies Press (US); The Evolution of telehealth: Where have we been and where are we going? https://www.ncbi.nlm.nih.gov/books/NBK207141/

Bohr, A., & Memarzadeh, K. (2020). Artificial intelligence in healthcare. Academic Press.

Bombard, Y., Baker, G. R., Orlando, E., Fancott, C., Bhatia, P., Casalino, S., Onate, K., Denis,

J.L., & Pomey, M. P. (2018). Engaging patients to improve quality of care: a systematic review. Implementation science: IS, 13(1), 98. https://doi.org/10.1186/s13012-018-0784-z

Bruce, G. (2023, November 10). Jury UPS Johns Hopkins hospital damages to $261M in Netflix case. Becker's Hospital Review - Healthcare News. https://www.beckershospitalreview.com/digital-marketing/jury-ups-johns-hopkins-hospital-damages-to-261m-in-netflix-case.html

Chung, C. C. Y., Ng, N. Y. T., Ng, Y. N. C., Lui, A. C. Y., Fung, J. L. F., Chan, M. C. Y., Wong, W. H. S., Lee, S. L., Knapp, M., & Chung, B. H. Y. (2023). Socio-economic costs of rare diseases and the risk of financial hardship: a cross-sectional study. The Lancet regional health. Western Pacific, 34, 100711. https://doi.org/10.1016/j.lanwpc.2023.100711

Clark, L. (2023, November 13). AWS staffer shows off former-prison offices on social media. The Register: Enterprise Technology News and Analysis. https://www.theregister.com/2023/11/13/aws_prison_offices/

Committee on Strategies for Responsible Sharing of Clinical Trial Data; Board on Health Sciences Policy; Institute of Medicine. Sharing Clinical Trial Data: Maximizing Benefits, Minimizing Risk. Washington (DC): National Academies Press (US); 2015 Apr 20. 2, Guiding Principles for Sharing Clinical Trial Data. Available from: https://www.ncbi.nlm.nih.gov/books/NBK285999/

Conrad, P., & Barker, K. K. (2010). The social construction of illness: Key insights and policy implications. Journal of Health and Social Behavior, 51(1_suppl), S67-S79. https://doi.org/10.1177/0022146510383495

Deloitte. (2022). 2022 Global Life Sciences Outlook Digitalization at scale: Delivering on the promise of science. https://www2.deloitte.com/content/dam/Deloitte/br/Documents/life-sciences-health-care/deloitte-life-sciences-outlook-2022.pdf

Edrees, H., Song, W., Syrowatka, A., Simona, A., Amato, M. G., & Bates, D. W. (2022). Intelligent telehealth in pharmacovigilance: A Future Perspective. Drug Safety, 45(5), 449–458. https://doi.org/10.1007/s40264-022-01172-5

Eglovitch, J. S. (2023, July 12). FDA sees rapid uptick in drug and biologic submissions with AI/ML components. Regulatory Affairs Professionals Society (RAPS). https://www.raps.org/News-and-Articles/News-Articles/2023/7/FDA-sees-rapid-uptick-in-drug-and-biologic-submiss

El-Sherif, D. M., Abouzid, M., Elzarif, M. T., Ahmed, A. A., Albakri, A., & Alshehri, M. M. (2022). Telehealth and Artificial Intelligence Insights into Healthcare during the COVID-19 Pandemic. Healthcare (Basel, Switzerland), 10(2), 385. https://doi.org/10.3390/healthcare10020385

Ethics and governance of artificial intelligence for health: WHO guidance. (2021). World Health Organization.

Faviez, C., Chen, X., Garcelon, N., et al. (2020). Diagnosis support systems for rare diseases: a scoping review. Orphanet Journal of Rare Diseases, 15(1): 94.

Feldstein Ewing, S. W., Wray, A. M., Mead, H. K., & Adams, S. K. (2012). Two approaches to tailoring treatment for cultural minority adolescents. Journal of Substance Abuse Treatment, 43(2), 190–203. https://doi.org/10.1016/j.jsat.2011.12.005

Frąckiewicz, M. (2023, June 3). The future of smart cities with AI and smart noise management systems. TS2 SPACE. https://ts2.space/en/the-future-of-smart-cities-with-ai-and-smart-noise-management-systems/#gsc.tab=0

Foucault, M. (1995). Discipline & punish: The birth of the prison. NY: Vintage Books, pp. 195-228.

Gómez-Díaz, B., Zamora-González, E. O., Miranda-Duarte, A., Roque-Ramírez, B., Vázquez-Cárdenas, N. A., Martínez-Gómez, G., Del Campo, J. M., Castillo-Jáuregui, E., Castro-Navarro, Á. R., Marín-Cruz, A., Rosas-Maldonado, S., Valdez-Anguiano, P. E., Barrera-López, R. A., & López-Hernández, L. B. (2023). Assessing knowledge, perceptions, awareness and attitudes on rare diseases among health care providers and health students in Mexico. Rare, 1, 100005. https://doi.org/10.1016/j.rare.2023.100005

Hand, S., Hund, M., Foundos, L., & Setty, L. (2023, October). Imagine the next 25 years of entrepreneurship [Conference session]. The meeting of TiE New York, New York.

Hayes, J. (2022). A tortured and deadly legacy: Kissinger and realpolitik in U.S. foreign policy. Ohio Capital Journal. https://ohiocapitaljournal.com/2022/12/15/a-tortured-and-deadly-legacy-kissinger-and-realpolitik-in-u-s-foreign-policy/

Johns Hopkins University. (2023). Data attack. https://www.jhu.edu/data-attack/

Johnson, K. B., Wei, W. Q., Weeraratne, D., Frisse, M. E., Misulis, K., Rhee, K., Zhao, J., & Snowdon, J. L. (2021). Precision medicine, AI, and the future of personalized health care. Clinical and Translational Science, 14(1), 86–93. https://doi.org/10.1111/cts.12884

Kafkas, S., et al. (2023). Starvar: Symptom-based tool for automatic ranking of variants using evidence from literature and genomes. BMC Bioinformatics. doi.org/10.1186/s12859-023-05406-w.

Kamei, T., Yamamoto, Y., Kajii, F., Nakayama, Y. and Kawakami, C. (2013), Meta-analysis of THMTN for COPD. Japan Journal of Nursing Science, 10: 180-192. https://doi.org/10.1111/j.1742-7924.2012.00228.x

Kaul, V., Enslin, S., & Gross, S. A. (2020). History of artificial intelligence in medicine. Gastrointestinal Endoscopy, 92(4), 807–812. https://doi.org/10.1016/j.gie.2020.06.040

Kuiler, E. W., & McNeely, C. L. (2023). Panopticon implications of ethical AI: Equity, disparity, and inequality in healthcare. AI Assurance, 429-451. https://doi.org/10.1016/b978-0-32-391919-7.00026-3

Kumar, A., Singh, A. K., Ahmad, I., Kumar Singh, P., Anushree, Verma, P. K., Alissa, K. A., Bajaj, M., Ur Rehman, A., & Tag-Eldin, E. (2022). A novel decentralized blockchain architecture for the preservation of privacy and data security against cyberattacks in healthcare. Sensors, 22(15), 5921. https://doi.org/10.3390/s22155921

Lindenbaum, S. (2013). Kuru sorcery: Disease and danger in the New Guinea highlands. 2nd Edition. Boulder: Paradigm Publishers.

Lynch, J., & Morrison, E. (2023). Deterrence through AI-enabled detection and attribution. The Kissinger Center. https://sais.jhu.edu/kissinger/programs-and-projects/kissinger-center-papers/deterrence-through-ai-enabled-detection-and-attribution

Narikimilli, N. R., Kumar, A., Antu, A. D., & Xie, B. (2020). Blockchain applications in healthcare – A review and future perspective. Blockchain – ICBC 2020, 198-218. https://doi.org/10.1007/978-3-030-59638-5_14

NORD Rare Insights. (2020). Ensuring access to telehealth for rare diseases. National Organization for Rare Diseases. https://rarediseases.org/wp-content/uploads/2020/10/NRD-2098-RareInsights-Telehealth-Report.pdf

Nwosu, A. U., Goyal, S. B., & Bedi, P. (2021). Blockchain transforming cyber-attacks: Healthcare industry. Advances in Intelligent Systems and Computing, 258-266. https://doi.org/10.1007/978-3-030-73603-3_24

Paul, A. (2021, November 17). Prisons are using Amazon transcribe and AI to monitor inmates' phone calls. Input. https://www.inverse.com/input/tech/prisons-are-using-amazon-transcribe-ai-to-monitor-inmate-phone-calls

Pedro, A.R., Dias, M.B., Laranjo, L., Cunha, A.S., Cordeiro, J.V. (2023). Artificial intelligence in medicine: A comprehensive survey of medical doctor's perspectives in Portugal. PLoS ONE 18(9): e0290613. https://doi.org/10.1371/journal.pone.0290613

Petryna, A. (2004). Biological citizenship: The science and politics of Chernobyl-exposed populations. OSIRIS 19, 250-265.

Pols, J. (2012). Care at a distance: On the closeness of technology. Amsterdam University Press. http://www.jstor.org/stable/j.ctt6wp5zw

Prainsack, B. (2017). Personalized medicine: Empowered patients in the 21st century? NYU Press.

Radanliev, P., & De Roure, D. (2022). Advancing the cybersecurity of the healthcare system with self-optimising and self-adaptative artificial intelligence (Part 2). Health and Technology, 12(5), 923-929. https://doi.org/10.1007/s12553-022-00691-6

Rice, T. (2003). Soundselves: An Acoustemology of sound and self in the Edinburgh Royal Infirmary. Anthropology Today, 19(4), 4-9.

SAMHSA. (2023). Overview of the impacts of Long COVID on behavioral health. https://store.samhsa.gov/sites/default/files/pep23-01-00-001.pdf

Secinaro, S., Calandra, D., Secinaro, A. et al. (2021). The role of artificial intelligence in healthcare: A structured literature review. BMC Med Inform Decis Mak, 21(125). https://doi.org/10.1186/s12911-021-01488-9

Sharma, S., Rawal, R., & Shah, D. (2023). Addressing the challenges of AI-based telemedicine: Best practices and lessons learned. Journal of Education and Health Promotion, 12, 338. https://doi.org/10.4103/jehp.jehp_402_23

Sharp, L. (2022). Death and Dying in carceral America: The Prison Hospice as an inverted Space of exception. Medical Anthropology Quarterly 36(2), 177-197. 10.1111/maq.12688

Shivers, M., Llanes, C., & Sherman, M. (2019). Implementation of an artificial immune system to mitigate cybersecurity threats in unmanned aerial systems. 2019 IEEE International Conference on Industrial Internet (ICII). https://doi.org/10.1109/icii.2019.00013

Taylor, K., May, E., Gupta, L., & Miranda, W. (2023). Seize the digital momentum: Measuring the return from pharmaceutical innovation 2022. Deloitte LLP. https://www2.deloitte.com/content/dam/Deloitte/uk/Documents/life-sciences-health-care/deloitte-uk-seize-digital-momentum-rd-roi-2022.pdf

Taylor, K., Properzi, F., & Joao Cruz, M. (2020, February 10). Intelligent clinical trials: Transforming through AI-enabled engagement. Deloitte Insights. https://www2.deloitte.com/us/en/insights/industry/life-sciences/artificial-intelligence-in-clinical-trials.html

Ulrich, R. S. (1984). View through a window may influence recovery from surgery. Science, 224(4647), 420-421.

van Wouwe, L., Rehm, H., Hoelzer, K., Alfano, S., & Gebel Berg, E. (2023, December). Advocacy in rare disease: Driving technology advances [Conference session]. The meeting of the Science/AAAS Custom Publishing Office. https://www.science.org/content/webinar/advocacy-rare-disease-driving-technology-advances

Vora, L. K., Gholap, A. D., Jetha, K., Thakur, R. R. S., Solanki, H. K., & Chavda, V. P. (2023). Artificial Intelligence in Pharmaceutical Technology and Drug Delivery Design. Pharmaceutics, 15(7), 1916. https://doi.org/10.3390/pharmaceutics15071916

Wang, C., Zhang, J., Lassi, N., & Zhang, X. (2022). Privacy Protection in Using Artificial Intelligence for Healthcare: Chinese Regulation in Comparative Perspective. Healthcare (Basel, Switzerland), 10(10), 1878. https://doi.org/10.3390/healthcare10101878

WHO issues first global report on artificial intelligence (AI) in health and six guiding principles for its design and use. (2021, June 28). World Health Organization (WHO). https://www.who.int/news/item/28-06-2021-who-issues-first-global-report-on-ai-in-health-and-six-guiding-principles-for-its-design-and-use

Wojtara, M., Rana, E., Rahman, T., Khanna, P., & Singh, H. (2023). Artificial intelligence inrare disease diagnosis and treatment. Clinical and Translational Science, 16(11), 2106-2111. https://doi.org/10.1111/cts.13619

Zhang, L., Losin, E. A., Ashar, Y. K., Koban, L., & Wager, T. D. (2021). Gender biases in estimation of others' pain. The Journal of Pain, 22(9), 1048-1059. https://doi.org/10.1016/j.jpain.2021.03.001

# Chapter 9:

## How AI is Weaponized Against Healthcare

**Ali Yousef HCISPP, CISSP, PMP, FHIMSS, CWNE**
*Director, Medical Device and Emerging Tech Security*

*Henry Ford Health*

### *Editor's Note*

Ali Youssef talks about his experience at Henry Ford Health in the 1980s. He has been an innovator across multiple domains of new technologies from electronic health records to IoT and AI, blockchain, and cyber security for the next generation of health technology for hospitals and healthcare systems. His excellent presentation from the Intelligent Health Symposium is the beginning of that conversation.

Health International Center. My name is Ali Youssef. I'm the Director of Medical Device and Emerging Technology Security at Henry Ford Health and I'm here to speak to you about how AI is weaponized or is being weaponized against health care.

So just to give you some background about myself, as I mentioned I'm the Director of Medical Device and Emerging Tech Security at Henry Ford Health. I have a little over 22 years of experience in biomedical engineering, health care IT, and cybersecurity. I'm a HIMSS fellow. I have a number of certifications and really my affiliation with the Intelligent Hospital Association is I am their wireless chair and more recently I've gotten more engaged in the cybersecurity area as well. I'm also involved with the AMI Healthcare Technology Leadership Committee as well as the Editorial Board. So, my claim to fame really dates back to 2014 when you know we first wrote our first book called Wi-Fi Enabled Healthcare. The book is still out there, and I think it's open now. You can read it without you know having to pay anything if you're interested in this particular topic. And I'm very excited about our upcoming book that we've done through the IHA which I wrote a chapter on medical device security in and that is the rise of the intelligent health system.

So, when we talk about AI specifically in healthcare and the promise of AI something comes to mind and really it has to do with, I'm not going to mention specific company names but a prominent AI research and deployment company that has been in the news recently and what really catches my attention about them is their mission statement. And their mission statement is our mission is to ensure that artificial general intelligence benefits all of humanity and if you really think about that it's a very altruistic and ambitious mission statement and it makes it so it's beyond a career it's more of a life goal is this laser focus on AI. So, when we shift this lens to healthcare specifically and the promise of AI in healthcare it really boils down to two main areas. AI is helping us automate routine mundane tasks and really augment our abilities so that we can do more in less time and when you start looking at that through the length of through the lens of clinical care you know one of the areas that comes to mind immediately is medical imaging. The ability to quickly process images, workflow automation whether it's clinical or non-clinical. So, looking at how do you triage or triage patients in an ED setting for example the different steps you have to go through, and which patients have a more urgent clinical need. These are areas where AI can be very beneficial.

Uncovering insights from mountains of data. We've been very good in healthcare about accumulating data and with the push towards meaningful use much of our data is consolidated and many health systems have some form of an EMR platform but really there are mountains of data that we need to sift through to get actionable insights and AI can be very helpful in that context. Of course, individualized treatment plans as I mentioned earlier and really looking at many different inputs and considerations when we're looking at treating a particular patient. And some of the other areas that are really exciting have to do with really automating administrative tasks. So instead of having a clinician needing them to update and populate EMR data or even capture the patient interaction AI does a really good job of filling that gap and I saw a statistic recently I think 40%of the clinician's time is being used towards administrative tasks like this. So, when we introduce AI into this equation it allows our clinicians more time to interact directly and focus on the patients.

And really last but not least is expansion of access. So, through the use of chat bots, through the use of automated methods like that, it allows us to reach out beyond our geographic area and really expand access at an affordable rate or price point.

So, to elaborate a little further on the promise of AI in healthcare this is one way to look at it and it really boils down into four different silos. Now if you really dig into this deeper you can expand this. This could be a much broader chart but at a very high level we're talking about patient-facing applications, telehealth applications, research applications, and doctor-facing applications. So, I mentioned medical imaging earlier. Some other benefits are data analytics, looking at drug discovery, information in the research realm, genetic research, being able to combine these mountains of data and make sense of the trends and come up with actions and really measures to take as a result of crunching the vast mountains of information. And really in the telemedicine space around disease management, lifestyle management, promoting wellness and well-being and automating a lot of those types of transactions. And from a patient-facing standpoint personalized genetics, looking at interacting in different ways with the patients like I mentioned earlier with AI chat bots and things of that nature. And then wearables of course that are collecting mountains of information about patients and sending that information back so it can be analyzed and trended over time. If you're interested in digging a little deeper into this, I've put the reference down here for this chart.

So, when we look at AI over the last year or year and a half, there's been a lot of press warning people about AI, warning the consumers about the dangers of AI. And as you can see here on the right hand side some of the headlines are quite dramatic. It's the end of the world as we It's the end of the world as we know it. Godfather of AI warns a nation of trouble ahead. Experts issue a dire warning about AI and encourage limits be imposed. And perhaps the most dramatic was this statement here you know mitigating the risk of extinction from AI should be a global priority alongside other societal scale risks such as pandemics and nuclear war. So, when you look at that it really makes you pause to try to understand why are these dire warnings being put out there and how is this relevant to health care. So, when I first started seeing these headlines, I thought people were alarmed about AI displacing different roles or job functions and I think that's a piece of the equation but it's not the whole the whole picture. And during this presentation I'm going to be going through why I believe some of these statements are being made at least in part.

But so why is health care relevant in this regard and why are we a target. So, one of the most prominent areas is the value of the data within health care systems. It's high value and it's persistent data. And it's combined and really in a centralized location. So, if you have a chronic condition for example, it's something that will not change drastically over time. And then you can get a lot of other information like you know addresses social security numbers etc. And much of that information is persistent it does not change over time. So, its value is not diminishing. As I mentioned earlier with the push towards meaningful use health care has become a lot more digital and it's comprised of many digital ecosystems that are very complex. Which makes it really difficult to defend. Health care revolves around life safety and there's life safety at stake. So, when bad actors look through that lens it's a lot more likely for a health care institution to pay a ransom because of this life safety aspect. And as you've read over the last several months health care is very resource constrained, especially non-profit health care. You've seen some of the numbers around the anticipated shortage of physicians. I think in the next 12 years it's anticipated I was reading in AMA that it's around 124,000 physicians. It's a shortage of physicians. And as we've seen in the nursing space it's a similar trend. Nurses are leaving that field in droves. I saw a statistic that 100,000 registered nurses were planning to leave that space between last year and this year. So definitely very drastic changes from that standpoint. And some severe constraints around resources and the resources that can be applied towards things like areas like cyber security.

So, I wanted to elaborate a little more about the AI risks in health care and that landscape. Essentially some of the things that are top of mind are concerning have to do with big data exploitation. So, this dependency on data lakes and when you start focusing in on that the integrity of that data is extremely important. And if the data is inaccurate to begin with it's a garbage in garbage out type scenario. We get much less value out of these

AI platforms. Of course, one of the topics that has been making headlines routinely is bias associated with AI or unfair outcomes. And that really has to do with the training data. If the training data includes societal biases to begin with that AI decision making process will also be biased and, in some cases, may amplify that bias. So, it's really important to be aware of that and to make sure that AI platforms are not exasperating unfair diagnoses or treatment for underserved communities. Cyber attacks are top of mind, and this is something I'll elaborate a lot more about in this in this presentation. And really it has to do with that augmentation and automation concept. If you take it and apply it towards cyber attacks, it makes them that much more effective and dangerous.

Disease modeling risk is another area that is of concern and that has to do with developing biological weapons, having the ability to create disease spread prediction models using AI. And this is certainly an area that can impact national security in a major way.

And really last but not least has to do with fakes and deep fakes. You've probably seen recently examples of voice emulators and video emulators where generative AI is used in ways to synthesize media and manipulate authentic media. And this is very concerning. It really blurs the lines between fiction and non-fiction.

So, the topic I really wanted to home in on and one that really has been getting a lot of attention lately has to do with offensive AI as it pertains to cyber security. This has been fueling the cyber arms race. I would say there's been a cyber arms race for decades now, but this is just catalyzing that. It's making it move so much more quickly. And just to give you a high level definition, when I refer to offensive AI, really what I'm referring to is it's a platform that's leveraging machine learning to supercharge cyber attacks. And it results in unpredictable contextualized speedier and stealthier assaults that can cripple organizations that are even prepared for this sort of thing. And by the way, threat actors are some of the earliest adopters in this space. Offensive AI has been used by the Department of Defense in areas like weapons making, but really, it's been getting a lot of attention lately in this specific space when it comes to cyber attacks. And on the right hand side here I have, I'm just illustrating several, it's an offensive AI tool compilation and there are many of these online. And they're readily available. They're easy to use. You don't have to be a subject matter expert in order to use these platforms, which makes them that much more dangerous. If you're interested in these specific ones, I have the link down here on the right. But as you can see, there are pen testing platforms out there, malware creation platforms, AI based botnet systems. The list goes on and on. Like I said, I mean, this is just a small sample of what's available.

So, if we dig a little deeper and look at specific cyber threats that have to do with AI, many come to mind, and these are relevant beyond healthcare. It's really healthcare and beyond. One of the most prominent has to do with phishing. And as I mentioned earlier, the lines between fiction and non-fiction are being blurred. And when you start having platforms that can underline, that can compromise that underlying trust system in our society, it's really something that we need to be paying attention to. So, in the case of phishing, we've seen phishing has been around for a while and it's concerning, but really automating the ability to create effective phishing campaigns to trick victims at scale is something that is of concern. Like I mentioned earlier, voice and image synthesis, where you can fool someone and impersonate someone to influence your targets. Intelligent reconnaissance has to do with collecting a bunch of information about a target very quickly. And that has to do with looking at images online. If they have a PC screen in the background, what is on that screen and being able to analyze information at that level and compile it to uncover vulnerabilities that can be specific to that individual or institution.

Rapid coding is another area that we've been paying a lot of attention to. And really the ability to deploy complex polymorphic malware that is specifically engineered to evade defenses. And I have a couple of examples on the right here. You can see Black Mamba. And there is a black hat sort of facing version of ChatGPT called warm GPT out there as well. But creating generative AI techniques and using techniques to dynamically create fakes that disguise malware, like I mentioned, and really automating the attack process and life cycle to make it really difficult for humans to defend or react against. And to that point, high volume and adaptive variation of high speed attacks can very quickly overwhelm static cyber defenses and manual threat hunting techniques that a lot of institutions are using.

So, if we dig a little deeper into phishing, this is one of the top concerns and often it's cited as the first point of entry. It's a low hanging fruit for bad actors. And it used to be that there were telltale signs to phishing emails. There were misspelling or grammar errors or the link URL would be inaccurate or the way that the email was addressed or written. You could quickly tell that it wasn't authentic. But now with the use of tools like generative AI, it's becoming much more difficult to discern these types of phishing emails. And on the right hand side here, you know, when you first interact with a platform like ChatGPT, let's say, and others, and you ask it to create a phishing email, there are guardrails that prevent you from doing that. But then if you're able to prompt it effectively, this was an output I was able to get out of the tool by prompting it effectively and asking it to craft an email to Robert Main, a made up name, essentially, trying to urge them to click on a link. And this is what it came up with. A strong sense of urgency. It has a placeholder for the link. And, you know, I thought it just did a brilliant job of using all aspects of psychology to try to coerce this individual to click on a link. So, you know, when you start using the tool in this manner, some of the outcomes can be diabolical. And in some cases, this link could be a legitimate link that is then going to a legitimate portal that is housing something nefarious where, you know, that's looking to take your credentials to take your credentials or for you to add your credentials. And we've seen this with automated phone phishing attacks as well. Like I mentioned, with the voice emulation technologies, it's becoming really difficult for humans to detect and react against these types of attacks. And this link here, for example, AI can be used to generate fake portals that look exactly like the legitimate portals to convince you to enter your credentials. Really, at the end of the day, the goal is to get the credentials of the healthcare workers to get an entry point onto the network. And then they go from there.

So, imaging attacks is another area that's been very prominent and has been getting a lot of attention. And this is really interesting, because when you start comparing images and the way an AI system deciphers an image versus a human, there are scenarios where you can manipulate images at the pixel level, where, you know, the human eye cannot detect the change, but it will throw off the AI algorithm completely to a point where it can mischaracterize something completely. It can go from a high level of accuracy to a very low level of accuracy in many cases. So, the examples that are given here really have to do with the radiology space, and this ability to show nonexistent abnormalities or hide evidence of actual disease, which ultimately will lead to a misdiagnosis or mistreatment. So, as you can see on the right here, this is an artificial intelligence reconstruct for an MRI scan. This is a legitimate use. Many software packages are designed now to, if you move slightly when you're in the MRI, and they need to clean up the image, AI is leveraged to do that. And these are algorithms that are, you know, built into these tools. So, imagine if you were to go in and compromise these algorithms, you can generate fictitious information and prompt action that is not, you know, merited.

So, the three main categories are, you know, natural scans with or without cancerous growth that would be untampered. The false benign category would be scans with artificially removed cancerous growth. And then, of course, the false malignant is scans with artificially injected cancerous growth. So, on the bottom right hand here, and I've cited the literature at the bottom, you can kind of see brain scans and the areas that are highlighted, these were added manually to trick a clinician into thinking something is there and look further into these images. So, when you start looking at how these machines work and their algorithms, even getting into the machine, the calibration system, it's a scary concept because now you can manipulate the output, you know, from these types of machines and impact clinical care directly.

And, of course, you know, last but not least, poisoning the training data set. So, now the system has intentional blind spots or within its code, there's programming for it to have false findings.

So, one other example I wanted to give has to do with the help desk. And this is really, was made prominent, more prominent, I would say, recently by the attack on MGM. But, essentially, many large healthcare and even smaller healthcare institutions rely on help desks. And this is where, you know, you call in if you have any customer service issues or if, as an employee, you need to reset your password, for example. But when you start looking at some of the emerging areas in the AI space and you put them in this context, it makes it very difficult to actually authenticate and validate that the person on the other side of the phone is actually the person intended to be there. And this has to do with the SIM swapping attack and voice emulation. It's becoming increasingly difficult to authenticate users. And, really, I think this concept of definitive authentication will be the next frontier where I can validate by several means and several authentication mechanisms that I'm, in fact, speaking with the person I believe to be speaking with. And, really, currently, the solution to this has to do with layering different authentication methods. That's been our best defense so far. So, essentially, that's something you know, something you have, and then something that proves who you are. So, biometrics, facial features, fingerprints, etc.

So, knowing all of this, now how can we defend against offensive AI? And I gave you the tip of the iceberg. There are many more examples that I did not mention. It would take, you know, hours to go through every scenario. But I gave you the ones that are most concerning, in my opinion. So, one key area is to acknowledge that this issue exists and that it's a growing concern. And with the rise of ransomware events, you know, almost on a daily basis now, it's difficult not to acknowledge this issue. Increased focus on risk management. You know, if you don't have a robust risk management practice in place today, definitely work towards setting one up. Because this is a key area, you know, as new platforms are being brought online, we really need to understand, and through threat modeling, understand what risks they could pose to the organization.

Leveraging defensive AI Leveraging defensive AI as much as possible. Like I mentioned earlier, with some of these offensive AI technologies, they're designed to overwhelm our systems. So, really, the only effective way to defend against it is through a defensive AI platform. So, having a robust security program in place, risk management would fall under that. And then, really, last but not least is focusing on business continuity. You know, if we were to have breaches and if we were to have cybersecurity events that impact the business or various business units, what will the reaction be? You know, how will we continue to operate? Having a solid business continuity plan in place. Because I do feel like, and you've heard this a lot lately, it's not a matter of if, it is a matter of when institutions are infiltrated. If someone takes a strong enough interest, they will find a way in eventually, whether it's through phishing or some other means. And with that, I'd like to conclude.

# Chapter 10:

## Investigating the Impact of Blockchain on Smart Cities and FinTech to Improve Healthcare

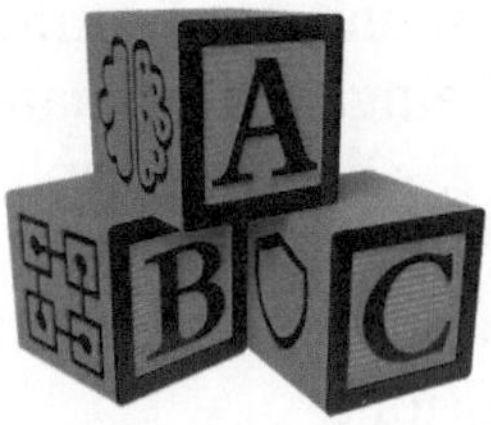


**A.J. Ripin**
*Chief of Staff*

*Merging Traffic*

### *Editor's Note*

In this chapter, A.J. Ripin draws on his experience in infrastructure investment and guiding scalable solutions that can have an impact on entire societies. This is the start of a conversation on the ability for AI, blockchain, and cyber security to have an impact on smart cities and the use of internet of things technologies. For the betterment of health care and other important aspects of society.

# Preface

The accelerating progression of urban development has seen an increased adoption of financial technology (FinTech) in Smart Cities, propelled by revolutionary technologies such as AI, Blockchain, and Cybersecurity. These technological advancements are revolutionizing city life, with blockchain playing a crucial role in this transformation process. By utilizing these cutting-edge technologies to tackle critical issues like congestion, resource allocation, and public safety, intelligent cities enhance the efficiency and sustainability of urban areas, significantly improving residents' quality of life. The successful deployment of Smart City models sets an example for future urban growth, demonstrating how technology can be seamlessly integrated into our lives to create more habitable, resilient communities that promote inclusivity, fulfillment, and human well-being. This dynamic interplay between urban expansion and smart cities across the marketplace highlights today's burgeoning, next-generation tech integration as an essential component to address challenges arising from rapid metropolitan nation alongside changing needs within growing populations:

- Accelerated Urban Growth – As per a report published by the United Nations, it's estimated that over two-thirds of the global population will reside in city regions by 2050.[1]

- Smart City Technology Investments – The global market size for smart cities is projected to increase from USD 410.8 billion recorded in 2020 to USD 820.7 billion by the year's end in 2025 at a CAGR rate of 14.8%.[2]

- Energy Management & Sustainability – Urban centers consume above two-thirds of total world energy while accounting for over seventy percent of worldwide CO2 emissions.[3]

- Intelligent Transportation Systems (ITS) – Expected ITS market value poised to reach around USD 30.65 billion by year-end -2026, at a CAGR rate of approximately 5.11%.[4]

- Public Safety & Security – Notable growth recorded in smart device networks and AI development for public safety tech applications.[5]

- Digital Governance Transformation – Increasing prevalence of digital governance within urban management; e-governance tools employed to enhance citizen engagement and improve efficiency in public administration while providing transparent services.[6]

- Healthcare Integration into Smart City Planning – The COVID-19 pandemic has necessitated healthcare integration into intelligent city planning, emphasizing innovative health infrastructure, such as telemedicine and remote patient monitoring, becoming vital components of modern urban expansion efforts.[7]

  The emergence of telemedicine and remote healthcare, particularly during the COVID-19 pandemic, has been a game-changer in the field of medical services. This rapid shift to virtual care platforms underscores the transformative power of technology in making healthcare more inclusive and far-reaching. Telemedicine has not only broken-down geographical barriers but also introduced a new paradigm in patient engagement and healthcare delivery. It has enabled real-time, remote consultations, diagnosis, and treatment, offering a lifeline to those in remote or underserved areas.

  The integration of these technologies into Smart City planning is pivotal. They complement the infrastructure of intelligent urban spaces, where connectivity and accessibility are paramount. Furthermore, with the ongoing advancements in 5G technology, the scope and efficiency of telemedicine are set to increase exponentially. This will enable more complex medical interactions, like remote surgeries and real-time monitoring of patients with chronic conditions, making comprehensive healthcare a reality for every urban resident. Thus, telemedicine and remote healthcare are not just temporary solutions for a pandemic-stricken world but fundamental components of future-oriented, smart urban healthcare systems.

- Emergence 5G Networks – The deployment of 5G technology is critical to supporting a wide range of IoT devices needed for innovative city operations. Ericsson predicts that by the end of 2025, this technology will have approximately 2.6 billion global subscriptions, enhancing connectivity and data processing capabilities crucial for implementing effective smart city solutions.[8] These deployments of innovations in sensing devices and communication networks enable cities to digitize their infrastructure and services, providing live data on various public aspects like traffic and public services.[9]

As we delve into the transformative role of technologies in Smart Cities, it's crucial to spotlight the revolutionary impact of blockchain in healthcare. This integration is not merely a technological shift, but a paradigm change in patient data management and pharmaceutical traceability. Blockchain's secure, decentralized record-keeping addresses the critical issues of data breaches and transparency in healthcare. It empowers patients with control over their medical data, facilitates seamless data sharing among healthcare providers, and brings unprecedented transparency to the pharmaceutical supply chain. This ensures drug integrity from production to delivery, reducing the risk of counterfeit medications. Moreover, blockchain's role in streamlining clinical trials by managing patient consent and data sharing accelerates medical research. In essence, this healthcare revolution, driven by blockchain, paves the way for a future where healthcare services are more efficient, safer, and more patient-centric, aligning perfectly with the ideals of Smart Cities - efficient, sustainable, and technologically integrated urban living.

# FinTech Application Within Smart Cities

The incorporation of FinTech within advanced cities fosters the creation of more inclusive, streamlined, cashless living spaces. As digitized payment options evolve, they offer significant improvements regarding cost savings and overall service enhancements. For example, Mastercard aspires to promote financial inclusivity plans to provide access to connect one billion individuals towards a digitized economy by 2025, the focus being enabling contactless payments, clicking small-scale businesses to accept consumer payments via mobile wallets and smart devices. These integrated payment solutions are also revolutionizing city infrastructure, especially within transportation, where contactless methods are gaining popularity. Citizens with government-issued ID cards also utilized essential functions around the city, including social payments, access grants, and initiatives. The proliferation of IoT devices and the advent of 5G driving growth in digitized wallet expenditure are estimated to reach $10 trillion by the end of the year twenty-twenty-five, making the possibility of a truly cashless society almost inevitable.[10]

It's accelerating beyond simply digitalizing financial transactions; blockchain, bolstered by AI advancements and reinforced with state-of-the-art cybersecurity, is revamping the entire economic framework. This integration elevates financial inclusivity from access to real-time processing security. Smart Cities stand at the forefront of technological adoption, operationalization, and scale, creating more efficient, inclusive, and secure economies and enhancing the quality of life within cities. The convergence of advanced technologies in Smart Cities is shaping the future wherein technology empowers and transforms urban fiscal services, heralding a new era of sustainable, equitable metropolitan development.

It is anticipated that these cities will evolve into intelligent hubs, and the role of FinTech will become increasingly critical, redefining what it means to live in an urban setting. Initially conceived as centers for enhanced and streamlined municipal services, Smart Cities are now expanding their scope to incorporate FinTech, in which Blockchain emerges as a key facilitator. This tech disrupts traditional concepts of conducting financial transactions beyond mere operational efficiency and reshapes the experience itself.

In the intricate design of Smart City development, where FinTech and blockchain redefine urban economic structures, the role of cybersecurity in healthcare technology emerges as a critical component. As healthcare systems advance with digital innovation, the imperative of robust cybersecurity measures becomes increasingly evident. The task at hand is not merely about safeguarding sensitive health information against cyber threats but constructing a resilient digital healthcare ecosystem. This ecosystem, underpinned by advanced cybersecurity protocols, ensures the sanctity and confidentiality of patient data, fostering a secure environment for technological healthcare advancements. By fortifying healthcare infrastructures against cyberattacks, we establish a foundation of trust and reliability, essential for the acceptance and success of digital healthcare solutions in Smart Cities. This intertwining of cybersecurity with healthcare technology is a cornerstone in building smart, sustainable urban spaces, where health data security is as paramount as financial transaction security, together driving towards a more secure, efficient, and human-centric urban future.

The core idea behind a Smart City involves crafting an ecosystem permeated by technology across all aspects of city living, including its finances. Integrating these elements aims to transform how residents interact with their surroundings via increased efficiency, ultimately reimagining what constitutes 'city life.' In this scenario, Fintech powered by Blockchain is a beacon innovation fundamentally altering how people engage financially within their communities. Blockchain's application in Fintech does far more than digitize monetary exchanges.

It completely overhauls existing structures, resulting in a financial revolution that enhances inclusivity, allows real-time transaction processing, and offers unprecedented security and trust. The role of blockchain is critical here. It symbolizes technological progress and represents a fundamental shift in how we perceive the structure of our fiscal interactions. Therefore, the evolution of Smart Cities is inexorably linked with the transformation of FinTech, wherein Blockchain serves as the center point of this development.

As cities become more technologically advanced, their monetary systems follow suit, becoming increasingly efficient, inclusive, and secure. This metamorphosis is crucial to improving the quality of life for urban dwellers, ensuring Smart Cities are interconnected, efficient, equitable, and financially empowering all residents. Blockchain Fintech paints an intricate yet harmonious picture in complex web modern metropolitan growth fusion Smart Cities. Smart cities epitomize the zenith of urban efficiencysustainability, leveraging data-driven decision-making to enhance living conditions in the town. Blockchain technology intertwines fabric with its unparalleled safety, transparency, decentralized nature-backed strength, immutable records, and intelligent contracts. FinTech threads through matrix innovative fiscal services expand accessibility, digitizing transactions and offering personalized, practical financial solutions. These elements form dynamic synergy fostering data-centric finance services, decentralized, resilient municipal economic structures, and automated, streamlined exchanges. This convergence lays the foundation for inclusive, sustainable metropolitan progression where tech isn't merely an enabler but a transformative force enhancing the financial health and overall lifestyle experience of people in these areas. This potent amalgamation of next-gen technologies within smart cities is only beginning. The immense potential exists for further transformations in the closer era of quantum computing. Quantum computing could further amplify these technologies, opening doors to incredibly productive, secure, creative urban finance ecosystems. Prospect quantum-enhanced intelligent metropolises invite us to envision future boundaries between technology and city existence continually redrawn, heralding extraordinary advancements in how live work interacts within our urbanscapes.

Blockchain technology within financial technologies (FinTech) drives smart city evolution, seamlessly amalgamating with advanced tech solutions such as artificial intelligence and cybersecurity. The potential for blockchain to revolutionize urban monetary systems cannot be understated due to its ability to democratize access to finances, thereby promoting inclusivity and equity within densely populated cities. Additionally, the indelible ledger feature inherent in this technology ensures that transactions remain secure and transparent – vital characteristics when dealing with complex urban fiscal interactions. Furthermore, combining blockchain with AI and cybersecurity establishes a strong base for delivering financial services while creating an efficient metropolitan network. As we approach an era dominated by quantum computing, these converging technologies offer intriguing possibilities that could boost smart cities' efficiency levels and security measures.

Smart Cities aim to foster access together with fairness, which forms part of their core mission statement- thus making accessible financing one primary goal they strive hard to achieve. Urban centers characterized by dense populations coupled with diversity prioritize inclusive finance initiatives heavily, where the role played via blockchain remains pivotal given its decentralized nature can act as a catalyst for breaking down traditional barriers obstructing entry into mainstream banking channels or any other form of essential financial service provision including loans etc., By leveraging power offered up via Blockchains; municipalities are now able to provide unbanked/under-banked citizens easier more equitable routes accessing critical money management tools aiding them greatly both financially socially but also contributing significantly toward overall health resilience local economies too.

The need for robust transactional safety mechanisms becomes paramount amidst intricate webs woven around multiple types of fiscal dealings within smart cities. Blockchain technology plays a crucial role in this context due to its immutable ledger feature, which ensures that each financial transaction is securely logged and resistant to manipulation. Such secure transactions are essential for densely populated urban areas where complex and high-volume fiscal exchanges occur regularly, thus necessitating increased user trust.

Interoperability in healthcare systems is not just a feature but a fundamental cornerstone for the effective delivery of modern healthcare services. This seamless communication and data exchange between diverse healthcare platforms and software goes beyond improving operational efficiency; it revolutionizes patient care by creating a unified, patient-centric healthcare ecosystem. This interconnected framework allows for comprehensive patient care, where medical histories, ongoing treatments, and potential health risks are accessible across various healthcare providers and institutions. Enhanced interoperability in Smart Cities, where diverse and intricate healthcare networks converge, means more than just data sharing – it represents a harmonious integration of healthcare services, ensuring that every individual receives consistent and informed medical care. This approach also aids in the early detection of diseases, streamlined management of chronic conditions, and more accurate prognoses, contributing significantly to the overall health resilience of local communities. In essence, interoperability is the key to unlocking a more inclusive, efficient, and effective healthcare system within the Smart City paradigm, ensuring that every citizen, regardless of their location or socioeconomic status, has access to the best possible healthcare solutions.

Blockchain's ability to integrate various financial services forms another critical aspect of building cohesive infrastructures within Smart Cities. The distributed ledger system intrinsic in blockchain enables seamless information flow regarding finances while facilitating smooth execution of transactions across different platforms ranging from digital payments up to insurance plus investment portals, thereby driving innovation by allowing these interconnected systems to adapt quickly according to changing needs and emerging trends shaping the future of landscape finance industry. These technological advancements offer unparalleled control over personal finance management and ease-of-use features, wherein blockchain guarantees swift, safe money transfers. In contrast, FinTech brings forth tools for efficient monetary planning, increasing accessibility of a diverse range of products, and enhancing overall economic literacy empowerment of individual households. The amalgamation between blockchain and fintech technologies fosters vibrant community economies marked by fairness and equality. By integrating such advanced solutions into their frameworks, smart cities can enhance efficiency levels while promoting transparency alongside resilience throughout their entire financial ecosystem – paving paths leading toward sustainable growth models, fostering innovative cultures, and consequently encouraging robust economic development initiatives on a large scale.

While the implementation of AI in healthcare signifies a leap towards personalized patient care and advanced diagnostics, it's equally important to recognize how blockchain technology is reshaping the financial landscape in Smart Cities. Blockchain's seamless integration in various financial services is pivotal in building cohesive infrastructures within these urban spaces. The synergy between blockchain's distributed ledger system and FinTech's innovative financial tools exemplifies a broader technological evolution. This evolution transcends beyond healthcare, encapsulating financial transactions, digital payments, insurance, and investment platforms in Smart Cities. As we witness AI revolutionize healthcare through tailored treatments and predictive analysis, blockchain and FinTech emerge as cornerstones in the financial sector, enhancing economic efficiency, transparency, and security. This holistic technological advancement across sectors is a testament to the dynamic and interconnected nature of modern urban ecosystems.

# A Paradigm for Blockchain Integration in FinTech

The rapidly evolving sphere of Smart Cities presents an opportunity to incorporate blockchain technology into the financial tech industry, marking a significant stride towards technological advancement and fiscal autonomy. However, this transition requires careful orchestration through methodical phased progression. The following cases offer a detailed guide for effectively incorporating blockchain mechanisms within the financial elements of Smart Cities. Creating a strategic blueprint for adopting blockchain is crucial for any city commencing on this path. This plan must be customized according to each city's distinctive regulatory backdrop, technical prowess, and socio-economic circumstances. Engaging various sector stakeholders - from governance bodies to businesses and community organizations - is vital during this phase as it ensures alignment with local laws while addressing specific urban needs comprehensively. Establishing robust technological infrastructure forms another critical component that sets the stage for successfully deploying and assimilating blockchain systems.

As cities worldwide spearhead public service initiatives involving blockchain integration, we can glean valuable lessons about their strategies' successes or challenges encountered along the way:

<u>*Decentralized Finance (DeFi)* has been embraced by various countries, each contributing to the field uniquely.</u>

- The U.S. is a leading hub for DeFi innovation, with numerous startups and established companies exploring DeFi applications. The country's robust technology sector and relatively favorable regulatory environment have enabled a thriving ecosystem of DeFi projects. Silicon Valley is a hotspot for DeFi startups.
- Known for its financial expertise, Switzerland has become a global leader in blockchain and DeFi. The country's "Crypto Valley" in Zug is home to numerous blockchain enterprises. Swiss regulators have also proactively created a supportive legal framework for DeFi and other blockchain technologies. Singapore has established itself as a friendly environment for DeFi and blockchain innovations.
- The city-state's Monetary Authority of Singapore (MAS) is known for its forward-looking approach to financial technology, and many DeFi

projects have chosen Singapore as their base due to its supportive regulatory framework and vibrant fintech ecosystem.

- Estonia's advanced digital infrastructure and e-residency program have made it an attractive destination for blockchain and DeFi projects. The country's progressive approach to digital technology extends to DeFi, which has pioneered integrating blockchain technology into its government services.
- South Korea is one of the most active countries in the cryptocurrency and blockchain space. The government has shown interest in regulating and integrating DeFi into its financial system, recognizing its potential for innovation in the financial sector.
- As one of Europe's largest economies, Germany has proactively created a legal framework for blockchain and DeFi. German regulators have been working on establishing clear guidelines for the industry, aiming to balance innovation with investor protection.

*The Tokenization of Assets*, a process where a digital token on a blockchain represents the ownership of a physical or digital asset, is being advanced by various countries worldwide.

- Switzerland is known for its financial market sophistication; Switzerland has been a leader in the tokenization of assets, particularly in real estate and fine art. Swiss law accommodates the tokenization of assets, making it a favorable environment for such innovations.
- In the U.S., there's a growing interest in tokenizing real estate, stocks, and even artwork. The U.S. Securities and Exchange Commission (SEC) has begun granting approvals for tokenized securities, indicating a regulatory openness to this technology.
- As a financial hub, Luxembourg has been at the forefront of legal frameworks supporting the tokenization of assets. Its progressive regulatory environment is conducive to the tokenization of various asset classes.
- Germany passed a law allowing electronic securities to be recorded on a blockchain, significantly facilitating the tokenization of assets like bonds and stocks.
- Singapore's forward-thinking approach to finance and technology has seen the country embrace tokenization, especially in the real estate sector.

- Australia has seen advancements in asset tokenization, particularly in commodities and real estate. The Australian Securities Exchange (ASX) is actively exploring blockchain technology.

- Estonia has been exploring the tokenization of assets through its advanced e-governance and blockchain initiatives.

These examples highlight the diverse and innovative ways countries adopt and regulate asset tokenization, paving the way for a more digitized and efficient financial future.

*Central Bank Digital Currencies Development* – Imagine a world where monetary transactions are faster, more secure, and transparent. These grand visions are the promise of Central Bank Digital Currencies (CBDCs), revolutionizing how we think about money in our digital age.

- Kaleido, a frontrunner in enterprise blockchain solutions, is at the forefront of this revolution, providing the essential tools for developing and managing CBDCs. Their platform offers robust, scalable, and secure blockchain technology tailored to the unique demands of digital currencies backed by central banks. With Kaleido's innovative solutions, the future of digital currencies is not just a concept but a rapidly approaching reality. This technology paves the way for more efficient financial systems, reduced transaction costs, and enhanced financial inclusion, bringing the transformative power of CBDCs to the fingertips of nations and their citizens. Embracing Kaleido's CBDC development tools means entering a future where financial transactions are seamlessly integrated into our digital lives. It opens possibilities for instant international payments, increased financial security, and a new era of monetary policy and economic management that could fundamentally reshape global finance.

*Blockchain and Fintech are at the forefront of enhanced security measures.* Several countries are leading in integrating blockchain and Fintech into smart cities, combining AI and cybersecurity as well as an eye toward future advancements in next-generation technologies.

- Known for its innovative city initiatives, Singapore integrates blockchain and Fintech extensively, focusing on AI-driven solutions for urban management and cybersecurity.

- The United Arab Emirates, especially Dubai, is a leader in using blockchain in government services, aiming to become a fully integrated intelligent city with a solid emphasis on cybersecurity and AI.

- South Korea, most notably Seoul, is investing heavily in smart city solutions using blockchain and AI, with a strong focus on cybersecurity.
- Known for its digital governance, Estonia integrates blockchain into its smart city initiatives, focuses on AI and cybersecurity, and is open to exploring quantum computing advancements.
- Tokyo and other Japanese cities are advancing intelligent city technologies, incorporating blockchain, AI, and cybersecurity, and showing interest in quantum computing.

These countries are setting benchmarks for integrating advanced technologies to create efficient, secure, sustainable smart cities. Additionally, these marketplace activities underscore the transformative potential of blockchain within urban financial ecosystems and serve as beacons of innovation and achievement in a constantly evolving field. Moreover, they offer a practical blueprint for blockchain application in urban economic contexts, providing invaluable guidance and inspiration for other cities looking to embark on similar ventures. A fundamental principle in implementing blockchain in Smart Cities' FinTech is ensuring scalability and adaptability. Smart Cities are diverse, each with distinct characteristics and evolving needs. Therefore, blockchain solutions must be flexible enough to accommodate this diversity and adaptable to the changing demands and scales of urban environments. The goal is to create blockchain systems that are effective at their inception and can grow and evolve alongside the city, ensuring long-term viability and relevance.

## Global Decentralized Finance (DeFi) Evolution

The financial sector is witnessing a transformative wave worldwide as Decentralized Finance (DeFi) takes center stage. This revolution goes beyond technological advancement; it represents a shift toward an equitable, decentralized, and accessible financial ecosystem. DeFi has the potential to redefine how individuals, communities, and societies interact with finance while also presenting unique challenges along with new opportunities. The global impact of DeFi platforms cannot be overstated - they are reshaping our approach to financial transactions and prompting us to reassess the risks and benefits inherent in this emerging economic evolution.

The United States showcases one advanced application of Decentralized Finance through MakerDAO's initiatives.

- MakerDAO is a leading player in the DeFi lending landscape. Proposals passed by MakerDAO include investments in U.S. Treasury and corporate bonds, alongside partnerships formed with traditional banking institutions for loan provision using Real World Assets (RWAs) as collateral security.

- Their proposed partnership with Huntingdon Valley Bank (HVB) is a notable instance of such integration. In this collaboration, a 100 million DAI vault for HVB will be created, which would serve within the MakerDAO Protocol framework, offering real-world loans via fully backed conventional institutions under the auspices of Maker Protocol.

- To ensure proper management of minting outflows from this vault and addressing commercial issues related directly to HVB, MakerDAO aims to establish a Multi-Bank Participation Trust, enabling capital flow from DAI into HVB coffers. This innovative arrangement sees an initial phase where half of the ownership rests on loans issued by HVB. In contrast, the remaining shares go to MBPTrust, leaving only about 5% stakeholder interest held by MakerDAO itself.

Such collaborations between traditional banks & defi platforms point toward growing convergence between these two sectors, thus bridging the gap between them further.[11, 12, 13, 14]

Estonia is leading the way in implementing blockchain and DeFi technologies with several innovative projects:

- Guardtime is a cybersecurity provider that leverages blockchain systems for data integrity assurance. Their KSI Blockchain technology provides proof of integrity and provenance for digital information and smart devices, offering transparent solutions across various sectors. Guardtime is a cybersecurity provider that uses blockchain technology to ensure data integrity. Their KSI (Keyless Signature Infrastructure) Blockchain, first developed in 2008 for the Estonian government, secures critical data in various sectors, including health, justice, and business. Governments and leading companies across telecoms, aerospace, defense, energy, financial services, and insurance have adopted this technology.[15] The KSI Blockchain Timestamping Service is notable for its compliance with the eIDAS regulation and inclusion in the European Trusted List, making it the first blockchain-based technology to receive such accreditation.[16]

  Using blockchain-based trust anchors allows for independent verification of timestamps without reliance on Guardtime or any third-party service provider.[17] Furthermore, KSI timestamps are stored and verified indefinitely, immune to quantum computing attacks, which makes them ideal for long-term archiving and future-oriented projects.[18] By implementing Guardtime's KSI Blockchain technology, the hope is that citizen healthcare and well-being are significantly enhanced through secure and transparent health data management. The technology's capacity to ensure the integrity and provenance of digital information guarantees that healthcare records are accurate and tamper-proof, thereby improving the quality and reliability of healthcare services. This leads to better-informed healthcare decisions and contributes to overall citizen well-being.

- CoinMetro, based in Tallinn, is one of Europe's fastest-expanding digital asset exchanges. Established in 2017, CoinMetro stands out as a unique financial platform that effectively bridges traditional finance with the innovative realm of blockchain technology. The company offers services that facilitate buying, trading, and investing in cryptocurrencies and provides real-time market analysis tools. CoinMetro's commitment to regulatory compliance and active engagement with regulators in various jurisdictions underlines its role in shaping and enhancing the regulatory framework of the blockchain industry.[19] CoinMetro's operations in Estonia, a nation known for its progressive stance towards digital technology, signify the country's significant contribution to the global blockchain ecosystem. Estonia has a reputation for being at the forefront of adopting and integrating digital technologies into various sectors, including finance and governance, making it an ideal environment for blockchain innovation.

These examples underline Estonia's progressive stance towards adopting digital technology while highlighting its significant contribution to the global blockchain ecosystem.

## Switzerland's Leading Asset Tokenization Initiatives

With an advanced financial market infrastructure, Switzerland has emerged as a frontrunner in tokenizing assets, especially within the real estate & fine art domain. The country's legal framework greatly facilitates such innovations: As per "Blockchain Law," which came into effect on February 1st, 2021, elements from Distributed Ledger Technology (DLT) regulations were incorporated, enabling creation of a new category called distributed ledger-based assets thus allowing shares etc. to be issued under this category & uploaded onto blockchains; The practice of asset tokenization has become commonplace within Swiss Financial Market facilitated by legislation like Federal Financial Market Infrastructure Act (FinfraG). This enables traders to directly link their investments, such as bonds or stocks, to tokens, thereby creating liquidity, making these investments more accessible, and generating market interest. The Swiss have extended the scope of tokenization to include luxury assets such as vintage cars, artwork, wine collections & watches. This approach democratizes the luxury market, allowing average investors to own a fraction of these typically illiquid and inaccessible assets.[20]

Switzerland's leading role in asset tokenization is facilitated by its advanced financial market infrastructure and a supportive legal framework - this can be seen as a guiding light for the evolution of smart cities. By adopting Distributed Ledger Technology (DLT) and Tokenization methodologies, Switzerland has paved the way toward a more inclusive economic ecosystem, which would play a crucial role in developing future smart cities where blockchain technology could enhance transparency and efficiency while increasing citizen engagement levels. Integrating AI alongside Cybersecurity further strengthens this infrastructure, ensuring data integrity and robust security.

These developments have extended the scope of tokenization in Switzerland to include luxury assets such as vintage cars, artwork, wine collections, and watches, democratizing the luxury market by enabling average investors to own fractions of typically illiquid and inaccessible assets. This approach reflects Switzerland's role in fostering innovation and accessibility in the financial market through supportive legislation and technological advancement.

## Central Bank Digital Currencies (CBDCs)

The overall emergence of Central Bank Digital Currencies (CBDCs) is a groundbreaking development in finance, with Kaleido leading the charge by providing enterprise blockchain solutions for their creation and management. Kaleido aids central banks in crafting flexible, secure infrastructures crucial for a thriving global economy.[21]

Their involvement spans over 100 countries, underlining their pivotal role in digitalizing payments, fostering financial inclusion, and propelling economies towards digital sophistication. CBDCs, facilitated by platforms like Kaleido, revolutionize monetary transactions by offering rapid, cost-effective, and streamlined processes.[22]

This evolution significantly affects everyday transactions, from local peer-to-peer exchanges to international trade, boosting individual and business financial operations. By leveraging blockchain, Kaleido enhances transparency in financial systems, bolstering accountability and improving fraud detection. Such clarity empowers citizens and communities to engage more actively with governmental initiatives, fostering a transparent economic environment. Integrating blockchain in CBDCs opens doors to new international settlement systems and payment ecosystems. This inclusivity enables a broader spectrum of people and businesses to engage in the global market, democratizing access to financial resources. While CBDCs herald numerous advantages, their implementation comes with challenges. Key concerns include safeguarding data privacy, fortifying cybersecurity measures, and tackling complex regulatory frameworks. Integrating blockchain in CBDCs opens doors to new international settlement systems and payment ecosystems, democratizing access to financial resources. A critical risk is the digital divide – ensuring that all segments of the population, regardless of digital literacy or technology access, are included in this financial revolution. Integrating AI, blockchain, and cybersecurity in CBDC development points towards a future where quantum computing could further revolutionize these systems. Quantum computing offers the potential for enhanced processing power and unparalleled security, transforming how financial transactions and policies are managed globally. Kaleido's contributions represent a transformative shift in financial system operations with profound implications for individuals, communities, and the global economy. However, realizing the full potential of CBDCs requires careful risk assessment and proactive strategies to address challenges, ensuring an equitable and secure financial future for all.

This partnership between Kaleido and Swift in CBDC development signifies a significant shift in financial systems, offering enhanced financial inclusion and efficiency. However, it also necessitates careful consideration of data privacy, cybersecurity, and regulatory challenges to fully realize CBDCs' potential; the integration of AI, blockchain, and advanced cybersecurity, along with the future potential of quantum computing, promises to revolutionize these systems, further offering unprecedented security and efficiency in global financial transactions.[23]

# Blockchain and Fintech Providing Enhanced Security and Technological Innovation for Smart Cities

Blockchain and Fintech have emerged as pivotal elements in enhancing security measures across the globe. Several forward-thinking countries are leading the integration of these technologies into their innovative city initiatives. By aligning blockchain and Fintech with advanced AI and cybersecurity strategies, these nations are bolstering their infrastructures and setting guidelines for operationalizing next-generation technologies. IoT, blockchain, and other computing technologies have been identified as key drivers in enhancing the efficiency of healthcare services within smart cities.[24]

- In Singapore's Punggol district project, enhanced security and new security models are being implemented by integrating blockchain, IoT, AI, and 5G technologies. The government agency JTC has collaborated with the research institution Wanxiang Blockchain to test new use cases centered around blockchain, IoT, AI, and 5G. Blockchain provides heightened security and transparency to data management, resulting in secure and immutable data records. IoT and AI technologies contribute to intelligent infrastructure management, enhancing real-time monitoring and decision-making capabilities. As a capstone, incorporating 5G technology ensures high-speed connectivity and supports the vast network of IoT devices, enabling a more robust and efficient urban digital infrastructure. This configuration represents a new approach to building a secure, interconnected, technologically advanced Smart City environment.[25]

- The Seoul Metropolitan Government (South Korea) has outlined an ambitious plan to invest USD 287 million on over 1,000 projects to kickstart the digital transformation for the post-COVID-19 era. This includes the establishment of a metaverse platform, the expansion of AI-powered CCTV, and the development of blockchain-based services. One notable initiative is developing a blockchain-based wallet application where citizens can store over 100 government-issued certificates. In Seoul's digital transformation project, enhanced security and new security models are primarily achieved through blockchain-based services and AI-powered technology development. The blockchain component is crucial for ensuring data integrity and security, especially in the blockchain-based wallet application, allowing citizens to store over 100 types of government-issued certificates securely. This application provides safe and private data storage and easy access for residents. Additionally, the expansion of AI-powered CCTV represents an advanced approach to urban surveillance, offering more efficient and intelligent monitoring capabilities for improved public safety and security management.[26]

- In Tokyo's "Smart Tokyo" initiative, enhanced security models are being implemented through a comprehensive use of advanced digital technologies. The initiative emphasizes creating a more connected, convenient, and comfortable city driven by cutting-edge information and communication technologies -- the integration of secure data management systems, intelligent monitoring solutions, and advanced communication networks to ensure public safety and efficient city operations. Additionally, "SMARTCITY × TOKYO" aim is to serve as a collaborative platform, bringing together various sectors to foster innovation in smart city technologies, further enhancing the security and resilience of urban infrastructures.[27]

Innovative healthcare solutions are reshaping the global healthcare landscape on a monumental scale, driven by technologies like blockchain, AI, and cybersecurity. These advancements represent a collective stride towards a healthier, more connected world. Healthcare systems around the globe are leveraging these technologies to enhance efficiency, bolster security, and cater to diverse health needs more effectively. This global adoption marks a significant move towards a universally elevated standard of healthcare, promising more equitable and accessible health services for all.

The integration of blockchain and Fintech within Smart Cities exemplifies not just a futuristic vision but a current reality, actively transforming urban life. These technologies are leading the charge in building cities that are secure, efficient, and sustainable. The application of blockchain and Fintech is a bold step in revolutionizing urban living, signaling a shift towards more inclusive, efficient, and technologically advanced urban environments. Looking to the future, it's apparent that these cutting-edge technologies will continually be instrumental in molding the smart cities of tomorrow. They open up a world of possibilities for improved security, economic growth, and enhanced quality of life for urban residents.

It continues to be a remarkable journey of healthcare innovation and its convergence with the evolution of Smart Cities. It highlights how these technological advancements are not isolated developments but part of a larger, interconnected framework transforming how we live, work, and maintain our well-being in an increasingly digital world. The future of healthcare and urban living, interwoven with these technologies, is a testament to human ingenuity and our relentless pursuit of better, smarter, and more inclusive living spaces. As we embrace this era of digital transformation, it's clear that these innovations will continue to shape our world, promising a brighter, healthier future for generations to come.

## References

1. https://www.un.org/en/development/desa/news/population/world-urbanization-prospects-2014.html
2. https://www.globenewswire.com/news-release/2020/12/17/2147132/
3. https://www.iea.org/reports/empowering-cities-for-a-net-zero-future
4. https://www.mordorintelligence.com/industry-reports/intelligent-transport-systems-market
5. https://www.mordorintelligence.com/industry-reports/smart-cities-market
6. https://fintechmagazine.com/digital-payments/smart-cities-how-finance-can-transform-urban-living
7. https://www2.deloitte.com/us/en/insights/focus/smart-city/building-a-smart-city-with-smart-digital-health.html
8. https://tnfsolutions.com/blogposts/the-future-of-iot
9. https://www.startus-insights.com/innovators-guide/digital-city-trends/
10. https://fintechmagazine.com/digital-payments/smart-cities-how-finance-can-transform-urban-living
11. https://blockworks.co/news/makerdao-opens-100m-dai-loan-to-huntingdon-valley-bank
12. https://tokeninsight.com/en/news/makerdao-partners-with-huntingdon-valley-bank

13. https://defiphilly.io/defi-philly-host-100m-makerdao-debt-vault-architect-from-huntingdon-valley-bank/

14. https://www.theblock.co/post/156301/makerdao-approves-100-million-stablecoin-loan-vault-for-151-year-old-us-bank

15. https://guardtime.com/timestamping#:~:text=,energy%2C%20financial%20services%20and%20insurance

16. https://guardtime.com/timestamping#:~:text=,conducted%20by%20T%C3%9CV%20Nord%2C%20Germany

17. https://guardtime.com/timestamping#:~:text=KSI%20Blockchain%20timestamps%20can%20be,media%20or%20decentralized%20public%20chain

18. https://guardtime.com/timestamping#:~:text=KSI%20timestamps%20can%20be%20stored,oriented%20projects

19. https://www.eu-startups.com/directory/coinmetro/

20. https://www.pwc.ch/en/insights/regulation/swiss-dlt-new-regulations.html

21. https://www.kaleido.io/industries/cbdc#:~:text=Central%20Bank%20Digital%20Currencies%20,to%20power%20the%20global%20economy

22. https://www.kaleido.io/industries/cbdc

23. https://www.kaleido.io/blockchain-blog/kaleido-and-swift-launch-cbdc-sandbox

24. https://pubmed.ncbi.nlm.nih.gov/35126961/

25. https://www.smartcitiesworld.net/news/news/singapore-announces-plans-for-blockchain-and-fintech-development-in-punggol-district-6684#:~:text=Punggol%20is%20being%20primed%20to,blockchain%2C%20IoT%2C%20AI%20and%205G

26. https://www.itu.int/hub/2022/02/seoul-metaverse-digital-transformation-ai-blockchain/

27. https://www.smart-tokyo.metro.tokyo.lg.jp/en/

# Chapter 11:

# The AI Simulation Prescription for Healthcare

**Richard Boyd**
*CEO*

*Ultisim*

## *Editor's Note*

In this chapter, Richard Boyd shares his years of expertise in AI from the perspective of gaming and simulation. To describe potential future uses and applications that will benefit health care and other aspects of society. His track record of bringing predictions into reality with both current state technologies and what we can expect in the near future holds great promise for showcasing the abilities of AI, blockchain, and cyber security integrated into scalable enterprise systems.

# The AI Simulation Prescription for Healthcare

Integrating Generative AI, Knowledge Graphs, and Simulation will revolutionize the healthcare industry. The profound impact of OpenAI's ChatGPT release on human civilization and the progress made through Large Language Models (LLMs) that power ChatGPT amplifies the need for caution and ethical considerations in developing such technologies.

AI-powered assistants, generative AI, knowledge graphs, and simulation technology will revolutionize the future of healthcare. On November 30, 2022, OpenAI released ChatGPT, taking us all by surprise. It was a momentous occasion that will be etched in our memories forever. A year on, we are still adjusting to this new reality. We were particularly taken aback by how our predictions were proven wrong, as we had expected it to be at least a decade before anything close to passing the Turing test would be possible. While large language models (LLMs) had shown great promise, they were still unsatisfactory and prone to errors in 2022. The technology industry was focused on large knowledge graphs (KGs) and neural nets that could solve narrow AI problems such as driving cars, logistics routing problems, or playing complex strategy games like Go or chess. Chatbots powered by LLMs were merely a way to ease interface issues with our big knowledge graphs and finite state machines in 2022, which showed promise but in 2022, were still unsatisfying and prone to error.

GPT, or generative pre-trained transform models based on natural language machine learning processing, has existed for almost a decade. Still, they had only surfaced for widespread use in 2018 with the introduction of BERT, Google's Bidirectional Encoder Representations from Transformers. This chapter will discuss how we employed some of these capabilities, up to and during COVID-19, and how LLMs paired with narrow AI knowledge graphs and sensor-fed digital twin simulation may be the right prescription to transform Healthcare in 2025 and beyond.

# Increasing Complexity in Healthcare:

We are in an exponential age of complexity and uncertainty. By advancing computer power, humans create systems thousands of times more complex than our comprehension of what emerges. In an interconnected world of such complexity, it should not be surprising to see events frequently spin out of our control and overwhelm us, to see "Black Swans" and unanticipated events appear more regularly. Grains of sand cause avalanches. Butterflies flap their wings and unleash hurricanes on distant shores. Financial markets crash, digital viruses wrack the Internet, and biological viruses take wing with air travel to sweep our planet. On the network-centric battlefield and in the technology-laden hospital, we ask humans to adapt to enormous complexity and perform flawlessly, where mistakes can lead to death. As complexity increases (and it shows no signs of abating), it becomes vitally important that we look for help from the machines who are becoming so much better than us at certain things.

Increasing complexity in Healthcare is compounding human errors, resulting in avoidable deaths and injuries. We address this complexity by recognizing that:

1. A stand-alone human being, however masterful, is no longer sufficient to diagnose and apply care

2. Healthcare is a team sport, requiring up to 14 FTEs per patient bed

3. Recent revolutions in sensors and AI provide superhuman capabilities and opportunities to extend life and avoid errors

4. More patient data is becoming available in digital, privacy-protected forms that permit deep-learning neural nets to extract insights unavailable to clinicians and healthcare providers (or even researchers).

In his 2011 commencement address at Harvard Medical School, Atul Gawande explained a central problem of medical practice today. He said that healthcare providers must learn a complex cooperative choreography akin to what pit crews perform during a Formula One race. Gawande explained that very few medical interventions were available to a practicing physician when designing modern medical practice. Therefore, it was conceivable for a single physician to hold himself forth as a master of all knowledge in the profession. He goes on to say that "Resistance ... surfaces because medicine is not structured for group work" ii Yet, the increasing complexity of the 4000 and growing surgical procedures and more than 6,000 drugs that an MD is legally allowed to inflict on a patient requires a cooperative team effort to avoid errors.

In 1975, a hospital patient required the care of 2.5 full-time equivalent caregivers (FTEs). Because of increasing complexity and advancing technology, a typical patient in 2023 requires as many as 14 full-time equivalents for complete care1.

At a minimum, Healthcare should adopt the engineering processes and technologies applied in aviation, engineering, construction, and virtually any industry that combines complexity with high risk. While Healthcare struggles to embrace checklists and basic systems engineering, Aviation, oil and gas, and other industries are adopting a new level of team integration: integrating teams of humans in cooperation and symbiosis with automation.

*"If being in a hospital bed made a difference, it was mostly the difference produced by warmth, shelter, and food, and attentive, friendly care, and the matchless skill of the nurses in providing these things. Whether you survived or not depended on the natural history of the disease itself. Medicine made little or no difference."*

*-Lewis Thomas in "The Youngest Science"*

Every year, more than 700 million passengers travel on over 10 million commercial flights in the United States. This requires a complex logistics, maintenance, and engineering system to ensure that all flights are safe. Despite the fact that aviation is subject to chaotic natural systems and human error, there were no fatalities last year. The last fatality from a commercial flight in the United States happened in 2009, when Continental Flight 3407 crashed into a house in Buffalo, killing 49 passengers due to human error. Checklists, safety interlocks, predictive maintenance, systems engineering, and simulation training are used in aviation to engineer human error out of the system and ensure safety. Furthermore, AI-powered machines are increasingly playing a role in achieving this safety outcome. By finding the right balance between humans and automation, we are engineering human error out of the system and saving lives daily. In contrast, approximately 39 million people checked into just over 7,500 hospitals in the United States last year. Medical errors are the third leading cause of death in the United States, according to a study conducted by Johns Hopkins University Medical School, with between 90,000 and 200,000 people dying each year due to preventable medical errors. This is equivalent to a 737 crashing into the ground every day. However, these deaths do not receive the same public outcry as aviation fatalities. Patients have an 18% chance of being harmed by medical care, according to a study of routine hospital visits to 10 hospitals in North and South Carolina. This error rate is unacceptable in any other industry. Yet, the healthcare industry is trailing behind in using available technologies and engineering approaches to reduce these errors dramatically. Surgeons have only recently started to use simple checklists to avoid mistakes in operating rooms, thanks to the efforts of Atul Gawande.

# Increasing intelligence

In order to provide patients with the best possible healthcare, we must become proficient in using automation technology. Patients deserve nothing less than exceptional healthcare. Fortunately, we do not need to rely on complex and expensive supercomputers like Watson to improve our ability to diagnose and prevent illnesses. Although the field of artificial intelligence has had its shortcomings in the past, it has since evolved and become an essential component in our healthcare teams. With the help of AI technologies like knowledge graphs, expert systems, and other elements, we can capture and utilize knowledge to assist human healthcare providers in various capacities. These systems are becoming more accessible and easier to use as they become more prevalent. It is crucial that we find the perfect balance between human expertise and automation to optimize outcomes. Those who master this balance and are comfortable using simulation, sensors, and analytics will outperform others and appear superhuman.

# The New Scientific Method

The use of Knowledge Graphs and LLMs has enabled us to enhance the scientific method. With the aid of AI, we can now examine a set of data, formulate our own hypotheses, conduct countless experiments, and gain fresh perspectives on the actions we can pursue.

At a TEDMED talk in California in 2010, Dr Rick Satava described what he calls a "new scientific method":

"Build the computer model, add the data from a real-world experiment, see if the results match real-world expectations, change the input data to more closely approximate the model, and run the next iteration. This is continued until there is concurrence with the evidence of real-world results. The result is that the world of science has (unknowingly) changed the scientific method to include an additional step when designing and experimenting with the experiment. The step is to model and simulate, by repeated iteration, to optimize the design of the experiment and then proceed to conduct the experiment."

Dr. Satava describes this change graphically, first in terms of the accepted scientific method:

**Figure 1**

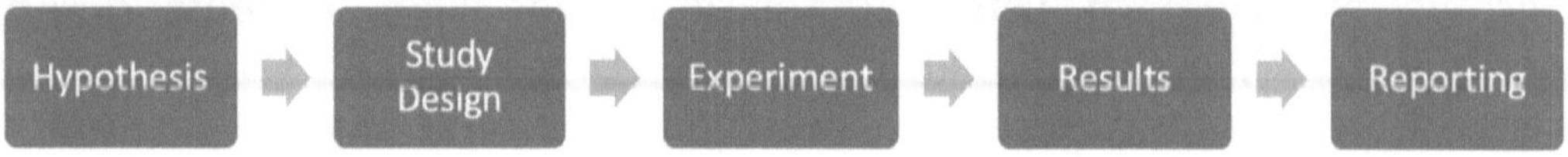


Dr. Satava then describes what he calls "the simulation method or the (new) scientific method:"

**Figure 2**

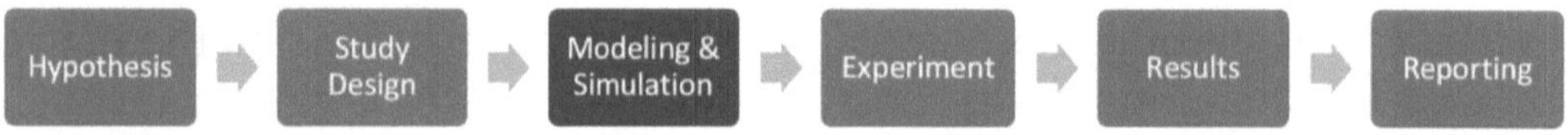


According to Dr. Satava, there is a shift in the scientific method towards incorporating modeling and simulation. This change has significant implications and provides vast opportunities in the field of healthcare. With the advent of Knowledge Graphs and large language models, these technologies can now participate in this methodology. Machine learning systems can tag relevant information with numerous conceptual node markers when constructing knowledge graphs. This holographic data fingerprint helps AI processing by matching information to the appropriate human or machine need.

So, our new scientific method now looks more like

**Figure 3** Machine learning scientific method courtesy of Tanjo Inc.

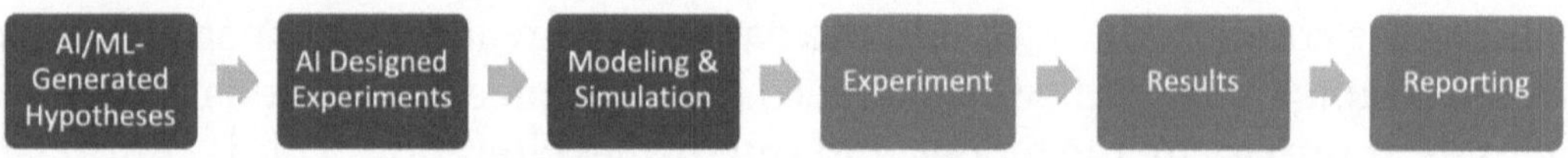

**Figure 4**

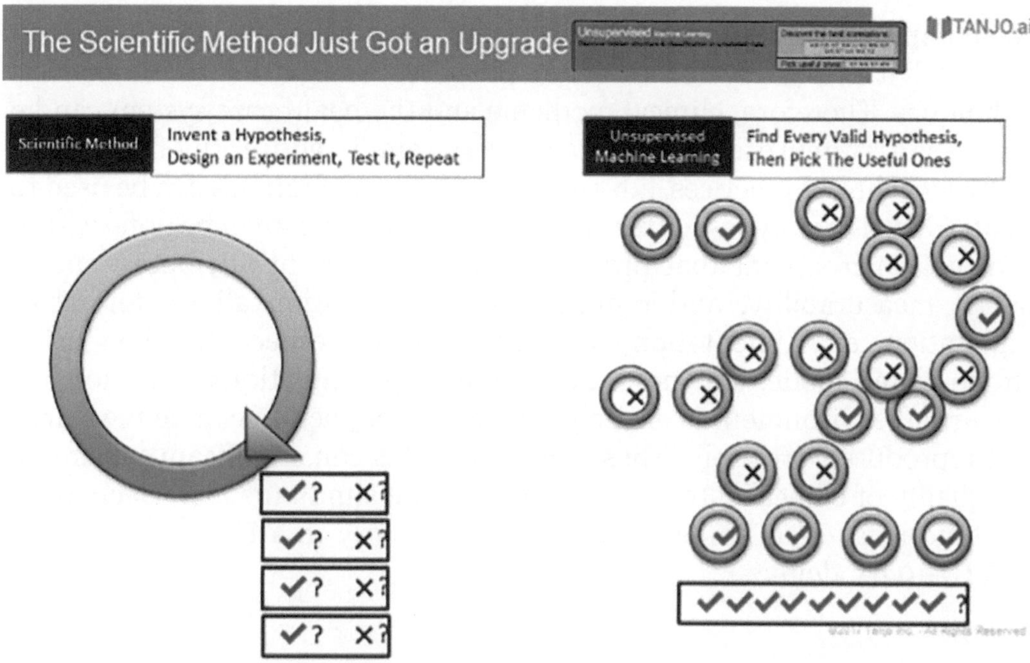


Boosman, Frank, Szczerba, Robert," Simulated Clinical Environments and Virtual System-of-Systems Engineering for Health Care," IITSEC proceedings 2010 "ICESTORM" I/ITSEC Proceedings, Orlando, FL (December, 2011)

# System of Systems Engineering with AI as Partner

It is essential to integrate systems engineering in healthcare. By leveraging AI, we can establish a system of systems engineering that can help us consider the various consequences of actions within the system for patient outcomes. Healthcare comprises of various elements, which include:

1. Devices that are usually electronic, often computer-based, and run complex software programs.
2. Processes utilized by clinicians in treatment, both formal and informal, and both individual and team-based.
3. Patients, specifically their physiology and its response to medical interventions, as well as their psychology and response to internal and external physical stimuli and clinician interactions.
4. Clinicians, primarily their psychology, including process following, clinical mistakes, and responses to interactions with patients and fellow clinicians.

5. Settings, or the surroundings in which clinical care takes place.

The complexity of clinical medicine at the point of care makes it difficult to model it effectively for research purposes using traditional analysis techniques. Therefore, clinical medicine and the healthcare system can be viewed as a "system of systems" or a meta-system. To address ineffective and inefficient clinical practices, advanced simulation techniques can be used to create virtual prototypes for testing improvements. This can be done within a virtual environment that provides four key inherent attributes: speed, safety, measurability, and reproducibility. Simulation allows for faster exploration, experimentation, and clinical trials, especially when using offline, batch mode, and non-man-in-the-loop simulations. Additionally, the virtual environment is entirely safe, and every action can be measured and reproduced precisely. These four attributes can significantly increase the quality of clinical care improvements while simultaneously decreasing the time it takes to implement them, particularly in a crisis such as the COVID-19 pandemic.

## The Simulation Century

We live in an age where we can model and simulate the past, present, and future using digital simulations. This technology gives us the power to review past events, gain better insights, make better decisions in the present, and even predict and design better futures. One essential aspect of simulation technology is its predictive ability. AI has significantly advanced over the last decade, and its primary focus has been to improve prediction. In healthcare, for example, AI is better than humans at analyzing a patient's current state and history, weighing the options for intervention, and predicting how the patient will respond. Chess is another example of how AI has surpassed human capability. AlphaZero, Google's chess AI program, taught itself the game by playing millions of games against itself, developing strategies that reflect the truth of chess rather than the priorities and prejudices of the programmers. Once again, we see the unique perspective of machines achieving insights not available to the human mind. AI is advancing beyond Moore's Law at an exponential rate, and the question remains: what simulations do our AI health partners need to fulfill this incredible promise?

# Digital Twin Hospitals and the Simulation Equivalency Principal

Modeling hospitals as systems will enable us to apply system engineering and render all processes and activities transparent to inquiry, digitally manifested, and ready for AI processing to produce better outcomes through simulation.

## *Digital Twin Humans*

The application of machine learning to vast digital data sets worldwide can provide valuable insights into better diagnoses, drug discovery, and individualized health management. Artificial intelligence (AI) has progressed through three stages of development. In the first stage, which spanned from around 1958 until 2009, we only asked computers to compute things that humans fully understood and could break down into logical gates and if/then statements. We then fed this information into computers as finite state machines or hierarchical behavior trees to run programs. The next phase is machine learning, where humans require assistance in teaching machines how to drive a car, for example. In this phase, we feed a massive training data set to a group of well-designed machine-learning libraries that infer understanding. Today, machine learning systems can watch hundreds of hours of video and drive autonomous vehicles flawlessly. At Tanjo, we used machine learning for short-term projects to provide banks, higher education institutions, and Fortune 2000 companies with intelligence amplification and automation to transform their operations. We routinely witnessed returns on investment of up to 10 times from machine learning implementations, which were usually an annuity. We have validated ROI measurements of as much as 600 times and one embarrassing result of 1600 times. However, we do not use the last one as a case study because it feels too hyperbolic. Our major breakthrough came when we realized that the machine intelligence systems we were building looked at people as they looked at information objects. We conducted an early experiment with training data from a popular dating app, and our machine learning algorithms created interest graphs and sentiment maps of each person from their data exhaust, resembling a Myers Briggs profile. Although we briefly considered creating a machine-learning dating app in 2014, we decided to call it the "Empathy Engine" and built "Tanjo Animated Personas" using these machine-learning patterns of human behavior.

When the graphical Internet was first born in 1993, a group of deep thinkers like Doc Searls and David Weinberger published The Cluetrain Manifesto http://www.cluetrain.com/

This central idea that the broadcast TV era was over and would yield to a world where individuals are empowered and "markets are conversations" was electrifying.

Sadly, the balkanization of the Internet into apps like Facebook and other social media walled gardens has dramatically diminished the hope behind that manifesto.

With our discovery that machine learning could model humans to help us better understand people's values, we realized what we had was "an empathy engine." Considering how much data exhaust from people is out there, we realized we could harness that to gain empathy. The next step is to figure out a business model where individuals will pay for the ability to control that exhaust and make it available to companies and government on their terms to communicate their interests, desires, and values without having to be subjected to focus groups and surveys and an endless onslaught of commercial ads.

In Doc Searls' book "The Intention Economy" and his lectures by the same name, he describes a world where individuals put out RFPs mediated by bots (in our model, they would be adaptive machine learning systems) that would engage with commerce and government when the individual is in a buying mode or wished to convey suggestions, values or complaints about government. In this world, companies only make products people want instead of creating products and trying to convince us to buy them. In this world, the government does not have to guess what their constituents want from them; they can poll the synthetic bot representations of those interests and know without having to do antiquated, misleading, and inaccurate polls and focus groups.

Alan Kay is fond of saying, "Perspective is worth 80 IQ points." Many technologies we use to create Tanjo Animated Personas have existed for a while. We used some of them to build game characters to make them more convincing. We built extensive constructive simulations of entire populations using agent-based models at Lockheed Martin. It was strange that people in market research were still doing surveys and focus groups to build five to ten segmentation models of everyone in a country or on the planet. Our unique history in gaming and building simulations for the DOD helped us see what now appears obvious. We need an entire synthetic population of customers or constituents, fueled by what they do, not what they say, to test future ideas without bothering actual people with robocalls and mail-in or e-surveys.

Our first thought was to create examples from rich open data stores that would allow people to see the appeal and value of being able to see through someone else's eyes. We had our system read everything written by Victor Hugo and everything written about him to "resurrect" Victor Hugo. We did Leonardo Da Vinci, Albert Einstein, and Harriet Tubman. We have over 100 of these animated personas from history living on our servers, devouring the web daily and rendering their opinions from their perspectives. We encourage educators to build curricula around these to increase empathy with history and culture.

Beyond that, we are still seeking the magic business model to have everyone managing and curating the data models they have to engage with companies and the government. For example, what if there was a model of interests and values allowed to ask questions and determine how to build products with the features and prices required? Instead of getting robocalled and surveyed to death, a bot is on the net, representing those interests and making money while we sleep.

## ANI vs. AGI

At the beginning of this chapter, we asserted that Artificial Narrow Intelligence paired with an LLM of our choosing and combined with a simulation digital twin would be an outstanding design to engineer human error out of the healthcare system and dramatically improve health outcomes. For our purposes, we will describe ANI as a narrow intelligence much like what was used by Deep Blue to win at chess against Gary Kasparov in 1997 and by Google's Deep Mind to win at the game of Go against Lee Sodol twenty years later in 2017.

*Artificial Intelligence* is a broad term that includes various capabilities.

In a 2019 article, Andreas Kaplan and Michael Haenlein described AI as a system with the "ability to correctly interpret external data, to learn from such data, and to use those learnings to achieve specific goals and tasks through flexible adaptation." The computer scientist Ben Goertzel coined the term Artificial General Intelligence to describe a flexibly adaptive and self-improving computer system that can pass any Turing test, win the Loebner Prize, and continue to improve and advance to develop its goals beyond our understanding.

## Following AI leadership

Combining better-tuned knowledge graphs with increasingly powerful large language models, AI will become the new UI for health healthcare management. Soon, it could be considered malpractice not to consult the AI on a radiology scan or other health intervention and diagnostic tools.

## HealthCare is a Team Sport

As late as 1975, Healthcare involved an average of 2.5 caregivers per bed. Today, it can be as many as 14. However, we still have an unacceptably high error/waste rate that kills over 100,000 people a year in the US unnecessarily. How do we harness AI and simulation with blockchain to provide secure and clear communication for the complex choreography of care?

*"The 21st-century imperative is determining how to achieve the right balance between humans and automation to optimize outcomes."*

Superhuman Healthcare provided by teams of humans in cooperation with increasingly powerful artificial intelligence, sensors, and automation may be our only hope for staunching the sucking chest wound of escalating errors and costs in Healthcare. Thankfully, the models for this cooperation and comfortable fluency exist and are now available to be adopted by Healthcare.

## Prompt Engineering

We are passing through the age of humans using LLMs and KGs, prompting them towards our goals. Soon, we will give the AI a goal, and it will call upon humans to assist in its work.

### *Knowledge Graphs: The Memex Resurrected*

In 1962, Douglas Engelbart wrote about his conceptual framework for augmenting the collective intelligence of humanity.

*"The system we want to improve can thus be visualized as a trained human being with his artifacts, language, and methodology. The explicit new system we contemplate will involve artifact computers and computer-controlled information storage, information handling, and information display devices. The aspects of the conceptual framework discussed here primarily relate to the human being's ability to use such equipment in an integrated system significantly."*

**Figure 5**

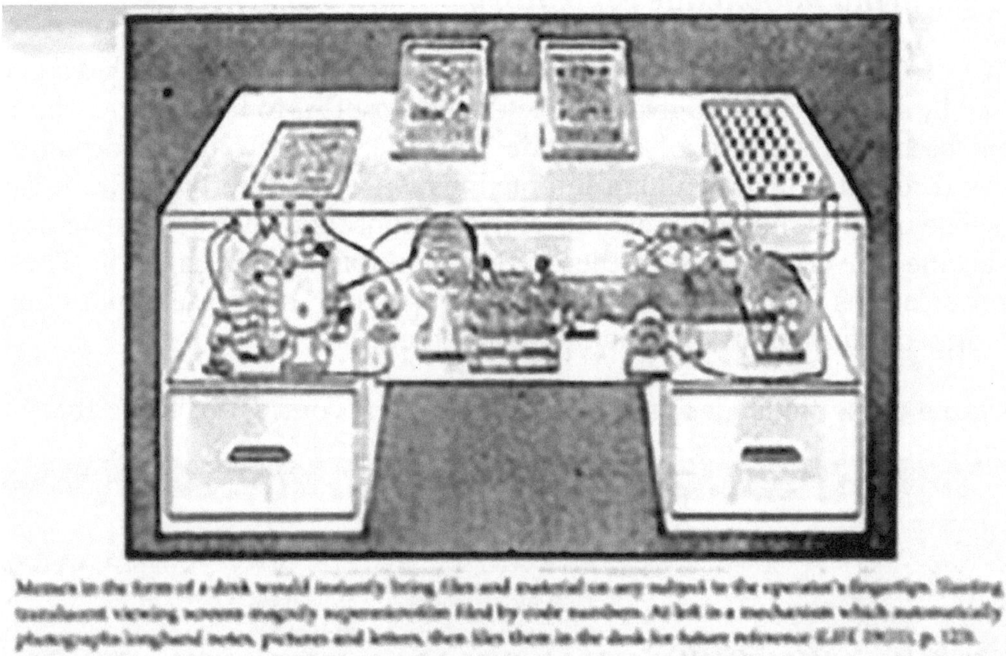

Memex is a portmanteau of Memory and Index.

## *Building a Covid Memex for Truth.*

Shortly after the COVID-19 epidemic began, we turned to applying the machine learning systems we had at our disposal to sort through the confusing barrage of information circulating the virus.

The cornerstone of the scalable system behind the Covid Brain was the creation of a machine-learning-derived capability of discernment, trained using a collection of example documents and structured data. Natural language processing (NLP) numerical methods, such as non-negative matrix factorization (NMF) and term frequency-inverse document frequency (tf-idf), helped to achieve discernment. We continuously evolved the platform by adding new cutting-edge models and approaches. At the time, ChatGPT, in its current form, did not yet exist. Instead, we employed a Bi-directional Encoders Representation with Transformers (BERT) system to allow researchers to interface directly and have a natural conversation with the Brain.

These maps include context and feature vectors, meaning the map is ***more accurate and superior to a human-manufactured*** taxonomy. The Enterprise Brain is ***continuously updated and improved with new content***, automatically integrating and categorizing this content to become an ***enduring knowledge repository.***

The ML Covid Brain fundamentally understands how content is related and used by specific roles. It gives people the power of AI to help curate, share, and become a steward of automatic, ongoing research and information served to individuals. Human interactions with the Enterprise Brain can include natural human-machine conversations and synthetic machine-machine conversations to further information for the learning loop. These conversations allow the COVID brain to get smarter and present more fully informed information without human intervention.

**Figure 6** A notional design for a Memex system, courtesy of Tanjo Inc.

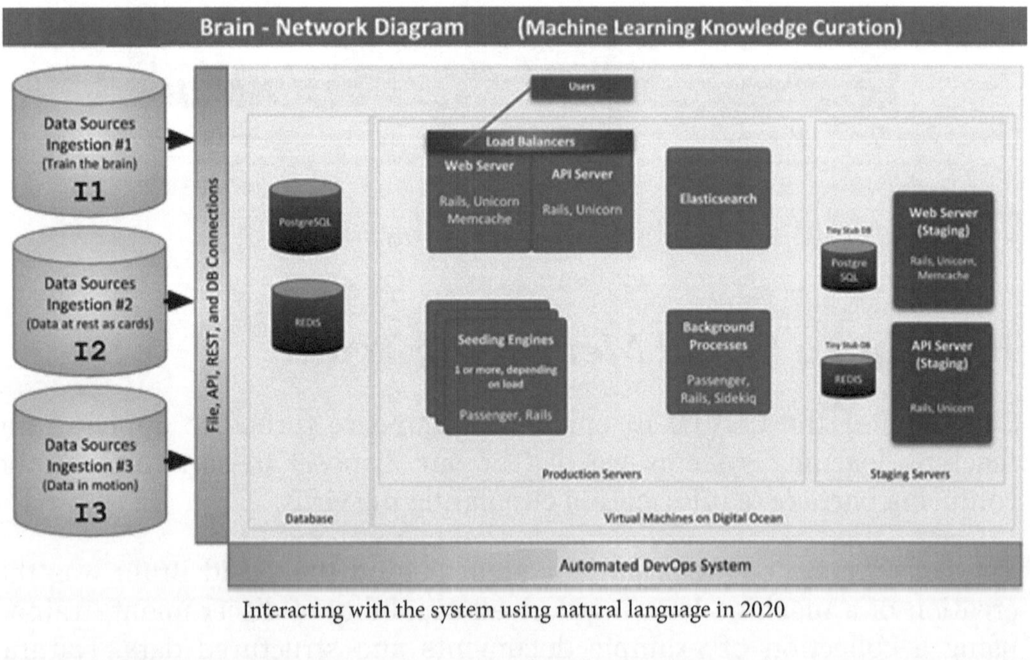


Interacting with the system using natural language in 2020

AI Personas create dynamic, simulated, machine learning-generated models of human behavior. AI Personas are powerful tools for creating deep customer understanding by simulating synthetic behaviors and interests. For example, an AI Persona SME scours the Internet for COVID-19-related topics or augments representative population behavior based on forcing function (such as imposed quarantine).

Depending on the available data feeds and desired outcomes, we leverage supervised and unsupervised methodologies for AI Persona training. We develop models based on demographics, interests, personality, sentiment, and behavior choice data. The greater the data, the more developed and accurate our personas are.

Dependingonthenatureofthedesiredpersonacharacteristics,wecanleverage Monte Carlo Tree Search, Hierarchical Finite State Machine (HFSM), utility systems with Markov models, n-grams, and influence maps. For content generation, we utilize Long Short-Term Memory (LSTM), Recurrent Neural Networks (RNN), Generative Adversarial Networks (GAN), and K-means clustering. Depending on the requirements, we integrate hill-climbing, gradient descent, and genetic algorithms for optimization tasks. Depending on the requirements, we utilize adversarial search and planning algorithms such as minimax and alpha-beta pruning and classification techniques such as perceptions, neural networks, and support vector machines. Finally, we deploy state-of-the-art AI architectural approaches, such as hybrid systems, subsumption architectures, and other ways to layer complex AI systems.

The steps in managing an AI/ML implementation:

1. *Process & Application Discovery* – Full assessment, rationalization, and documentation of the software, processes, data, and standards for each application, platform, or system

2. *Data Acquisition* – The DataOps Lifecycle allows an understanding of data interdependencies, system access requirements, and management across the entire data fabric.

3. *Design and Disposition* – Develop and determine the interface architectures for to-be deployment while assessing data, software, and systems transformation patterns.

4. *AI Training* - Leverage advanced computer vision, native DLLs and VDI intercept techniques, legacy code bases, SOPs, and historical data when available for training each model.

5. *Integration* - Transition to on-site systems, perform load testing, and interface communication optimization.

6. *Deployment* - Deploy into the production environment and final testing.

7. *Performance Monitoring* – Assess outcomes (user experience, SLAs, scalability) to continuously improve the product throughout the sustainment lifecycle.

**Figure 7**, The Tanjo Covid Memex mapping information in real-time in 2020

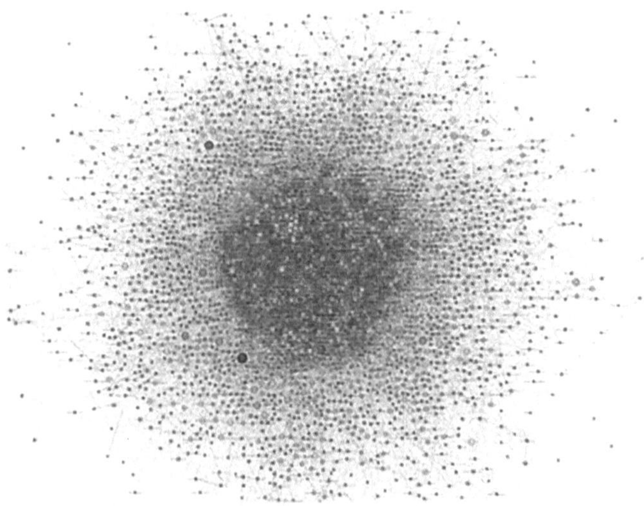

**Figure 8,** Curated content from the Covid Memex. 2020 Courtesy of Tanjo Inc.

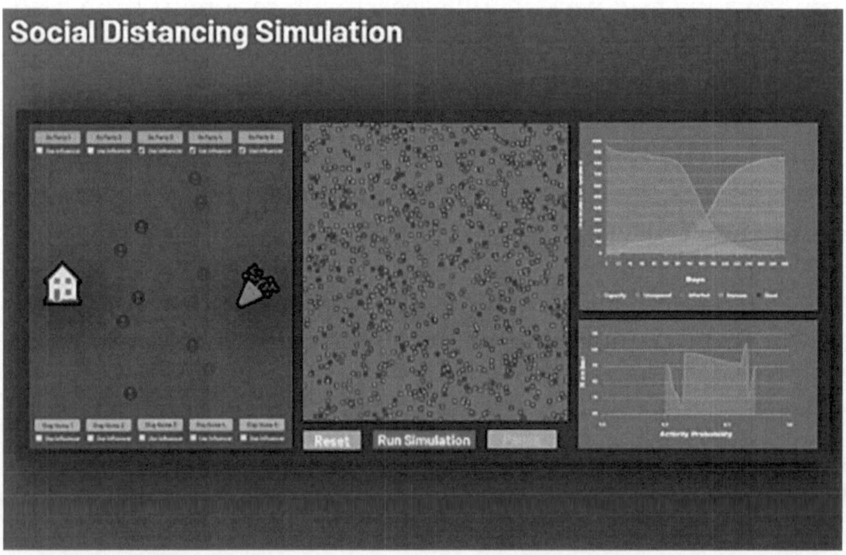

# Considerations Before Attempting to Implement AI.

We must perform an AI readiness check or assessment before implementing anything.

First and foremost, it is essential to understand that machine learning is unlike other enterprise software. It is opaque in how it makes its determinations; there is no machine learning debugger, and it is subject to hallucination and model collapse. Implementing machine learning systems on company data in a controlled training setting is prudent, with the system housed behind a firewall, whether on-premise or in a controlled cloud environment. Understanding that current ML systems cannot transcend their databases is essential. Also, it is optional to create a single data lake. Data can be left in its various data pools, whether at rest or in motion and can be harvested by the system as needed in a process we call data fusion.

ChatGPT has just passed its one-year birthday. There are rumblings about Q*, a secret program underway at OpenAI, rumored to be the next giant leap toward what AI researcher Ben Goertzel calls Artificial General Intelligence, or AGI. If it becomes a genuinely adaptive and self-improving AI as Goertzel conceives it, he says it will be the last invention humanity will, or need, make. From then on, he expects these AGIs to run and operate all our companies.

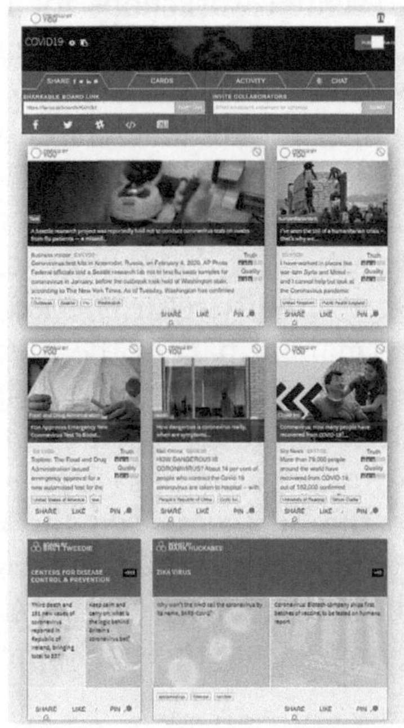

Lockheed Martin ICESTORM brochure 2010

# Conclusion

Every organization should now focus on creating ambient interfaces to the increasingly intelligent network of humans and machines cooperating. There is a revolution in sensors and computing capacity that, when ultimately paired with the active and passive sensors in the "Internet of Things," will render virtually everything and everything and every person on the planet transparent to discovery and inquiry and ultimately to some level of automation. We know that the Internet and search make an already intelligent person more intelligent. This new capacity we are developing will make anyone wielding it superhuman. Anyone not completely fluent with these new abilities will not only be outperformed by those who are but will be considered handicapped.

Every organization should deeply analyze every activity to determine the balance between human effort and attention (and intelligence) and machine intelligence, effort, and attention. Achieving the correct machine and human balance to optimize outcomes is a 21st-century imperative.

Even before the unexpected advent of ChatGPT 3, companies had awakened to the incredible return on investment from machine learning implementations. From 2014 to 2016, Richard Boyd and his team presented workshops for blue-chip companies like Cisco, Cigna, Lenovo, and JP Morgan. These companies had yet to recognize the value of simple process automation (RPA), much less fully implemented knowledge graphs connected to machine learning decision support systems and market research models of their customers. When ROI case studies that showed 10x to 100x returns began to emerge, companies had no choice but to start investigating their options. Moreover, when they understood that the returns were annuity returns, they realized that machine learning would become a permanent part of the business strategy and infrastructure. Those trends are only accelerating with large language models like ChatGPT, Llama, and Orca. AI becomes an even more potent ally when paired with LLMs and Knowledge Graphs (KGs), contextually trained on a narrow focus pertinent to the business. Add the ability to model and simulate from natural or synthetic data in an Internet of Things (IIOT) sensor-fed Digital Twin of the world, and new capabilities will emerge. We are only now beginning to glimpse what this could mean.

The applications that make the low-hanging fruit list for Healthcare include

1. Process automation. As noted above, someone should analyze every activity in an organization to determine the level of AI Robotic Process Automation (RPA).

2. Decision support: AI/ML combination systems trained on symptom/ diagnosis pairs can weigh the benefits and downsides of actions and recommend the optimal course of action. Until we have achieved AGI,

there should always be a human in the loop informed by these tailor-made systems.

3. Digital twins are of a hospital's systems, devices, processes, clinicians, and settings to estimate the current state, analyze past and future possible actions, and simulate future states.

4. Digital Twins of patients to model health journeys, improve awareness around the social determinants of health outcomes, and improve patient records and communication.

5. Create a Vannevar Bush-like machine learning memory (or Memex) of the company's organizational knowledge to address silver tsunami issues and analyze how information enters an organization, is processed, and makes decisions.

6. Prompt engineering for augmenting information work.

A few projects focus on modeling aspects of human physiology and anatomy, though there does not seem to be a single unified "human physiome" model. Here are a few notable efforts:

1. The Virtual Physiological Human (VPH) project: A large EU-funded effort to develop computational models and tools for modeling the human body. Focuses on organ systems, disease modeling, drug effects, etc. The VPH Institute coordinates associated research and data.

2. The Physiome Project: An NIH-funded project, with a database of computational models spanning molecular, cellular, tissue, and organ physiology. Models are quantitative, validated with experimental data. Access requires free registration.

3. The Digital Human Project: Aimed at modeling human physiology, biomechanics, neuroscience etc. Focuses on integrated whole body models. Some freely available datasets and tools, but much of the data seems proprietary or requires collaboration/involvement in the project itself.

4. Various individual university and industry labs are also working on computational physiology models of specific organ systems (e.g. Cardiac Physiome, Respiratory Physiome projects). Data availability and access vary.

In summary, extensive modeling efforts and associated datasets exist, but access and integration across different sub-fields pose challenges. Assessing efficacy involves validating models against empirical physiological data, but systematic evaluations across models still need to be improved.

## References

Centers for Medicaid and Medicare Services. (2009). 2007 National Health Care Expenditures Data. Office of the Actuary, National Health Statistics Group.

Fox, M. (2009, March 2). US Hospital Profits Fall to Zero: Thomson Reuters. Retrieved June 23, 2010, from Reuters.com: http://www.reuters.com/article/idUSTRE5216G320090302

Gawande, A. (2009). The Checklist Manifesto: How to Get Things Right. New York, New York: Metropolitan Books.

Greenberg Quinlan Rosner Research. (2009, November 10). American Public Supports Investment in Prevention as Part of Health Care Reform. Retrieved June 23, 2010, from Trust for America's Health: http://healthyamericans.org/assets/files/TFAH-RWJFPreventionSurveyII.pdf

HealthGrades. (2004). Patient Safety in American Hospitals. Golden, Colorado: HealthGrades.

High Confidence Software and Systems Coordinating Group, Networking and Information Technology Research and Development Program. (2009). High-Confidence Medical Devices: Cyber-Physical Systems for 21st Century Health Care. Arlington, Virginia: National Coordination Office, NITRD.

Kaushal, R., Bates, D. W., Franz, C. S., Soukop, J. R., & Rothschild, J. M. (2007). Costs of Adverse Events in Intensive Care Units. Critical Care Medicine, 35 (11), 2479-83.

Kohn, L. T., Corrigan, J. M., & Donaldson, M. S. (2000). To Err Is Human: Building a Safer Health System. Institute of Medicine, Committee on Quality of Health Care in America. Washington, DC: National Academy Press.

Murray, C. J., & Frenk, J. (2010). Ranking 37th-Measuring the Performance of the US. Health Care System. The New England Journal of Medicine, 362 (2), 98–99.

Nolte, E., & McKee, C. M. (2008). Measuring the Health of Nations: Updating an Earlier Analysis. Health Affairs, 27 (1), 58-71.

PricewaterhouseCoopers Health Research Institute. (2008). The Price of Excess: Identifying Waste in Healthcare Spending. New York, New York.

Quigley, P. (2009, September/October). F2761 and the Integrated Clinical Environment. ASTM International Standardization News.

Reid, T. R. (2009). The Healing of America: A Global Quest for Better, Cheaper, and Fairer Health Care. New York, New York: The Penguin Press.

Sabik, L. M., & Lie, R. K. (2008). Priority Setting in Health Care: Lessons from the Experience of Eight Countries. International Journal for Equity in Health, 7 (4).

Saunders, T., Croom, C., Austin, W., Brock, J., Crawford, N., Endsley, M., et al. (2005). System-of-Systems Engineering for Air Force Capability Development. Washington, DC: United States Air Force Scientific Advisory Board.

Singer, P. (2009, July 15). Why We Must Ration Health Care. The New York Times.

The Leapfrog Group. (2008, March 27). Fact Sheet: Never Events. Retrieved June 23, 2010, from Leapfrog Group.org:

Armed Forces Journal – Nearer the holodeck. http://armedforcesjournal.com/nearer-the-holodeck/

The Download: Richard Boyd, Co-Founder and CEO, Tanjo Inc. – GrepBeat. https://grepbeat.com/2020/06/30/the-download-richard-boyd-co-founder-and-ceo-tanjo-inc/

OLIVEIRA MATEUS, JOÂO VASCO DE. "Prototipagem Digital 3D No Contexto Do Ensino Do Design. Seu Papel Na Fase Conceptual De Desenvolvimento De Produtos Industriais." 2016, https://doi.org/10.4995/Thesis/10251/63671.

https://www.unite.ai/richard-boyd-the-co-founder-ceo-of-tanjo-inc-interview-series/

"More Than 27 Million Americans Will have Untreated Hearing Loss in 2010, Says Hearing Exec." The Hearing Review (Online), vol., no. , 2010, p. n/a.

https://www.nbcnews.com/health/health-care/could-medical-errors-be-no-3-cause-death-america-n568031

https://mymedicalscore.com/medical-error-statistics/

# Appendix 1

What are TAPs?

A Tanjo Animated Persona (TAP) is a synthetic model of human interests and values. These synthetic models, or personas, represent individuals but are not tied to any specific individual and, therefore, protect privacy (GDPR compliant). By modeling attitudes and interests and permitting simulations to test ideas, TAPs offer a compelling new approach to market research.

Our offering is grounded in two theses:

Thesis #1: Humans have distinct personalities with unique interests and value models.

Thesis #2: By leveraging data, we can simulate these interests and values and allow experimentation and testing with them that is as valid as – and in some cases superior to – results from focus groups and surveys. We perform this testing at scale for less effort than qualitative research with humans.

In the sections below, we will outline what goes into creating these animated personas and how to employ them in research.

## *Why use TAPs in research?*

Modeling and Simulation: TAPs are agent-based models that can be placed in simulated environments to see how their models react to different stimuli.

The models use three methods:

1) entirely derived from data,

2) Derived partly from data and partly hand constructed using a set of assumptions, and

3) entirely created by hand from assumptive models.

Each of these methods can be useful for testing ideas and predicting outcomes.

We typically seek to create a model of a persona from data such as purchase patterns or social media interaction, then augment that model with assumptions about other possibly unknown variations such as geography, political beliefs, and other psychographic models to generate subtypes of a persona (for example, Soccer Mom at 25 living in Jacksonville vs. Soccer Mom at 43 living in Seattle). The level of detail of the persona, and therefore the nuance of responses to stimuli, increases the diversity of data used to construct it. In the simulated TAP environment, brands can run tests to see how each subtype of persona might react to new product offerings or messages, allowing for unprecedented scale and granularity in market research.

## *The Problem with Focus Groups, Surveys, and ePanels*

When Netflix sought to improve its recommendation system, it issued a $1 million grand challenge. It had people worldwide compete to improve its recommendations. The winning team improved on Netflix's algorithms by only 10%. Before the challenge, however, they had determined that asking people a set of survey questions yielded very different recommendation results from actual user activity, including ratings.

*In other words, there is a marked difference between what people say and what they do.*

The best indication of a person's real interests is what they do with their attention. Therefore, TAP models created from robust historical data can be superior in their predictions to models based on questionnaires. For example, past buying behavior predicts future buying behavior better than surveys reveal.

## *How we create a TAP*

**Step 1:** Gather as much data as possible on the target population: demographic, psychographic, sentiment (writing samples or surveys?), and choice model data from either a discreet choice model experiment on the target population or Federal and commercial health behavior purchase and watch data sources.

**Step 2:** The Interest Graph. The machine learning system and a human analyst generate a list of topics, areas of interest, specific interests, sentiments, and choice preferences. Those are correlated and clustered into pattern groups. The Interest Graph includes predictable concepts, such as civil rights, and unexpected concepts only the machine detects. The persona model comprises this map of interests, concepts, and sentiments.

An interest graph is what makes up the "brain" of the persona—visualized like the photo above, with hierarchies of interests and concepts that make up the larger whole.

**Step 3:** If we have sample writing or other social listening data from the target population, we can also build deep psychographic models into the personas, and they will demonstrate preferences for specific language in written (and later spoken) conversations.

Beyond just what a persona is interested in, psychographic models can determine what sentiment they prefer in a given text (visualized above).

**Step 4:** A configured and server-activated persona model interprets online content, articles, and videos for information objects that match their interests and preferences. They will read those items or "Watch" the videos (initially, they would read the closed captioning text of a video) or listen to podcasts and rank the content they encounter with an interest score, revealing to the researcher preferences for media forms, communication models, language and topics.

**Step 5:** The scanning and scoring in Step 4 repeated for the number of topics defined in Step 2.

**Step 6:** A word cloud is generated based on a scoring system of all the topics.

We now have a persona with a complete hierarchy of interest graphs. The Tanjo system scrapes thousands of sources daily to pull in the most popular and relevant content. Each content is held up and scored against the interest graphs of the personas and the persona's topic maps.

In this way, the personas "experience" new information and current events, and – if desired – their attitudes and interests can evolve. One of Tanjo's earliest personas, a simulation of Victor Hugo, was created in February of 2017. Based on the content read over the past year, we have observed that the Victor Hugo persona has diverged in its interest graph and preferences from the persona initially created. It is of philosophical interest that his exposure to media has influenced his goals. Typically, consumer marketing clients prefer that the personas not change so that we can lock the interest graph upon initial creation.

## *Research Applications*

Here are three key benefits to healthcare researchers:

1. **Test messaging**
   Beyond just watching the personas to see how their interest graph changes as they react to current events, Tanjo's toolset allows them to present new writing to the personas and have them respond with their interest scores. The personas will react in real-time with interest scores from their perspectives. Testing before sending emails or launching ad campaigns – and tuning messaging for each segment – can dramatically improve response.

2. **Circumvent marketing and sales bias.**
   A very illustrative and valuable exercise is to build persona models based on a survey of the marketing personnel to reveal who they think their different customer segmentation models are; then create persona models from data or customer segmentation models and compare the two to see where there are differences between perception, and what the data reveals, informing a new approach to messaging.

3. **Model future behavior and choices and affect those future behaviors and choices**
   The basic framework of this architecture is a modular, hierarchical decision making approach, similar to the popular Behavior Tree (BT) architecture used in games, called the Component Reasoner. It can support many approaches to decision making, but we rely primarily on a utility-based approach called the Weight-Based Reasoner created at Lockheed Martin by Kevin Dill at Virtual World Labs.

## *Natural language discussions*

In 1997 members of the Tanjo team worked on a game with science fiction writer Douglas Adams (Hitchhiker's guide to the Galaxy) called Starship Titanic. In that game we attempted to create a means to converse with characters in natural language. Our entire Velocitext dictionary contained about 500 words, and yet some of the resulting interactions during gameplay caused Douglas to coin the term "Spookitalk" to describe the eerie feeling of interacting with a synthetic character. Today we have the means to go far beyond those early attempts and expect to permit TAP users to speak freely and convincingly with their customer persona models in the future.

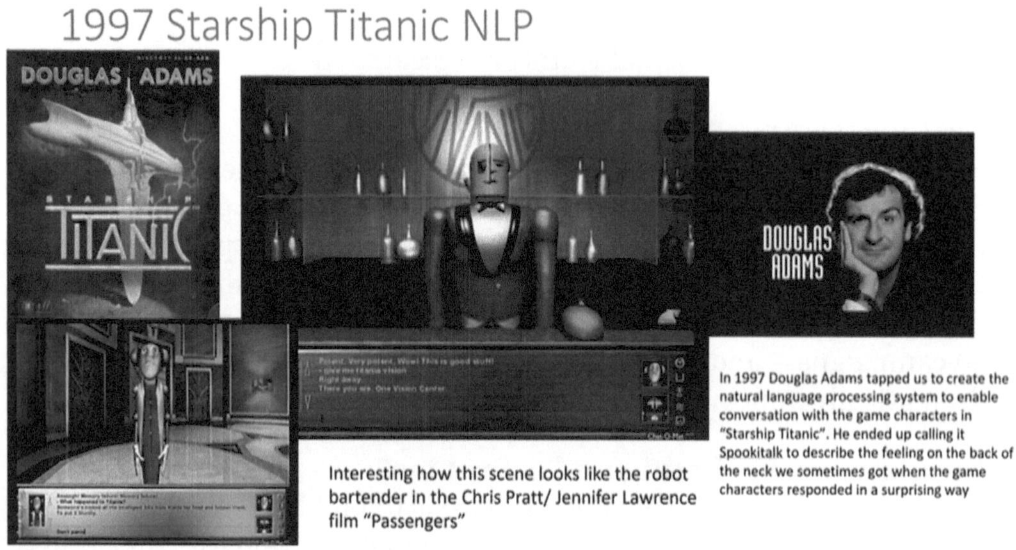
1997 Starship Titanic NLP
DOUGLAS ADAMS
STARSHIP
TITANIC
DOUGLAS
ADAMS
Interesting how this scene looks like the robot bartender in the Chris Pratt/ Jennifer Lawrence film "Passengers"
In 1997 Douglas Adams tapped us to create the natural language processing system to enable conversation with the game characters in "Starship Titanic". He ended up calling it Spookitalk to describe the feeling on the back of the neck we sometimes got when the game characters responded in a surprising way

# Chapter 12:

## ABC's as Accelerators for Societal Impact

*ROI, Rapid Response, Case Examples*

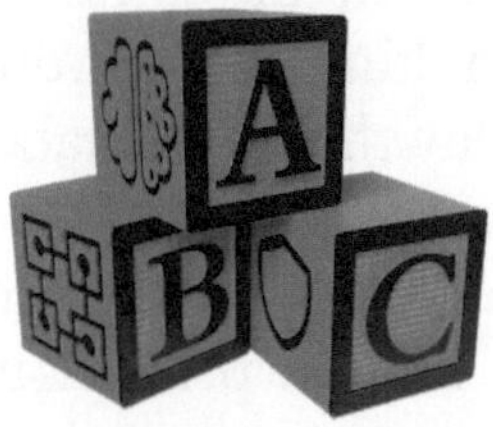


**Eric Kant**
*Founder*

*Kant Consulting Group*

### *Editor's Note*

Eric Kant has been on the front lines of healthcare as a first responder ever since 9-11. His understanding and embrace of technologies for disaster, crisis, and mass casualty events has lead to the creation of real time operational systems, like trusted ops, that leverages, predictive analytics, verification of mission, critical records, using blockchain and other technologies on a secure infrastructure with good cyber hygiene. This chapter provides an overview of some of those systems and their practical applications in real world use, as well as next generation *ABC* solutions for emergency response and front line health workers.

Artificial intelligence, blockchain, and cybersecurity are often considered revolutionary concepts in the healthcare industry. However, these technologies have been utilized to effect outcomes for many years. Embedded in different variations in different hardware. While primary healthcare has benefited from research and innovation, the pre-hospital and post-disaster environments have not seen the same level of progress despite their significant societal impacts.

Pre-hospital care is the vital link between the scene of a medical emergency and the hospital. There is no greater immediate social impact, as saving someone's life and returning them to be part of their community. Paramedics are often the first responders who face the critical life-or-death situations. Artificial intelligence has the potential to improve patient outcomes by providing instant support to paramedics in decision-making. AI-powered wearable devices can monitor patient vital signs and relay this information to medical personnel in real-time. Furthermore, AI can analyze the patient's medical history to provide tailored treatment plans and medication recommendations. AI-powered triage systems can also help in prioritizing emergency patients based on the severity of their condition.

However, the full potential of AI in pre-hospital care relies not only on the integration of blockchain and robust cybersecurity measures but also on the adoption of decision intelligence as a critical framework. This approach is essential in making the entire system valuable to decision-makers. Decision intelligence provides a holistic view, integrating multiple AI inputs to enhance decision-making processes. Blockchain technology will serve as a foundation, instilling trust in the data used by AI.

Using analytics to save lives in pre-hospital care is not a new concept. In the late 90's, technology was still not very common in the fire services. However, our department was young, progressive, and open to implementing new technologies. This is where we learned that well-implemented technology could save lives and change the outcome. The impact of saving a life extends far beyond the individual; it resonates within the entire community and has implications for the future.

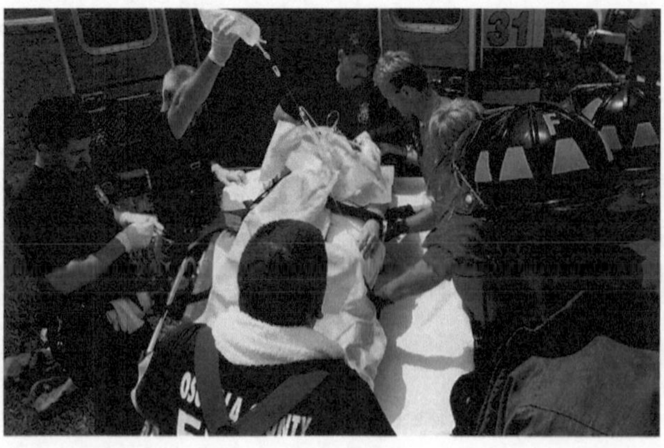

The shift towards incorporating technology in the fire services began in the mid 90's when our team deployed pen-based EMS data collection software. The EMS tablets provided every paramedic with a device that they could use to fill out their EMS report and upload it to HQ and the hospital via modem. This allowed us to mandate and ensure that required fields were being followed by the paramedics. Furthermore, we could analyze the data collected to understand how a medic or unit was performing in the field. Running a paramedic scorecard on the database was an invaluable element in understanding overall field performance.

Implementing this technology was not an easy feat as it was cutting-edge in terms of what was available at the time. The year was 1994, there was no Wi-Fi, no iPhones, and no real internet. Our tablets had the biggest memory card we could buy, which was only 5mb. Despite this, our department recognized the potential of technology and its role in improving operations.

Zoll Medical Company eventually acquired an EMS reporting company, which provided us with access to cutting-edge 12-lead capture and analysis software. As paramedics, we understood the critical importance of time when it comes to a heart attack. The ability to perform a 12-lead EKG in the field had the potential to significantly reduce "door-to-drug" times, a crucial factor in saving lives. "A heart attack is all about time," as paramedics we understood this intimately.

This technology revolutionized our ability to capture, diagnose, and transmit results to the emergency room (ER) right from the patient's side. It was groundbreaking because clot busters (TPA) and door-to-drug times for cardiac patients were just being utilized in the ER. Early scans meant earlier treatment, which is vital in saving lives during a heart attack. The efficiency of this new system was evident in how quickly the patient's condition was evaluated, significantly reducing the time to treatment. Dr. Kenneth Byerly, an emergency room doctor, emphasized, "We can save 15 to 20 minutes of evaluation time with this system. That's a long time when you're talking about a heart attack."

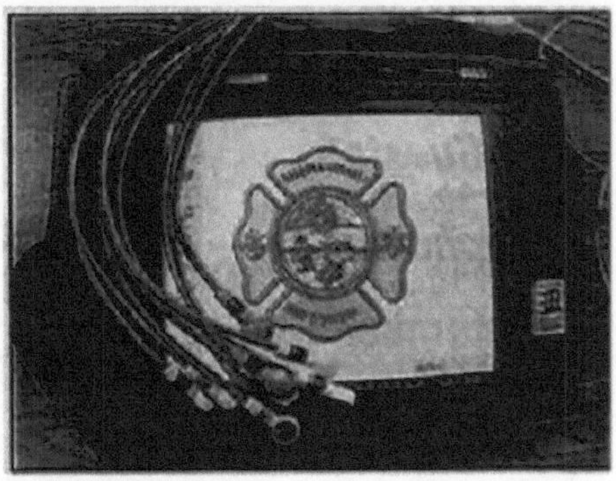

(Source: Savino, Lenny. "Laptop Ekg Speeds Up Race To Save Lives." Orlando Sentinel, 12 Sept. 1999https://www.linkedin.com/pulse/20140718130650-18612069-realizing-early-on-that-well-implemented-technology-could-save-lives/.)

In the rapidly evolving landscape of technology and public safety, the future entails a dynamic interplay of artificial intelligence (AI), blockchain, cybersecurity, and crucially, decision intelligence as a guiding framework. Decision intelligence is an emerging discipline that combines elements of decision science with advanced data analytics. It provides a structured approach to making informed decisions, considering the complex interplay of various data inputs, outcomes, and feedback loops. By integrating decision intelligence, the potential of AI in enhancing pre-hospital care and emergency response becomes even more profound. AI, with its advanced algorithms, can significantly augment human efforts in various aspects of emergency management. For instance, at the dispatch level, AI can analyze conversations, ask pertinent questions, and translate speech to ensure clarity and precision in emergency communication. In triaging, AI's ability to assess patients before they arrive at the hospital offers invaluable insights to medical teams, while its predictive models can identify patients at higher risk of adverse outcomes, a significant leap in prognostication.

The full realization of AI's benefits in pre-hospital care, however, hinges on the effective integration of blockchain and robust cybersecurity measures, along with decision intelligence. Blockchain technology, serving as a foundational element, instills trust in the data utilized by AI systems. This trust is vital when AI depends on extensive databases for critical life-saving decisions, ensuring that AI systems are based on reliable and authoritative sources—a necessity in healthcare where precision is crucial.

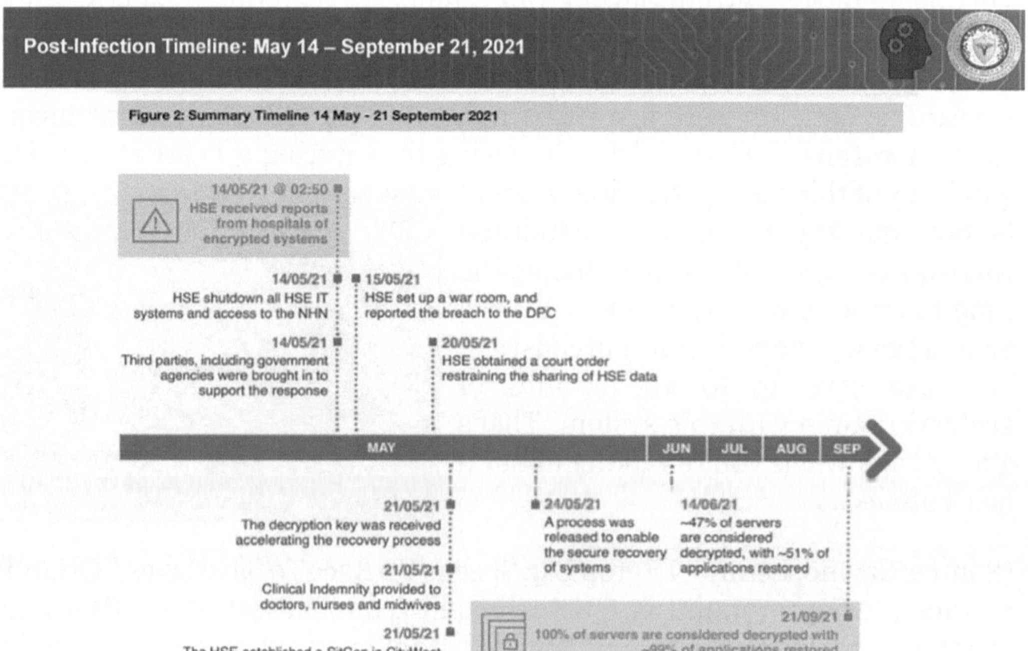


Source: HSE/PwC

In tandem with blockchain, cybersecurity safeguards the infrastructure and interactions essential to emergency services. As AI increasingly merges with the Internet of Things for continuous patient monitoring, the protection of sensitive medical data and systems from cyber threats is paramount. It is imperative to rigorously test these technologies, particularly in light of the latest advancements in large language models and generative AI. In a sector where human lives are at risk, ensuring the reliability, safety, and ethical application of AI and blockchain can become essential.

By incorporating decision intelligence, we enhance our ability to make well-informed, data-driven decisions, a vital aspect in the complex and high-stakes field of healthcare. This comprehensive approach, which integrates state-of-the-art technologies and decision intelligence, has the potential to redefine emergency management. It aims to make it more efficient, responsive, and, above all, aligned with the needs of individuals. One of the key findings stemming from the cyberattack was the absence of a single responsible owner for cybersecurity within the HSE at the time of the incident. Additionally, there was no dedicated committee providing guidance and oversight for cybersecurity measures or addressing the vulnerabilities and gaps in key controls.

During large-scale disaster, like pandemic, the structure and effectiveness of healthcare delivery systems become crucial. A notable example of this occurred in May 2021 when Ireland's Health Service Executive (HSE) fell victim to a ransomware cyberattack. As Ireland's publicly funded healthcare system under the Department of Health, the HSE encompasses both public hospitals under direct HSE authority and voluntary hospitals utilizing national IT infrastructure. This centralized healthcare system, which is characterized by a unified approach and coordination, differs from more fragmented systems like those in the United States. In the United States, healthcare is provided by multiple autonomous providers, leading to a diverse landscape of healthcare delivery and decision-making. The centralized system, on the other hand, ensures a more streamlined and cohesive approach to healthcare provision, with a focus on efficiency, accessibility, and coordination among various stakeholders.

The HSE cyberattack, the most significant attack on an Irish state agency and the largest known attack against a health service computer system, had far-reaching implications. It resulted in a nationwide shutdown of all IT systems, causing severe disruption in healthcare services. Access to diagnostics, medical records, and the exposure of private information of thousands were among the consequences. Unfortunately, the response to the attack was hindered by a failure to promptly identify and contain it, despite early warning signs. The HSE, heavily reliant on third-party assistance, faced significant challenges due to a lack of pre-planning for high-impact technology events.

The impact on the HSE's IT environment was substantial, with 80% of its systems being encrypted. The use of on-premise email systems, which were also affected, severely impacted communications. To contain the attack, the HSE took action by powering down systems and disconnecting from the internet. This incident highlighted the importance of proactive measures in safeguarding healthcare systems against cyber threats. In this situation AI capability that staff may have come to rely on to provide critical health care assessments would be completely ineffective and unusable.

The recent ransomware cyberattack on the HSE has shed light on a critical vulnerability in centralized healthcare systems. This incident underscores their susceptibility to cyber threats, which can cause disruptions to essential services and have prolonged social impacts on individuals and communities. One potential mitigation option could involve the integration of blockchain technology, which has the potential to play a significant role in mitigating ransomware attacks and enhancing the overall security of healthcare IT infrastructure. Ransomware attacks, such as the one encountered by the HSE, typically involve encrypting critical data and systems, rendering them inaccessible until a ransom is paid. The centralized nature of the HSE's IT infrastructure, with interconnected data and systems, made it an attractive target for such an attack, resulting in widespread disruption. (source: Health Service Executive. (2021). Lessons Learned from the HSE Ransomware Attack. [PDF file]. https://www.hhs.gov/sites/default/files/lessons-learned-hse-attack.pdf)

In this context, blockchain technology presents a promising solution. With its decentralized and distributed ledger system, blockchain can securely store data in a decentralized manner. This ensures that even if a part of the system is compromised, the entire network does not necessarily suffer the same consequences. The decentralized nature of blockchain inherently mitigates attacks that exploit centralized systems. This is especially true when it comes to securing IoT (Internet of Things) devices using blockchain technology. By leveraging the decentralized and tamper-resistant nature of blockchain, IoT devices can be protected against unauthorized access and ensure the integrity and privacy of the data they generate. The integration of blockchain technology brings an additional level of security and trust, serving as a supplementary layer in the comprehensive security process for IoT device security.

Additionally, blockchain can facilitate secure, transparent, and efficient access controls. In a healthcare setting, where access to sensitive patient information is critical, blockchain can provide a secure way to manage permissions and identities, ensuring that only authorized personnel can access specific data. This helps prevent unauthorized access, which often serves as an entry point for ransomware attacks.

As we embrace the transition to blockchain technology as a part of our layered cybersecurity approach, we encounter a heightened level of complexity that necessitates new capabilities. This complexity arises from the need to comprehend the intricate strategies employed by adversaries, analyze vast amounts of data, and meticulously scrutinize detailed logs from ledgers, among other critical multimodal information sources. It is precisely in this context that AI assumes a pivotal role, empowering security personnel with advanced tools and capabilities to effectively tackle these challenges and enhance overall cybersecurity resilience. By harnessing the power of AI, we can enhance our understanding, streamline operations, and fortify our defenses in the ever-evolving landscape of cybersecurity.

(Source: Endale Mitiku Adere, Blockchain in healthcare and IoT: A systematic literature review, https://www.sciencedirect.com/science/article/pii/S2590005622000108)

The intersection of artificial intelligence (AI), blockchain, cyber and healthcare presents new opportunities, as well as complex challenges. These technologies have significant potential to improve healthcare outcomes, but the complexity of their inter-dependencies introduces new risks. In such a complex environment, it's essential to have a decision-making process that not only transcends cybersecurity but also uses decision intelligence to understand the risk of cascading interdependences.

As technology advances, different industries must learn to adapt, particularly in the current age of AI, blockchain, and healthcare. One essential aspect of adapting to these technological advancements is through decision intelligence driven capabilities-based assessments, which allow organizations to evaluate their structure, work processes, and capabilities. These assessments provide valuable insights into how different components interact with each other to understand risks and make effective decisions.

Capabilities-based assessments are assessments that evaluate an organization's abilities to achieve a mission, considering the environment, resources, and other factors. Capabilities based assessments using a decision intelligence framework provide a repeatable methodology to understanding the complexities of AI, blockchain, healthcare and cyber. The integration of these technologies requires a high level of analysis and evaluation to identify potential risks and provide a reasonable way to manage them.

Decision intelligence, as a term of art, is a way of incorporating human judgment into decision-making processes that use data and algorithms. It helps to balance the differences and perspectives of decision-makers while considering the interrelationships between various factors. (source: 4Cast AI. (n.d.). Ireland Case Study. Retrieved from 4Cast AI Ireland.)

Artificial Intelligence, blockchain and cyber are powerful tools that have the potential to revolutionize healthcare, especially in the pre-hospital and post-disaster environments. While research in these areas is relatively limited, the potential benefits are significant enough to warrant a more in-depth study and investment. The applications of AI and blockchain in pre-hospital and post-disaster care are not just limited to improving patient outcomes. They can also reduce the workload of medical personnel, improve supply chain management, and enable better resource allocation. By investing in research and innovation in these areas, we can ensure that pre-hospital and post-disaster care will be more efficient, effective, and save more lives.

# Chapter 13:

# Case Study Collection

**Dexter Hadley, MD, PhD**
*Chief of Artificial Intelligence*

*University of Central Florida, College of Medicine*

**Jacob Braun**
*Doctoral Student*

*University of Central Florida*

## *Editor's Note*

This chapter provides several examples of early adoption of AI and blockchain in action, enabled by a secure cyber security infrastructure. Early examples of consortia and networks from the early days of the pandemic. Dr. Hadley's clinical research and health disparities evidence, along with the power of associations, consortia, and and multi-institution networks from Kaleido and their partners. Point the way to next-generation ABC solutions.

# Introduction

AI in healthcare stands at the forefront of a technological revolution, seamlessly merging advanced computing with medical acumen to elevate patient care and operational efficiency. Its influence spans from predictive patient analytics to administrative streamlining, symbolizing a significant shift in healthcare delivery and management. In this evolving scenario, insurers have integrated AI algorithms into their frameworks, notably through the nH Predict AI algorithm by NaviHealth, a move that has sparked both interest and controversy.

The nH Predict algorithm, crafted by NaviHealth, serves as a sophisticated AI tool aimed at optimizing healthcare resource allocation for insured individuals. This AI-driven model scrutinizes patient data, identifying hospitalized Medicare Advantage members suitable for discharge to lower-acuity post-acute care settings. It evaluates clinical factors—diagnosis, comorbidities, vitals, procedures, and complications—to assess whether a patient requires continued hospitalization or can transition to rehabilitation, skilled nursing, or home health care with remote monitoring. This approach seeks to reduce unnecessary hospital stays without compromising patient recovery and outcomes.

When the nH Predict system identifies a patient as ready for discharge from acute care, insurers such as UnitedHealthcare assess these recommendations through their utilization management teams. If they agree with the discharge decision, a coordinated plan is activated to transfer the patient, ensuring efficient and smooth transition to ongoing care after hospitalization. This process focuses on both operational efficiency and the well-being of the patient.

However, the implementation of nH Predict has not been without controversy. Allegations suggest the algorithm may pressure premature discharges, leading to care denial, highlighting the need for unbiased audits, peer-reviews, patient-focused oversight, and transparency in AI integration within healthcare administration and clinical practice.

This case study navigates the delicate balance between AI-driven efficiency and the imperative of patient-centric care, delving into the complex roles and challenges AI presents in modern healthcare.

# United Healthcare Case

UnitedHealthcare (UHC), a major player in the U.S. health insurance sector, serves as a critical case study for examining the integration of AI in healthcare practices. In 2019, UHC's Medicare Advantage division initiated the use of the nH Predict[3].

After using the algorithm, multiple lawsuits were filed against UHC, with claimants alleging that the nH Predict algorithm encouraged premature termination of hospital services, disregarding the actual health status of patients. These accusations pointed to an unsettling trend: AI-driven decisions reportedly resulted in unwarranted denials of essential healthcare, appearing to favor financial savings over patient well-being, and prioritizing profit margins over the health needs of individuals. Audits of these decisions revealed that over half of the service denials influenced by AI were later overturned upon appeal, casting doubt on the algorithm's accuracy in predicting discharge risks.

# Humana Case Study

UHC isn't the only major insurer using the controversial nH Predict algorithm; Humana, a leading health insurance provider in America, faces a lawsuit[2] filed on December 12, 2023, alleging misuse of this AI model. The lawsuit accuses Humana of exploiting the nH Predict's high error rate, which led to a significant number of wrongful denials of necessary post-acute care. It claims that Humana's strategy hinged on the fact that only a small fraction of policyholders (about 0.2%)[1] challenge these denials, leaving most either paying out-of-pocket or forgoing care. This practice allegedly resulted in financial benefits for Humana at the expense of elderly patients' health, contradicting doctors' care recommendations.

The lawsuit goes on to paint a disturbing picture of AI misuse in healthcare. According to the legal documents, the nH Predict AI Model, used to assess post-acute care needs, often contradicts the medical opinions of treating physicians. Similar to the allegations against UHC, the nH Predict Algorithim has reportedly led to widespread and premature discharge of elderly patients from care facilities, causing significant health risks and financial burdens. The suit further alleges that Humana's rigid adherence to AI predictions, rather than individual patient needs, is a strategic move. By limiting employee discretion and penalizing deviations from AI recommendations, Humana ensures policy compliance. This strategy, plaintiffs argue, has not only increased the denial rates of necessary care but also shifted financial responsibilities to patients and American taxpayers, as Humana cites Medicare eligibility as a reason for coverage denials. The case raises critical questions about the ethical use of AI in healthcare and the responsibility of insurers towards their policyholders.

## Ethical Considerations

Incorporating broader ethical principles into healthcare AI is crucial to ensure that patient-centered care is maintained, especially considering cases like UHC and Humana. This involves carefully balancing the efficiency offered by technological advances with the core human elements of empathy and understanding inherent in healthcare.

One of the primary ethical tenets in healthcare is the principle of non-maleficence and beneficence, which dictates the duty to do no harm and to act in the best interest of the patient. While AI in healthcare, like in the UHC and Humana cases, offers significant efficiencies in data processing and predictive analytics, it must not compromise patient safety or the quality of care. The alleged premature discharge of patients influenced by AI in the cases raises concerns about prioritizing cost savings over patient welfare, potentially violating these ethical principles.

Another essential topic is transparency and accountability in AI systems. It's crucial for both professionals and patients to understand AI's decision-making process, ensuring trust and effectiveness. For example, if an AI tool contradicts a doctor's recommendation, the algorithm's reasoning should be traceable for necessary review or override. This ties into informed consent, as patients must understand their treatment, including AI's role. If healthcare providers cannot comprehend an AI suggestion, it challenges their ability to inform patients adequately.

Furthermore, addressing racial bias in AI development is also a significant ethical consideration. The principle of justice demands equitable treatment for all patients. However, AI can perpetuate racial biases, as evidenced in cases where medical algorithms exhibit differential performance among racial groups. This issue often stems from using training datasets that lack diversity, leading to inaccuracies in diagnosing or treating patients of color. Ethical AI deployment necessitates diversifying training data and rigorously evaluating systems across varied populations to ensure equitable healthcare outcomes.

Finally, continual monitoring and improvement are essential for ethical AI use in healthcare. AI systems require regular assessments to check for accuracy, biases, and their impact in real-world settings. The frequent upholding of appeals against AI-driven decisions in the UHC exemplifies the need for ongoing evaluation and refinement of these systems.

# Impact on Patients

The integration of AI-driven decisions in patient care, particularly in the context of UHC and Humana, has yielded a complex landscape with both promising advancements and significant concerns. AI's capacity to streamline healthcare processes is undeniable, yet its application in insurance claims and treatment approvals, as evidenced in the cases, has raised critical issues.

In UHC's case, a significant number of AI-driven claim denials later reversed on appeal suggest flaws in AI decision-making. This is not merely a statistical concern but has real-world consequences for patients. AI's erroneous denials can delay essential treatments, worsening health outcomes and causing emotional and physical strain for patients and families. Similarly, in Humana's case, the knowledge that few patients would appeal denials indicates a deliberate exploitation of this tendency, further jeopardizing patient welfare.

Moreover, these overturned decisions underscore the necessity of a human-centric approach in healthcare AI. AI's proficiency in managing large datasets and predicting trends cannot yet fully grasp the nuances of individual patient cases, which often require human judgment and empathy. Both the UHC case and the Humana case vividly illustrates this point, showing that while AI can aid in healthcare management, it must be balanced with a focus on patient welfare.

The promise of personalized, preventative care through AI is another area of potential impact. Industry leaders envision a future where AI, through analyzing population health data, could identify risk factors for various conditions well before symptoms appear. At an individual level, AI could analyze biomarkers and genetics to tailor prevention plans, leading to significantly improved outcomes compared to generalized approaches. However, this potential must be weighed against real-world examples, such as the UHC case, where AI's shortcomings were evident.

Furthermore, amidst AI's drive for optimized efficiency, maintaining the emotional and psychological aspects of care is crucial. AI tools like chatbots and virtual nurses cannot replace the empathy and understanding provided by human healthcare professionals. Both cases serve as a reminder that while AI can augment healthcare delivery, it should not replace the human connection that is central to patient care.

## Conclusion

In conclusion, looking at AI's role in healthcare, particularly in UHC and Humana cases, reveals a complex landscape. AI's potential in healthcare is indeed vast, with benefits that include enhanced diagnostic accuracy, more personalized treatment options, and increased operational efficiency. This potential springs from AI's capacity to rapidly process large datasets, recognize complex patterns, and make recommendations based on sophisticated algorithms.

On the other hand, real improvements need to be made in its integration include the necessity of algorithmic transparency for trust-building, the urgency of addressing AI biases for equitable healthcare, and the critical need for accountability in AI-driven decisions. Central to these insights is the imperative to prioritize patient welfare in AI integration, ensuring that technological advancements enhance, not hinder, patient care. At the end of the day, health care is about helping people and those people must be prioritized over profit margins. AI has transformative potential; it is up to the healthcare community to decide what that transformation will look like.

## Works cited:

1. Karen Pollitz, et al., Claims Denials and Appeals in ACA Marketplace Plans in 2021, KFF (Feb. 9, 2023) https://www.kff.org/private-insurance/issue-brief/claims-denials-and-appeals-in-aca-marketplace-plans/ (last visited Nov. 13, 2023).

2. For Each Person, HUMANA, https://www.humana.com/about/impact/

individual (last visited Nov. 30, 2023). Plaintiffs v. Humana Inc. (2023). United States District Court for the Western District of Kentucky. No. 3:23-cv-736. Retrieved from https://storage.courtlistener.com/recap/gov.uscourts.kywd.128636/gov.uscourts.kywd.128636.736.0.pdf

3. Estate of Doe et al. v. UnitedHealth Group Inc., et al. (2023). United States District Court for the District of Minnesota. Civil Case No. 0:23-cv-01637. Retrieved from https://cdn.arstechnica.net/wp-content/uploads/2023/11/class-action-v-unitedhealth-and-navihealth-1.pdf

# Blockchain-Backed Mortality Monitor Provides a Model for the Future of Automated Insurance Claims

## Provided by Kaleido and Partners

## *Executive Summary*

The life insurance sector faces a challenge due to the absence of a centralized system for managing death benefits and claims. To address this, Riskstream developed the Mortality Monitor proof of concept, which provides a unified digital platform for information needed in claim processing. This system enables insurers to promptly identify potential deaths, easing the process for beneficiaries and expediting claim settlements. Further, the integration of smart contracts allows for immediate payment of claims, setting a precedent for more efficient and automated claims processing in the industry.

In the United States, the prevalence of life insurance policies are highly prevalent, with almost 260 million policies for about 330 million people as of 2022. The intricacies of these policies, combined with Americans' participation in retirement plans and annuities, pose a significant challenge to insurance providers, especially when processing claims after an individual's death. An individual is often listed in various databases across multiple organizations, further complicating the process of notifying carriers about the death of a policyholder and getting beneficiaries paid in a timely manner.

This not only creates an enormous administrative burden for providers but also complicates an already difficult time for the bereaved. If a person passes away, their relatives may need to reach out to each individual provider, provide a paper copy of proof of death, then wait weeks, months, and sometimes years for claims to be processed.

The Institutes RiskStream Collaborative™ recognized that this was a difficult situation made worse by current, cumbersome processes. As a consortium of major insurance providers, they saw an opportunity to bring a new, automated solution to the market to connect competing providers and provide a single source of truth for claim processing.

## Transforming the Inefficient Death Notification Process

Currently, death notification is a cumbersome and inconsistent process. It involves multiple carriers and requires the collection of various documents, leading to data duplication, potential errors, and difficulties for beneficiaries. This inefficiency not only delays the delivery of death benefits but also adds to the emotional burden on beneficiaries during their time of grief. A family member, Riskstream recognized, may need to call multiple providers, prove the death of a relative, and do so on multiple occasions.

What if all these Life & Annuity (L&A) providers had a single source of death records that they could trust, query against, and use to process claims efficiently?

The Institutes RiskStream Collaborative™ chose Kaleido to build the Mortality Monitor. Founded by the team who led IBM's early blockchain development, Kaleido's team realized early on that distributed ledger technology could change the way we live and work—if only it was easier for businesses to adopt.

Founded in 2015, Kaleido's mission is to speed up enterprise and government adoption of blockchain, digital assets, and asset tokenization through a radical simplification of the technology. They built a platform that allows companies to instantly spin up blockchain networks, plug-in familiar development tools, and reach production on solutions in weeks, instead of years. This inherently scalable platform is at the heart of many leading global consortia, and provided the foundation for the Mortality Monitor.

Mortality Monitor used Kaleido to quickly stand up a multi-party system on a blockchain and begin onboarding members who shared the goal of streamlining the death claims process. The vision was for a secure, permissioned database wherein a single death certificate could be uploaded to the system and automatically be available to all providers. Kaleido made this possible by leveraging the inherent strengths of blockchain—security, transparency, and efficiency—in the Mortality Monitor to serve as a centralized and reliable source of decedent information. Kaleido also made it easy for members to conduct business around the blockchain with tools like secure messaging and document exchange.

Like any consortium or collaborative business network, members of the consortium could be invited, onboarded, and given access to the available records. Events, like the upload of a new record, could trigger alerts to providers and prompt them to query their own records for any claims that may apply to that record. Essentially, when a person passed away the death would be noted and ping each member with a long-term vision of automating claims against those events. Real-time, secure, and transparent access to data about deceased individuals, along with digitized and automated claims processing, would dramatically reduce settlement times, lower operating costs, and enhance support for beneficiaries.

Administrative staff allocated to back-end claims paperwork could spend time supporting customers or building the business. According to one estimate, private insurers spend 17% of revenue on administrative costs, the bulk of which would be eliminated if back-office systems were digitized. RiskStream's own analysis suggested that the Mortality Monitor could save up to $603 million dollars by 2025 for consortium members by eliminating redundant administrative processes[3].

# Challenges and Considerations in Implementation

The implementation of Mortality Monitor involved analyzing overlapping policyholders and the time gap between claims paid dates across different companies and sectors. This analysis used SHA-256 hashed social security numbers and additional data for privacy.

Once data is securely shared among providers, it becomes clear how smart contracts could be used to enable business processes to operate based on the available death certificates and protected social security numbers.

For example, the business logic might tell the system to query for a social security number in our policy database each time one is uploaded and if one is found, trigger an alert to process the claim. Further automation could be added based on how much the data was trusted. With confidence in the system, payments could automatically be sent to beneficiaries based on these events.

A viability study conducted after the Mortality Monitor was launched revealed a surprising level of inter-carrier overlap, as much as 4% across providers[4]. They found that the initial hypothesis that people have policies with multiple providers was correct. They also found that this overlap led to significant delays in payments for policyholders with multiple carriers. This highlighted the efficiency gains achievable through the Mortality Monitor wherein the full claims process could be automatically triggered by a blockchain-based application.

The successful implementation of Mortality Monitor opens doors to broader applications of blockchain in the insurance industry. Similar sharing of data and automating of processes off that shared data could improve underwriting and risk management, optimize claims management across home, auto, and health insurance, simplify finance and accounting processes, and transform regulatory and compliance practices.

A blockchain-backed application that operates as a single source of truth could interact with fraud protection tools. The Reinsurance Group of America cites risk profiling, underwriting, claims processing, and fraud monitoring as places where AI-backed tools can enable stronger controls for providers[5].

# The Promising Future of Blockchain in Insurance

Blockchain technology promises to revolutionize various processes in the insurance industry, making them more efficient, transparent, and secure. By addressing key challenges, it stands to significantly enhance the overall experience for policyholders and beneficiaries alike.

Blockchain offers a decentralized, tamper-proof ledger that ensures the integrity and traceability of transactions and policyholder data. Applications backed by this technology bring trust to previously competitive environments, creating opportunities to build more collaborative and efficient systems.

They also have the potential to transform the back office, automating previously cumbersome, labor-intensive processes. Smart contracts take simple if-then logic and turn them into enormous cost savings when applied to industries that remain paper-based and redundant.

The possibilities of blockchain technology in transforming the insurance claims process become even more exciting when matched with emerging AI tools. As processes are put on the blockchain and trusted data is collected and shared, AI can operate on top of that data to provide additional risk management and fraud protection. It can identify patterns or anomalies in the claims process and alert providers to potential fraud. Generative AI tools can also learn from incoming data and react to events, reaching out to customers to communicate the status of a claim and answering questions about the claims process. AI's predictive capabilities can further improve the customer experience and generate revenue for providers with personalized policy recommendations, dynamic pricing, and entirely new products designed to match market needs.

Blockchain, operating as a secure, shared database, along with automated business logic and AI tools, has the potential to change the way insurance companies operate. When the technology is matched with business and customer needs, it becomes a wonderful tool for business and a way to solve real problems for real people on a truly global scale.

# References


1. Rudden, Jennifer. (2023, December). Total number of life insurance policies in force in the United States from 2008 to 2022. Statista. https://www.statista.com/statistics/207651/us-life-insurance-policies-in-force/

1. Archer, D. (2011, September 20). Medicare is more efficient than private insurance. Health Affairs Blog. Retrieved from https://www.healthaffairs.org/do/10.1377/hblog20110920.013390/full/

1. The Institutes RiskStream Collaborative. (2021). Mortality Monitor Viability Study [PDF file]. https://f.hubspotusercontent30.net/hubfs/2449883/2021_MortalityMonitor.pdf

1. The Institutes RiskStream Collaborative. (2021). Mortality Monitor Viability Study [PDF file]. https://f.hubspotusercontent30.net/

hubfs/2449883/2021_MortalityMonitor.pdf

1. Parkin, Neil. (2023, August). Artificial Intelligence and Insurance Fraud: Four dangers and four opportunities. Reinsurance Group of America. https://www.rgare.com/knowledge-center/article/artificial-intelligence-and-insurance-fraud-four-dangers-and-four-opportunities

# How Synaptic Health Alliance is Transforming the Healthcare Back Office

## *Executive Summary*

The Synaptic Health Alliance built a consortium that allows leading insurance companies to update and share provider data, reducing the costs of maintaining this data, eliminating redundancies across the industry, and bringing a level of collaboration to a competitive space. The consortium incentives participation with tokens, opening new revenue streams for participating companies and providing a model for further collaborations in the insurance space.

The healthcare industry is undergoing a transformative phase thanks largely to blockchain technology. One of the industry leaders helping to define this transformation is the Synaptic Health Alliance, a consortium formed by some of the biggest names in healthcare.

Founded in 2017, the Synaptic Health Alliance leverages blockchain to address some of the most pressing challenges in healthcare. With a vision for a connected, interoperable healthcare space that dramatically cuts costs and improves patient outcomes, the Alliance began its blockchain journey by tackling a redundant, back-office process that costs insurance carriers an estimated $2.1 billion each year[1].

# The Provider Data Exchange Platform

Members of the Synaptic Health Alliance include large industry players like Humana, MultiPlan, UnitedHealth Group, Cognizant, Corvel, and ProCredEx. All of these insurance carriers are required by law to maintain a directory of providers. This directory includes the names of doctors, current addresses, and contact information for each office.

The challenge with maintaining this information lies in the fact that it is always changing. Providers move, phone numbers change, key contacts leave, yet each provider must keep all these records up to date on an annual basis.

Traditionally, maintaining these provider databases required a back-office staff to call provider locations and verify contact information or an outside agency. Contract agencies charged high fees to keep data up-to-date for insurance carriers. All of this was redundant across the industry, as each carrier had to maintain a record for each provider. There was no way to share this data.

That was the issue that the Synaptic Health Alliance solved with the Provider Data Exchange platform. The platform was created to ensure that provider demographic information in health plan directories is up-to-date and accurate and shareable between Alliance members. By leveraging blockchain technology, the platform enables carriers to join the consortium as members, share validated data, and subscribe to updates for other carrier's data. This collaborative approach means that only one carrier would need to create a provider record that could be shared with the group.

The exchange was developed using Kaleido's blockchain platform, enabling the creation of a collaboratively managed, synchronized distributed ledger. This allows members to seamlessly share updates to provider data. With the consortium in place, the Alliance used tokens, representative of real dollars, to incentive participation in the Exchange.

Essentially, when an insurance carrier uploaded a record that was validated they were paid by the other members for completing the record for them. This payment was a fraction of the administrative costs to update the record, which encouraged carriers to subscribe to data updates, and it turned the creation of provider record into a revenue opportunity instead of a revenue cost for the carrier that provided accurate data.

Another layer of trust was added to the system when a carrier could be docked tokens for uploading an inaccurate record, meaning the token economy inside the exchange worked to reward and deter, ensuring the best possible data at all times. The accuracy of the data is holding, as today members report 94% agreement with data as they make provider outreach calls.

The consortium proved the business value of reaching across competitive lines to share the work of provider outreach, as each participating carrier was able to eliminate administrative redundancy. Michael Kim, SVP/CIO of Multiplan, said the "shared ledger improves productivity and reduces costs for every Alliance member. Thus far, Alliance participation has resulted in a 500% ROI annually for Multiplan." This type of ROI, or return on collaboration, to put it another way, is the real value of blockchain-backed multi-party systems.

By "sharing the work," Alliance members save on data maintenance, and in some instances turn what was once a cost into a revenue opportunity. But the Exchange also saves time on the provider side, as offices aren't responding to a regular flow of calls from carrier call centers or data agencies to verify contact information.

Benefits extend to patients as well, as the 94% accuracy of data means customers can obtain current, accurate information that they need to access care through their health plan websites.

## Building on an Enterprise-Grade Platform with Room to Scale

The Synaptic Health Alliance selected Kaleido as its blockchain infrastructure provider because the platform has a history of operating in regulated industries, from healthcare and government, to finance and supply chains. The Alliance trusted Kaleido to build a secure, hardened blockchain that was simple for members to use and allowed administrators to easily scale.

"We've proven the business value of a shared ledger for keeping care provider data up to date and accurate," said Kyle Culver, Co-Founder of Synaptic Health Alliance and Director of Emerging Technology at Humana. "The next step in our strategic roadmap is to continue onboarding additional members. Kaleido makes that onboarding process quick and simple for us without sacrificing the quality of our network."

The Exchange leverages Hyperledger FireFly, an open-source blockchain middleware that Kaleido developed for the Hyperledger Foundation, data streams, messaging, and advanced security measures to guarantee network performance and safety. The platform also conforms to ISO27K and SOC 2 Type 2 standards, providing critical high availability and disaster recovery options for large-scale enterprise applications. This hardened platform is important for the Exchange, as it ensures always-on access to data that is required by law, but it also offers a secure and scalable platform for innovation.

Using the platform to prove the business value of collaboration, allows members to think about what data could be shared next and how that data could further enable business and empower customers.

## Sharing Accurate Data Securely is Only the First Step

"The efficacy of blockchain grows by network effect and the value of it is really relational to who's participating," said Kyle Culver. "The more people we have contributing data, the better it is going to be. The faster we get the data, the more elements we can get, the more accurate that information is going to be."

Culver is clear that the value of a blockchain application is as valuable as the amount of data it shares and the number of collaborators who participate. This is true for provider data and potentially even more impactful as we find ways to introduce other forms of data, like health outcomes, health and lifestyle studies, and treatment plans.

Imagine extending the model provided by the Provider Data Exchange to include disease information or health outcomes. Now layers on top of this health data geographic and lifestyle factors.

What patterns might we see emerge if this information was reviewed using AI tools, adept at finding anomalies and patterns in outcomes. Could AI tools review a universe of patient data, securely anonymized to protect privacy, and return to a doctor a treatment plan? And if these treatment plans were intelligently informed and therefore more trusted by patients, potentially complete with an expected statistical outcome if followed, how might these treatment plans improve health and what savings would that bring to the healthcare space?

The Provider Data Exchange, an early, successful application of blockchain in the insurance space, is exciting proof of the value of collaboration. But it is also only a preview of the potential when blockchain, secure sharing of sensitive data, and AI come together to help improve the lives of people.

The transformative capacity of blockchain in altering how organizations exchange data is immense, with pioneers such as the Synaptic Health Alliance at the forefront of this evolution.

# References:

1. CAQH. (2011, December). Issue Brief: Administrative Provider Data. [Analysis completed by Booz & Co., now Strategy&, Inc.]. https://www.caqh.org/sites/default/files/solutions/events/2011/q4/IssueBrief.pdf

## *Jacob Braun*

Jacob Braun is a first-year PhD student in computer science at the University of Central Florida. His research interests include deep learning, AI ethics, and medical AI. Jacob is committed to pushing the boundaries of knowledge at the intersection of AI and Medicine. His dedication extends to navigating the ethical challenges that accompany these advancements in technology.

# Chapter 14:

## The Future of Artificial Intelligence in Healthcare: Is Your Healthcare Organization AI Ready?

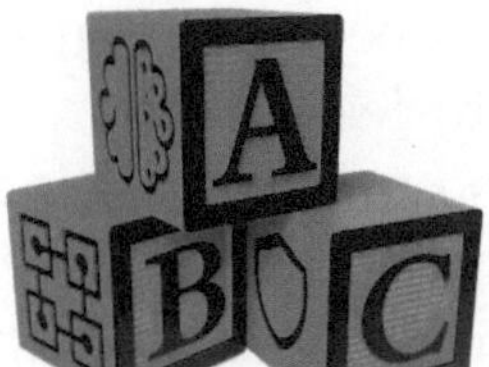


**Anthony Chang, MD, MBA, MPH, MS**
*Chief Intelligence and Innovation Officer,*

*Children's Health of Orange County*

*Chair, American Board of AI in Medicine (ABAIM) and Alliance of Centers of AI in Medicine (ACAIM)*

*Associate Scholar*

*Stanford AIMI*

### *Editor's Note*

Dr. Chang kicks us off by starting what will be an ongoing conversation with his excellent, intelligent, health, and social science professor, Dr. Chang. Symposium presentation highlighting best practices in the use of AI in healthcare research and precision medicine.

We're all, we're all learners and on this journey of AI and healthcare.

So, what I thought I'd do is share with you some of my personal reflections on AI in healthcare and I think it would be nice to start off with the Model T and you're wondering why. It's because I think, you know, when Henry Ford thought of the Model T and solved the assembly line and all of those issues, he forgot one thing, which is just the public did not know how to drive. So, technology adoption, and this has a lot of relevance to

Artificial Intelligence, is that we need to learn the technology, even though the technology is here with us.

Also, this is the first picture of the automatic elevator without a human operator, and it was only because of a strike of human operators that the people were willing to take the risk of riding an operatorless elevator. So, sometimes an external threat or inconvenience can also push technology. Of course, we know that desktop computing took several decades before it really became popular because of the need for programming, which many, many people did not know how to do. So, think about these technology adoptions and it's usually over a period of decades, but we don't have that luxury with Artificial Intelligence with the speed that it's moving.

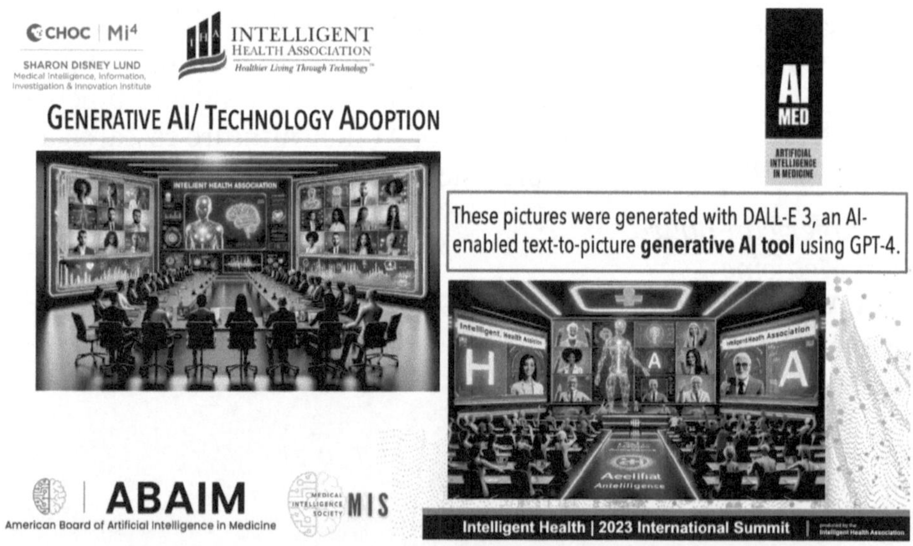


So, I used DALL-E 3, which is an AI-enabled text-to-picture Generative AI tool and wanted the picture of an Intelligent Health Association, note the misspelling there from the Artificial Intelligence, and with our audience and I said, well how about with more enthusiasm? And here is what it would look like with more enthusiasm. So, Generative AI is defined as new content or data from having been trained with big databases. And I kind of call it AI 2.0 because it's a truly exciting period.

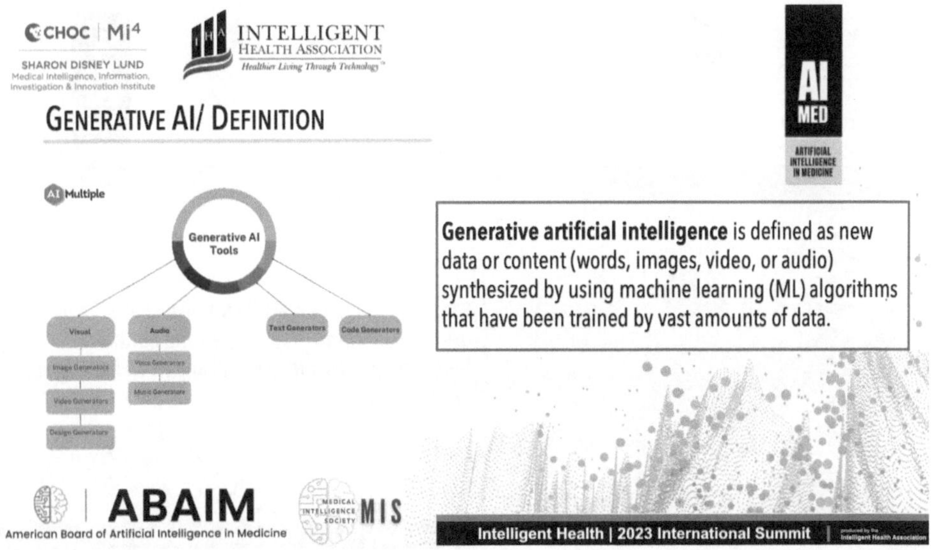


Now I got asked one time at a meeting giving a talk like this, what is ChatGPT? Is it information or knowledge? I think I would call it super information because it's not quite knowledge. It might be parroting knowledge but it's I don't think it's quite capable yet of giving us true knowledge, although it's debatable. But I think that at the end of the day it's nice to have super knowledge and then faster perhaps journey to wisdom that we all could use more of. So, I think ChatGPT and its Large Language Models, and Gemini, just got released by Google, is really providing us with super information but probably not wisdom yet.

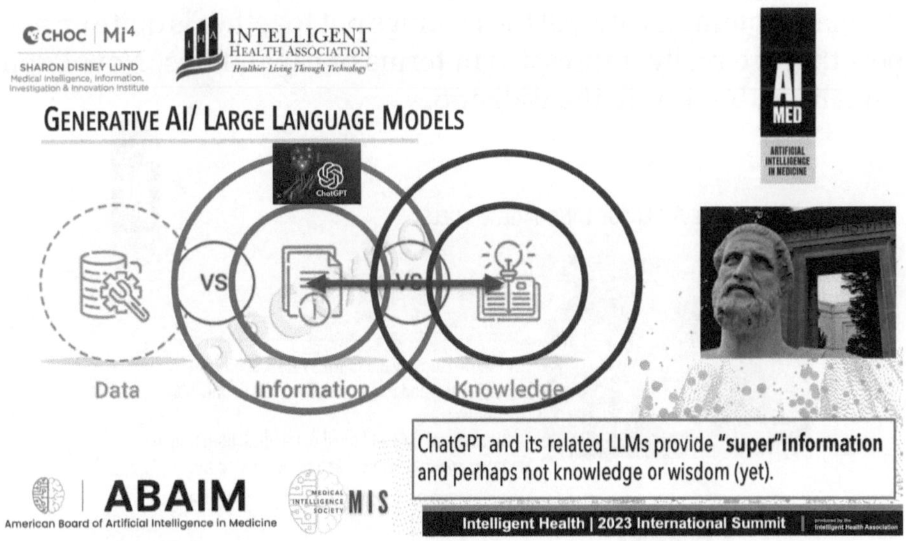

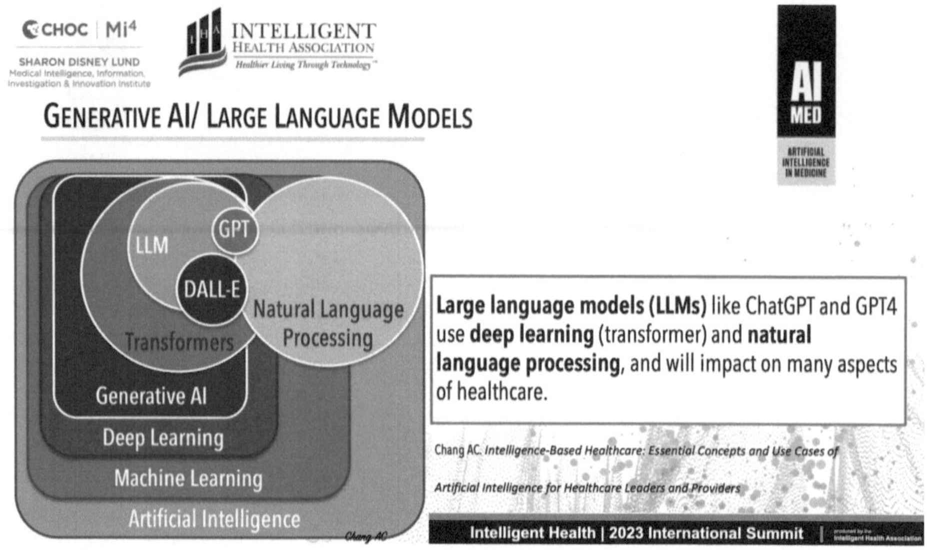


I was trying to describe to my colleagues where I think Transformers and Generative AI sit. So, there's really no good diagrams. I have to synthesize them myself. Of course, using AI was was not adequate, but if you think of Generative AI as a subset of Deep Learning, which is AI mimicking the brain, it's basically powered by Transformers. That's the AI architecture. That's really, excuse the pun here, but transforming the AI world right now. And so, it's aptly named and then combined with Natural Language Processing is where GPT and Large Language Models sit. So, in other words, GPT then is a sort of a convergence of Large Language Models and Transformers and Deep Learning, and Natural Language Processing, which is how computers and humans communicate. All these things put together is quite an assembly of tools that are really impressive in terms of capabilities. Now I don't just talk to talk on, but I walk the walk too.

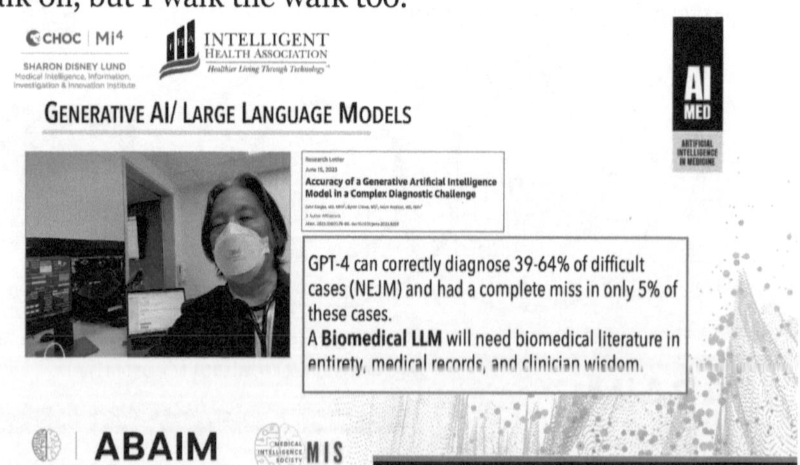


Here is myself in clinic using a Large Language Model as part of my clinic. I'm going off to see about 25 families today in clinic and I'll have a laptop open next to me using a Large Language Model that has AI capabilities to just help me have perhaps an even better feel for how patients are doing and what else I can do to improve my care. So, I think part of AI is being humble enough to know that we have more to learn from other resources that are available. And the biomedical Large Language Models are getting better all the time.

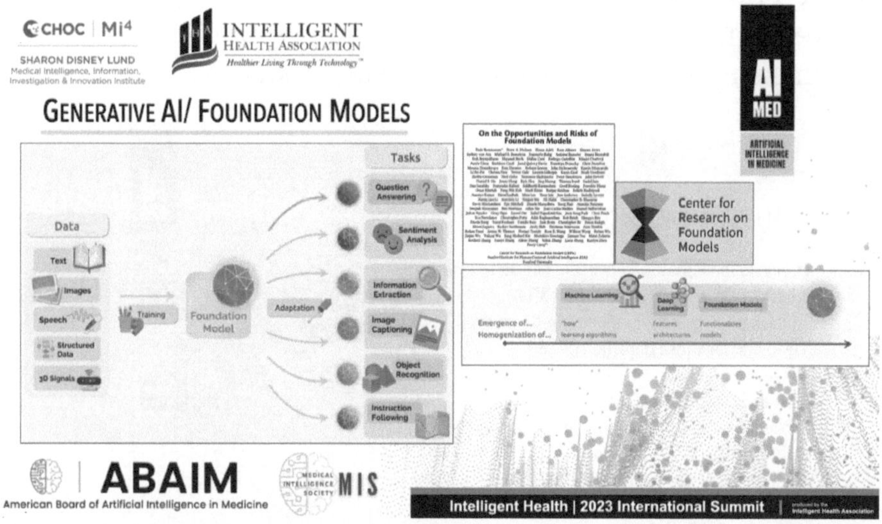


Now the one of the exciting developments is the concept of a foundation model which is taking multiple data types and be able to use AI to give us multiple outputs. So, Generative AI, if you think about it, is the beginning of the era of foundation models that I think will really be very exciting for healthcare. And here is an example of such a foundation model. So essentially, we'll be taking all sorts of data from the EHR, from images, etc. and also wearable technology in the future and it will be helping us to take care of complex patients and acute chronic care management. So very, very exciting future for clinicians.

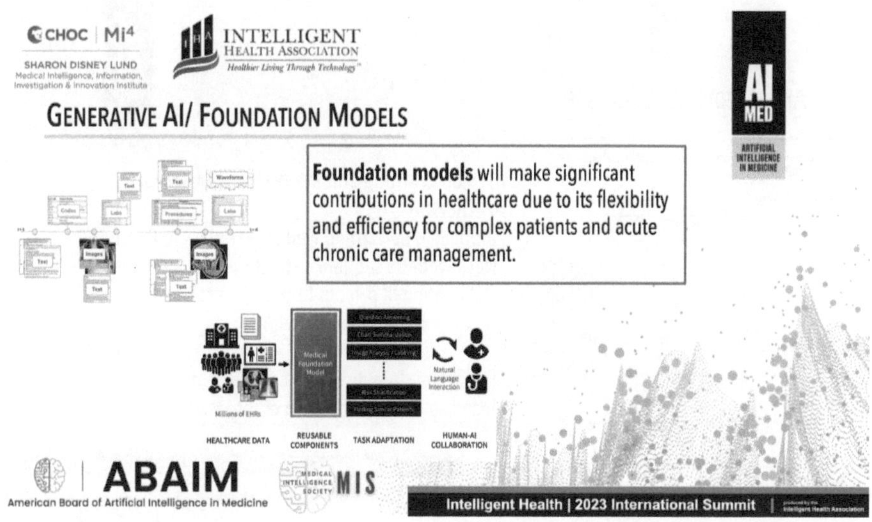

So, if I look back on the past decade, so let's look retrospectively and and look at the successes and the disappointments and then as we look into the future. So, I would say the past decade some of the major accomplishments of AI has been won on the area of medical imaging. Quite mature, can supersede the performance of even human experts in certain areas and importantly now has quite a few FDA cleared and approved algorithms now and we're moving into the era of using AI for moving images even and there's even payment available now for certain tools.

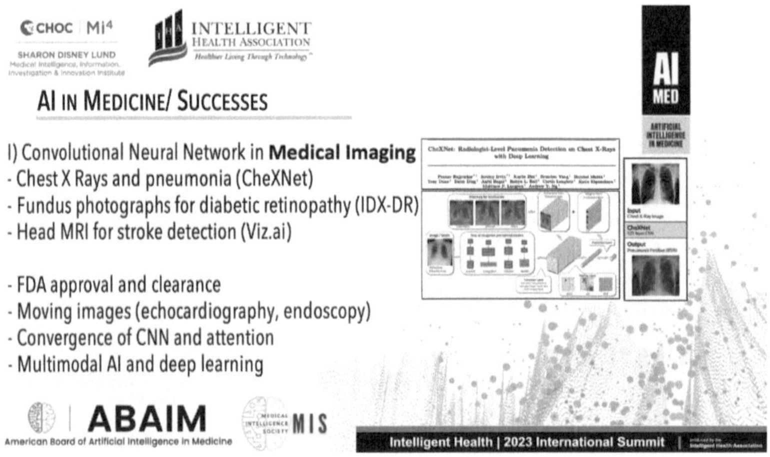


Number two, in terms of success, I think is the impressive use of Deep Learning for 3D Protein Structure Prediction based on genomic sequencing. It used to take months and years. Now it takes hours, maybe not hours quite yet, but they're capable of hours and certainly days and weeks now. So, this is going to be huge for drug discovery and vaccine design. And it has been already because the vaccine is going to be very useful for the virus that's mutating so quickly at so many different sites.

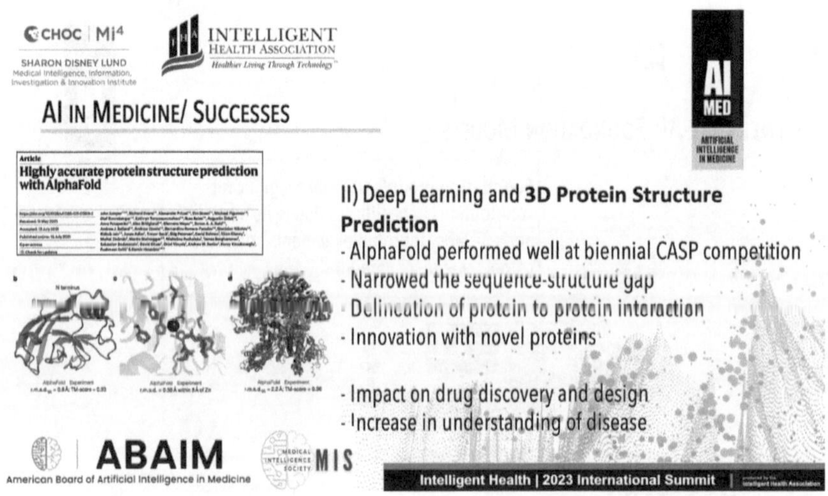

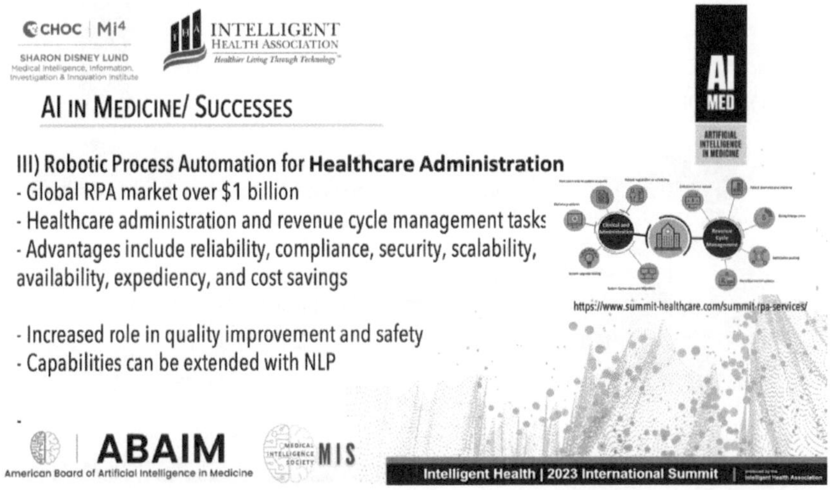
CHOC | Mi4
SHARON DISNEY LUND
Medical Intelligence, Information, Investigation & Innovation Institute
INTELLIGENT HEALTH ASSOCIATION
AI MED
AI IN MEDICINE/ SUCCESSES
III) Robotic Process Automation for Healthcare Administration
- Global RPA market over $1 billion
- Healthcare administration and revenue cycle management tasks
- Advantages include reliability, compliance, security, scalability, availability, expediency, and cost savings
- Increased role in quality improvement and safety
- Capabilities can be extended with NLP
https://www.summit-healthcare.com/summit-rpa-services/
ABAIM
American Board of Artificial Intelligence in Medicine
MIS
Intelligent Health | 2023 International Summit

Robotic Process Automation for Healthcare Administration has been quietly reducing cost of healthcare. So that's a very important development as well.

While there are plenty of disappointments, perhaps more than successes, on the right is a picture of DALL-E 3 responding to my query to have a picture of myocarditis. So somehow the cells are shaped and heart-shaped and which is obviously very comical. So, I think that wasn't a success.

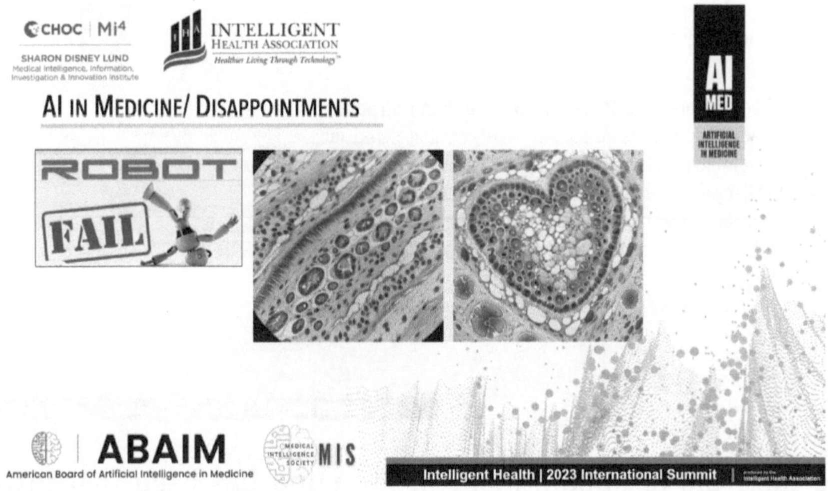


So, three main disappointments and there are many more. One is AI having continual issues with access to healthcare data that's accurate and complete. So that's sort of the foundation of AI. So, if you don't have good data and data sources then that's a a problem.

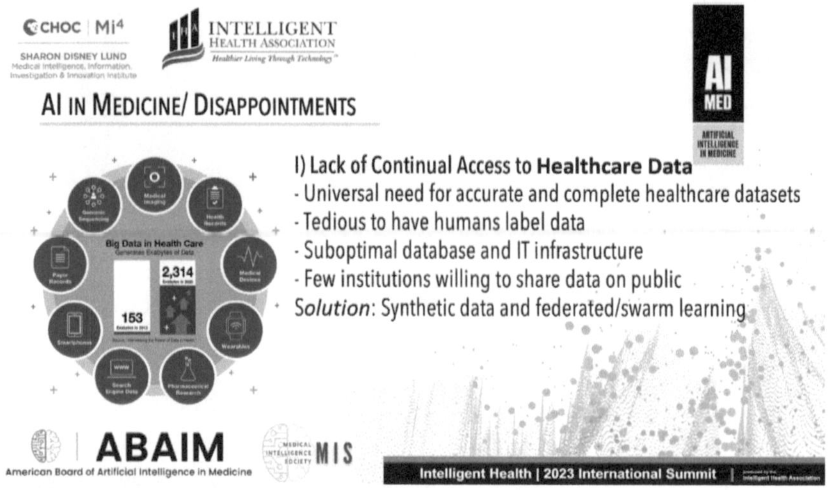


The second, I think, main disappointment has been the relatively poor performance of AI-enabled decision support and one of the very, very well publicized one is out of Michigan that when they looked at some of the EHR sepsis models. So, I think we, we really need to get the clinicians even more involved from the inception of the project and guided.

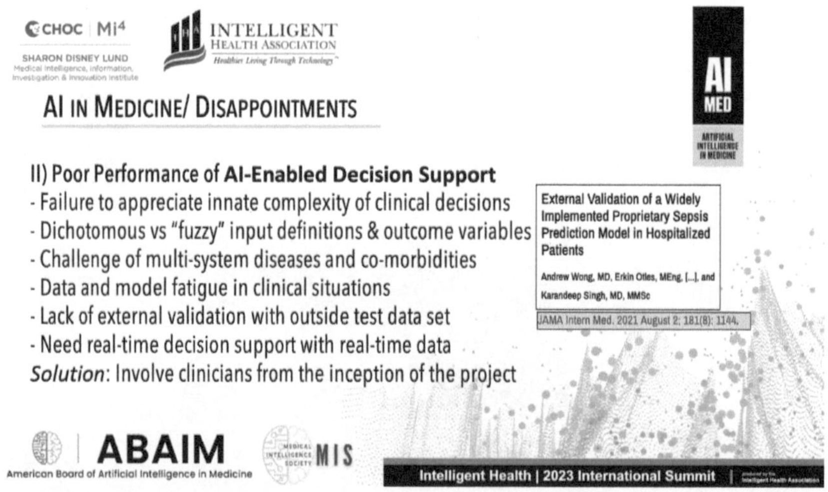


And the third big disappointment in my mind has been that insufficient clinical relevance and impact over the AI projects. So, we have this publication to practice schism that is very, very sizable and that needs to be narrowed. Again, I think getting clinicians involved from the very beginning is going to be part of the solution.

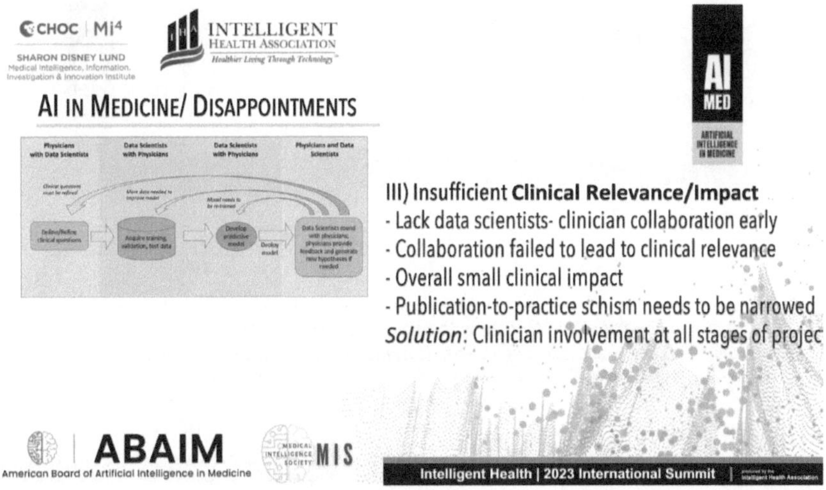


So, let's look to the future of AI with a positive mindset and I think one is with a wearable technology, genomic information as well as a recent emphasis on social determinants of health. We're going to move from evidence-based medicine to intelligence-based healthcare, which I think is truly very exciting for the future.

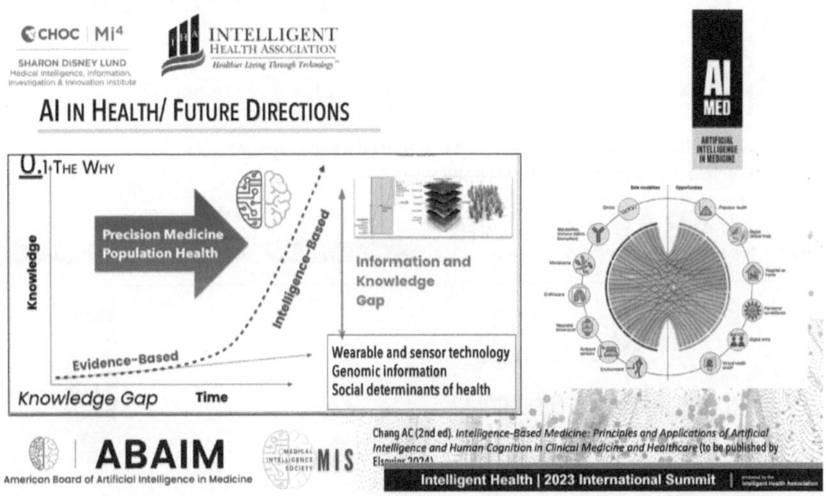


In addition, I think we're going to get around some of the data sharing headaches that hospitals and health systems have by more and more decentralized Federated learning, which means that you actually share the insights from the data without actually sharing the raw data, which I think is a technological go around for working together. I think another direction in the future that's relevant for AI is that we'll have more and more real-world data and experience that AI will be relying on rather than traditional randomized controlled trials. Also, future research and AI will be focused on the use of synthetic data, which I think will add to the capabilities AI in the future.

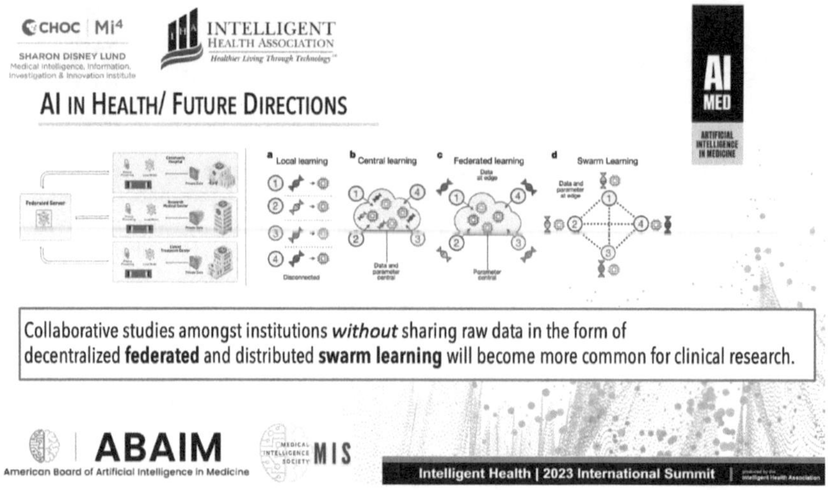
CHOC Mi4
SHARON DISNEY LUND
Medical Intelligence, Information, Investigation & Innovation Institute
INTELLIGENT HEALTH ASSOCIATION
Healthier Living Through Technology
AI IN HEALTH/ FUTURE DIRECTIONS
AI MED
ARTIFICIAL INTELLIGENCE IN MEDICINE
a Local learning
b Central learning
c Federated learning
d Swarm Learning
Disconnected
Data and parameter central
Parameter central
Data at edge
Data and parameter at edge
Collaborative studies amongst institutions without sharing raw data in the form of decentralized federated and distributed swarm learning will become more common for clinical research.
ABAIM
American Board of Artificial Intelligence in Medicine
MEDICAL INTELLIGENCE SOCIETY MIS
Intelligent Health | 2023 International Summit

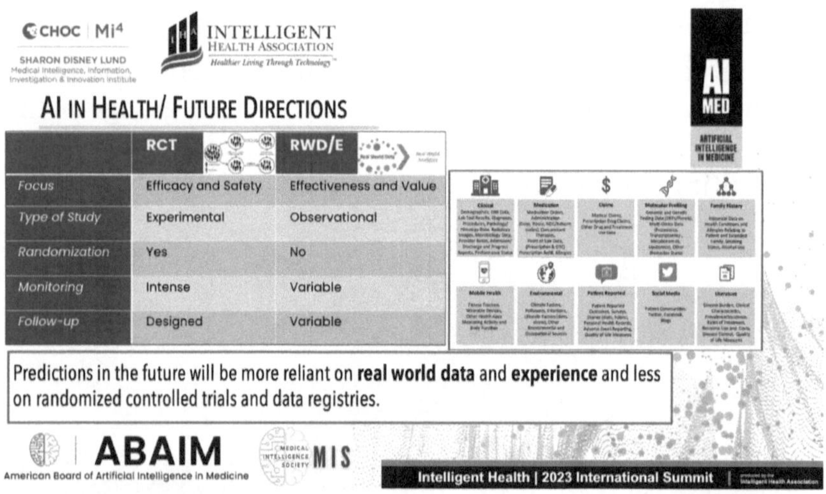
CHOC Mi4
SHARON DISNEY LUND
Medical Intelligence, Information, Investigation & Innovation Institute
INTELLIGENT HEALTH ASSOCIATION
Healthier Living Through Technology
AI IN HEALTH/ FUTURE DIRECTIONS
AI MED
ARTIFICIAL INTELLIGENCE IN MEDICINE
RCT
RWD/E
Focus
Efficacy and Safety
Effectiveness and Value
Type of Study
Experimental
Observational
Randomization
Yes
No
Monitoring
Intense
Variable
Follow-up
Designed
Variable
Predictions in the future will be more reliant on real world data and experience and less on randomized controlled trials and data registries.
ABAIM
American Board of Artificial Intelligence in Medicine
MEDICAL INTELLIGENCE SOCIETY MIS
Intelligent Health | 2023 International Summit

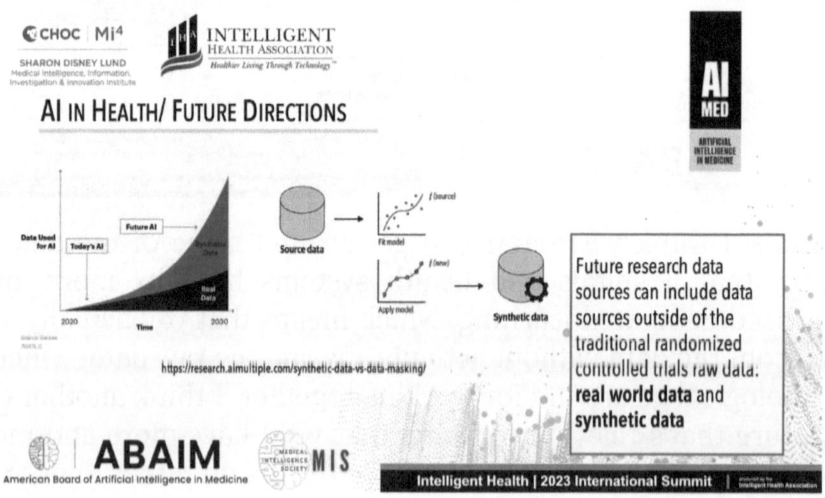
CHOC Mi4
SHARON DISNEY LUND
Medical Intelligence, Information, Investigation & Innovation Institute
INTELLIGENT HEALTH ASSOCIATION
Healthier Living Through Technology
AI IN HEALTH/ FUTURE DIRECTIONS
AI MED
ARTIFICIAL INTELLIGENCE IN MEDICINE
Data Used for AI
Today's AI
Future AI
Synthetic Data
Real Data
2020
2030
Time
Source data
Fit model
Apply model
Synthetic data
https://research.aimultiple.com/synthetic-data-vs-data-masking/
Future research data sources can include data sources outside of the traditional randomized controlled trials raw data: real world data and synthetic data
ABAIM
American Board of Artificial Intelligence in Medicine
MEDICAL INTELLIGENCE SOCIETY MIS
Intelligent Health | 2023 International Summit

So, if I were getting close to holiday time, if I were to have 3 wishes for humankind in terms of AI and healthcare, one would be the availability of a real-world, real-time learning system that's connected by all the capabilities of the AI. So, essentially a healthcare brain for the future where we can all learn together and in real-time. And this is the beginning of that long journey towards that. If you want to equate that to go into Mars, it's similar in terms of the ambitious goal and vision. This is and echocardiogram that's performed at my hospital that's simultaneously seen and interpreted by a hospital in Rome, Italy. So, the beginning of the journey is to connect all of us.

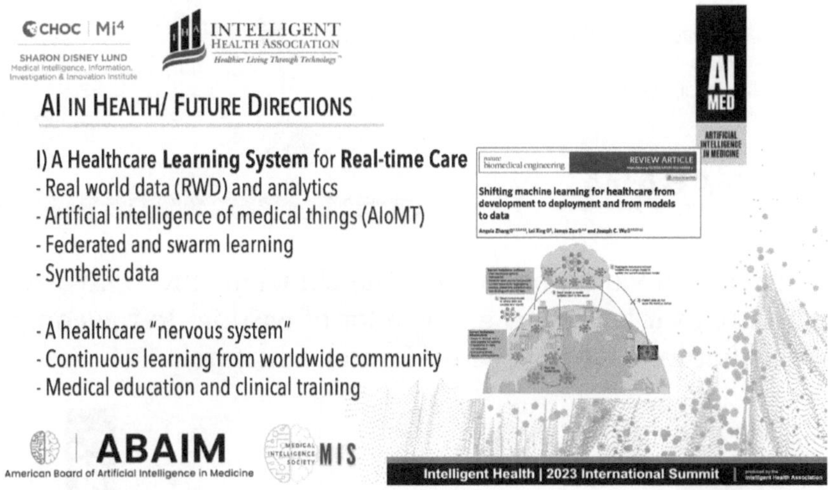
CHOC | Mi4
SHARON DISNEY LUND
Medical Intelligence, Information, Investigation & Innovation Institute
INTELLIGENT HEALTH ASSOCIATION
Healthier Living Through Technology
AI IN HEALTH/ FUTURE DIRECTIONS
AI MED
ARTIFICIAL INTELLIGENCE IN MEDICINE
I) A Healthcare Learning System for Real-time Care
- Real world data (RWD) and analytics
- Artificial intelligence of medical things (AIoMT)
- Federated and swarm learning
- Synthetic data
- A healthcare "nervous system"
- Continuous learning from worldwide community
- Medical education and clinical training
nature biomedical engineering
REVIEW ARTICLE
Shifting machine learning for healthcare from development to deployment and from models to data
ABAIM
American Board of Artificial Intelligence in Medicine
MEDICAL INTELLIGENCE SOCIETY MIS
Intelligent Health | 2023 International Summit

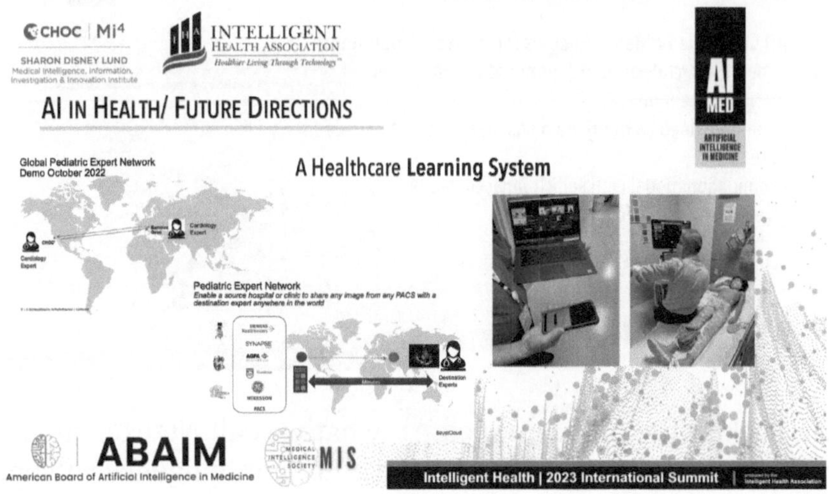


My second wish would be for all of us to have a digital health twin, virtually so that all of our medical records and images can be converging and combined into a virtual twin. So, we have a virtual copy of ourselves so that we can perhaps try different medications for the conditions that we have without a basically a trial and error that we do now. So, I think that's very exciting. Perhaps the concept of randomized controlled trials will be different in the future.

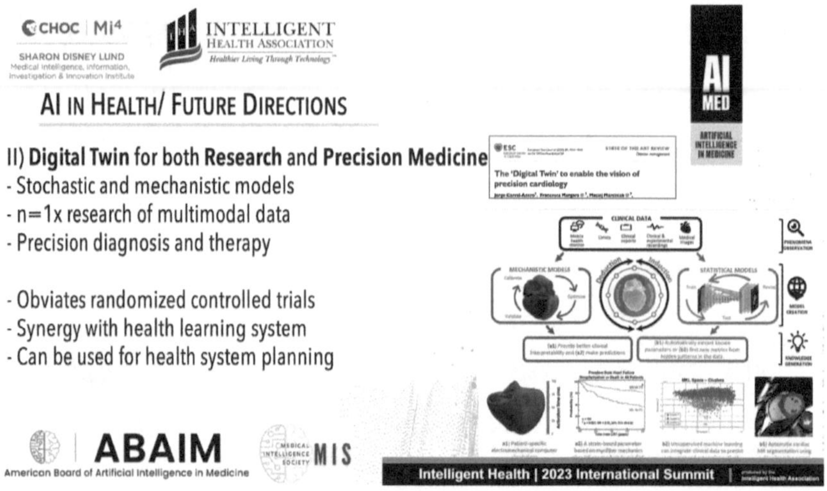
CHOC Mi4
SHARON DISNEY LUND
Medical Intelligence, Information, Investigation & Innovation Institute
INTELLIGENT
HEALTH ASSOCIATION
Healthier Living Through Technology
AI IN HEALTH/ FUTURE DIRECTIONS
II) Digital Twin for both Research and Precision Medicine
- Stochastic and mechanistic models
- n=1x research of multimodal data
- Precision diagnosis and therapy
- Obviates randomized controlled trials
- Synergy with health learning system
- Can be used for health system planning
The 'Digital Twin' to enable the vision of precision cardiology
CLINICAL DATA
MECHANISTIC MODELS
STATISTICAL MODELS
AI
MED
ARTIFICIAL INTELLIGENCE IN MEDICINE
ABAIM
American Board of Artificial Intelligence in Medicine
MEDICAL INTELLIGENCE SOCIETY
MIS
Intelligent Health | 2023 International Summit

And my third wish would be to have the clinicians more involved with AI and healthcare as it is now by giving a lot of wisdom to the computational intelligence that we have now with AI and healthcare.

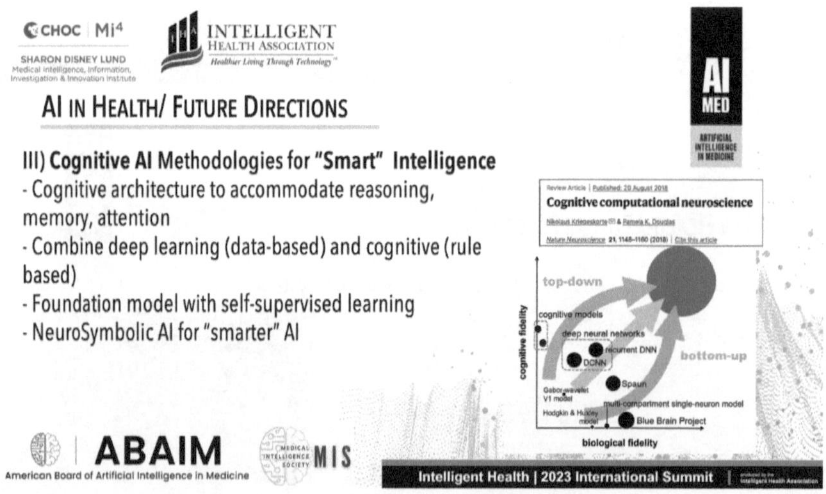


So going back to the old fashioned AI, what we call NeuroSymbolic AI. So, the AI will become smarter because the human intelligence will enable it to be smarter. So, in the future, I think clinical research and clinical care as well as everything we do, safety, education will all be wrapped into one bundle instead of being separated as silos that we have now, which I think creates a lot of lack of information and knowledge. So, in the future everything will be bundled together similar to the brain. We don't do many, many things separately. We do it all together.

So, in esscense, we're kind of in the period of being a teenager behind the wheel for the first time. It's a very powerful revolution in AI right now. So, it's just a matter of us learning to drive, learning to be able to handle this capacity of AI.

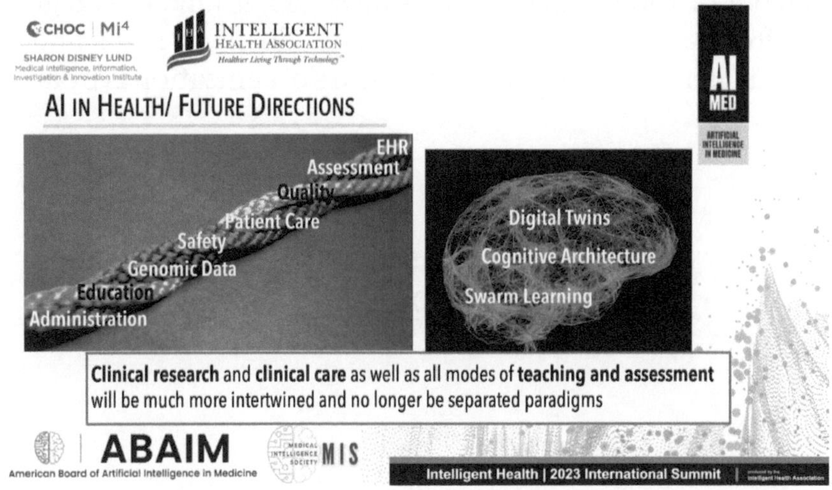


So, I was asked to comment on how I recommend that we assess the AI readiness of a healthcare organization. So, this is part of a research study that we've been doing looking at assessing healthcare organizations for AI readiness. So, I know there are a few AI maturity models, but I happen to respectfully disagree with that way of assessing AI and the healthcare organization. I think we need to start with just seeing where you are.

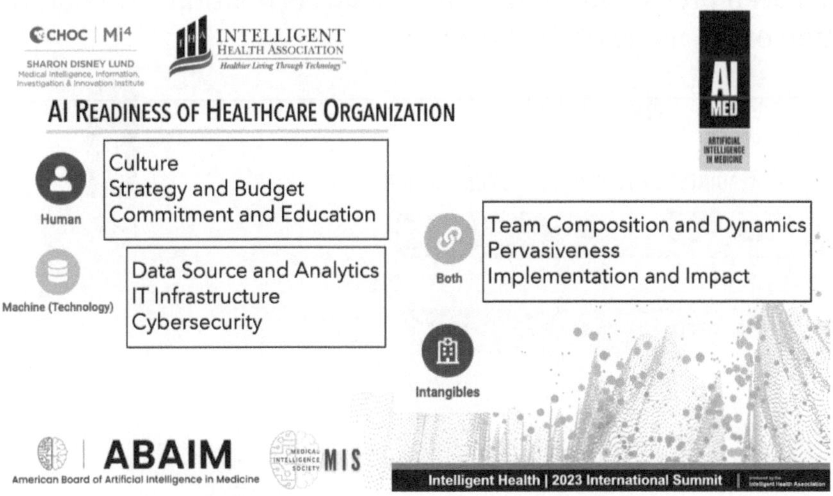


So, there are four different areas, human, so that's like culture and education, the machine or the technology, so that's where you assess your IT infrastructure and data sources. When you combine them, both is looking at things like team composition and implementation and impact and lastly the intangibles.

So, this is a typical healthier organization that we did a spider diagram of in terms of the human technology and the area that both. You can see that this hospital has enough human and technology but not but needs to develop the the sort of the intersection of these two areas. And this particular hospital scored a 55 out of 100 for their AI readiness. So, it kind of categorized the continuum from nascent and aware to ready, finally to focus and enabled. So, this is a snapshot of where your healthcare organization is by an 11 sector assessment tool.

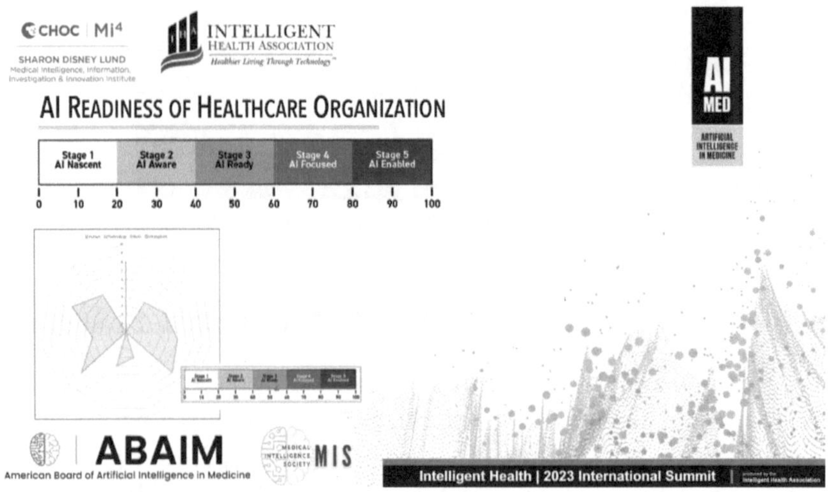


And when you look at the hospitals that we've looked at so far, we've looked at 12 now, and it takes a while to assess the hospital, and the range from 0 to 100 has been pretty wide and there was no correlation to the brand or the recognition of the name of the hospital.

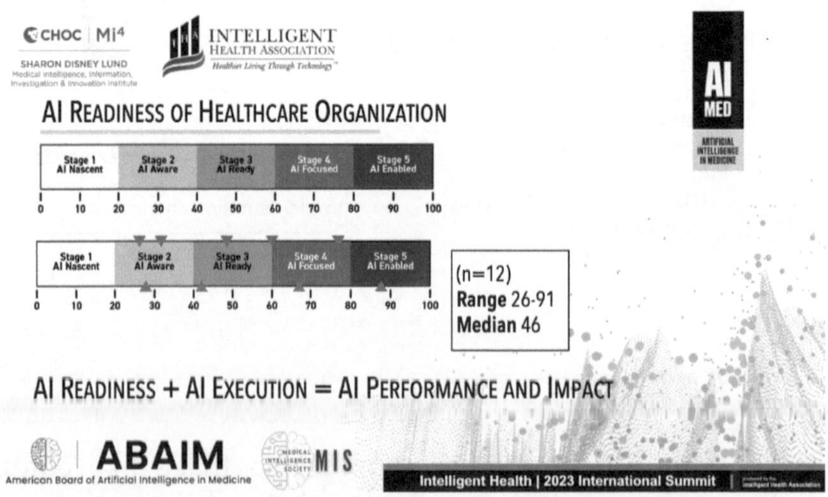


So, the range is 26 to 91 in terms of AI readiness and the median score is about 46. 46 would put you in the AI-ready category, which is I think improving from hospital to hospital. So, I think the take home message here is that AI readiness is the beginning of the journey, sort of what you have. It's sort of like your natural IQ. How you do in school is how you execute and study. So, I think that instead of AI maturity, which doesn't uncouple the two important elements, I think AI readiness has a beginning plus AI execution, which is essentially assessing your execution of the AI projects is going to give you AI performance and impact. I think the beginning of the journey again is AI readiness, and then AI execution gives you AI performance and impact.

So, I love this Charles Darwin quote. Very apropos for AI. “It's not the strongest and most intelligent, but the most adaptable to change species that will survive.”

Here are some books if you're interested in learning more. There's a journal now called Intelligence Based Medicine which has clinician friendly articles. And if you really want to have a crash course in AI that's healthcare focused, this is a monthly course that we offer that's backed by 50+ organizations and companies and you basically double your knowledge going through that one or two day course as proven by assessments. And also, the privileged convener of an Alliance of Centers of AI Medicine called ACAM that's been in existence since 2021. We have close to 100 now, including a pediatric subgroup. So, it's truly very exciting to have everyone together. We convene once a month virtually and once a year in person. And Harry and Sherry will be a part of AI Med Global Summit that's coming up next year in May of 29th - May 31st 2024.

And I want to thank my smart colleagues and mentors at Stanford for always being such a great resource for me to learn from. And my home team at Children's Hospital of Orange County who give me coverage and support for talks like this.

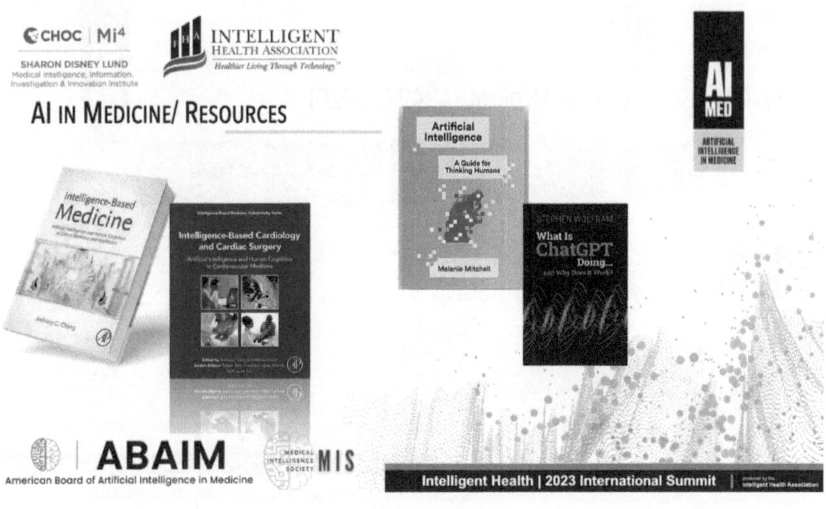

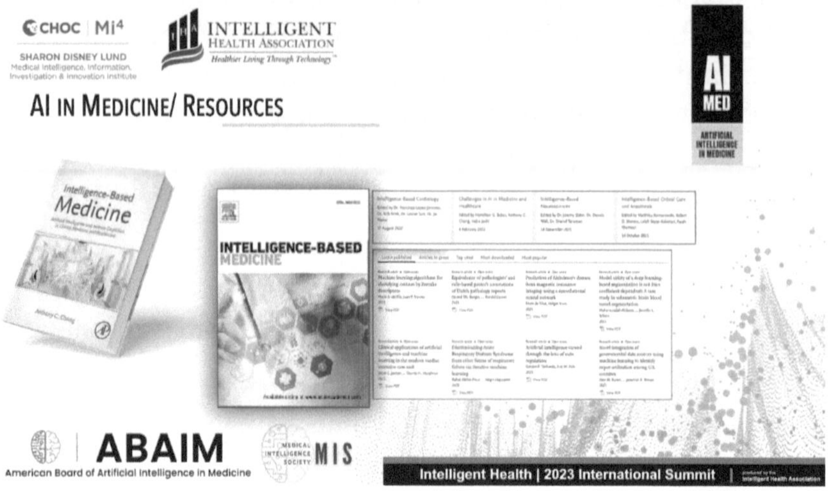
CHOC | Mi4
SHARON DISNEY LUND
Medical Intelligence, Information, Investigation & Innovation Institute
INTELLIGENT HEALTH ASSOCIATION
Healthier Living Through Technology
AI IN MEDICINE/ RESOURCES
AI MED
ARTIFICIAL INTELLIGENCE IN MEDICINE
Intelligence-Based Medicine
INTELLIGENCE-BASED MEDICINE
ABAIM
American Board of Artificial Intelligence in Medicine
MEDICAL INTELLIGENCE SOCIETY
MIS
Intelligent Health | 2023 International Summit

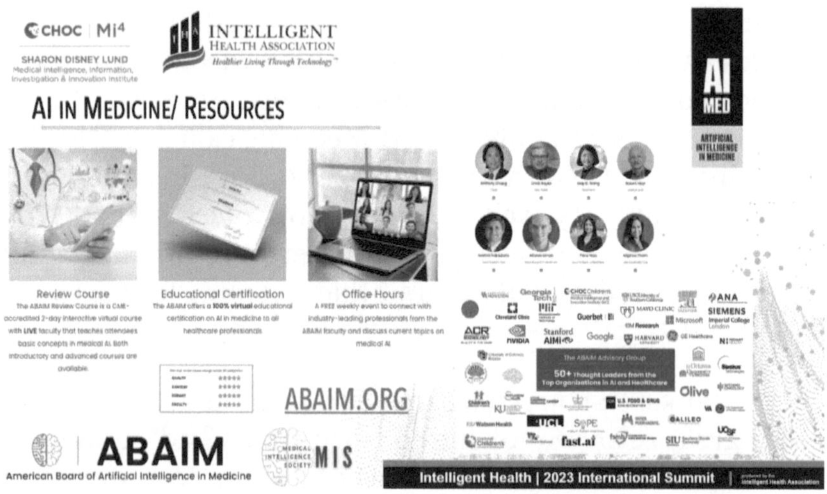
CHOC | Mi4
SHARON DISNEY LUND
Medical Intelligence, Information, Investigation & Innovation Institute
INTELLIGENT HEALTH ASSOCIATION
Healthier Living Through Technology
AI IN MEDICINE/ RESOURCES
AI MED
ARTIFICIAL INTELLIGENCE IN MEDICINE
Review Course
The ABAIM Review Course is a CME-accredited 2-day interactive virtual course with LIVE faculty that teaches attendees basic concepts in medical AI. Both introductory and advanced courses are available.
Educational Certification
The ABAIM offers a 100% virtual educational certification on AI in medicine to all healthcare professionals
Office Hours
A FREE weekly event to connect with industry-leading professionals from the ABAIM faculty and discuss current topics on medical AI
The ABAIM Advisory Group
50+ thought leaders from the Top Organizations in AI and Healthcare
ABAIM.ORG
ABAIM
American Board of Artificial Intelligence in Medicine
MEDICAL INTELLIGENCE SOCIETY
MIS
Intelligent Health | 2023 International Summit

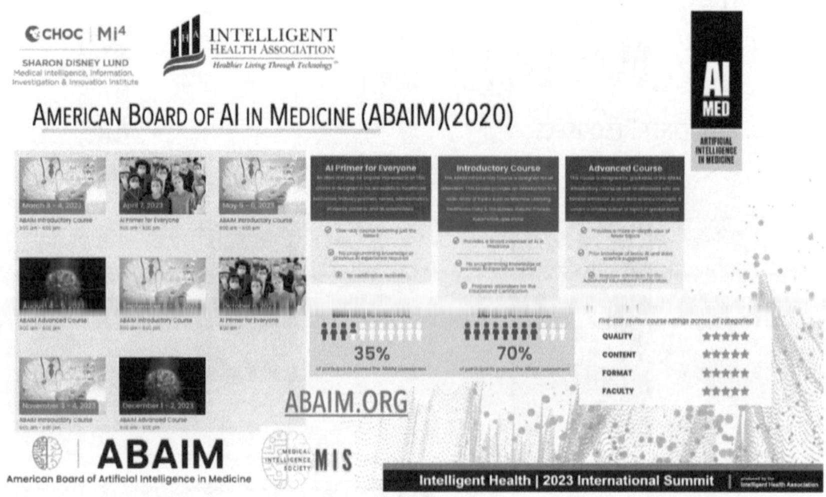
CHOC | Mi4
SHARON DISNEY LUND
Medical Intelligence, Information, Investigation & Innovation Institute
INTELLIGENT HEALTH ASSOCIATION
Healthier Living Through Technology
AMERICAN BOARD OF AI IN MEDICINE (ABAIM)(2020)
AI MED
ARTIFICIAL INTELLIGENCE IN MEDICINE
AI Primer for Everyone
Introductory Course
Advanced Course
35%
70%
QUALITY
CONTENT
FORMAT
FACULTY
ABAIM.ORG
ABAIM
American Board of Artificial Intelligence in Medicine
MEDICAL INTELLIGENCE SOCIETY
MIS
Intelligent Health | 2023 International Summit

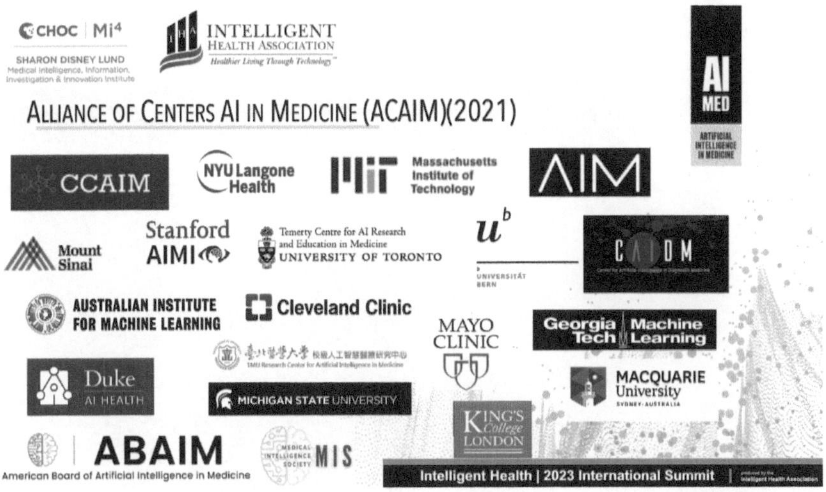
CHOC Mi4
SHARON DISNEY LUND
INTELLIGENT HEALTH ASSOCIATION
ALLIANCE OF CENTERS AI IN MEDICINE (ACAIM)(2021)
AI MED
CCAIM
NYU Langone Health
Massachusetts Institute of Technology
AIM
Mount Sinai
Stanford AIMI
Temerty Centre for AI Research and Education in Medicine
UNIVERSITY OF TORONTO
AUSTRALIAN INSTITUTE FOR MACHINE LEARNING
Cleveland Clinic
MAYO CLINIC
Georgia Tech Machine Learning
Duke AI HEALTH
MICHIGAN STATE UNIVERSITY
MACQUARIE University
KING'S College LONDON
ABAIM
American Board of Artificial Intelligence in Medicine
MIS
Intelligent Health | 2023 International Summit

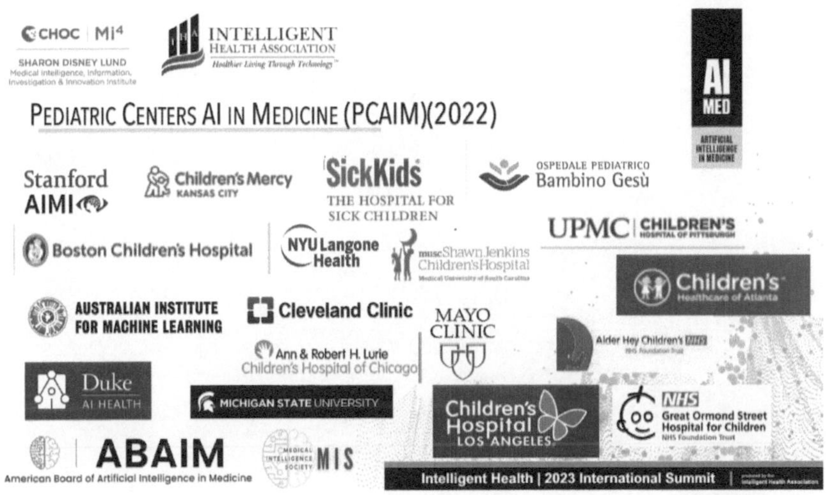
CHOC Mi4
SHARON DISNEY LUND
INTELLIGENT HEALTH ASSOCIATION
PEDIATRIC CENTERS AI IN MEDICINE (PCAIM)(2022)
AI MED
Stanford AIMI
Children's Mercy KANSAS CITY
SickKids THE HOSPITAL FOR SICK CHILDREN
OSPEDALE PEDIATRICO Bambino Gesù
UPMC CHILDREN'S
Boston Children's Hospital
NYU Langone Health
Shawn Jenkins Children's Hospital
Children's Healthcare of Atlanta
AUSTRALIAN INSTITUTE FOR MACHINE LEARNING
Cleveland Clinic
MAYO CLINIC
Ann & Robert H. Lurie Children's Hospital of Chicago
Alder Hey Children's NHS
Duke AI HEALTH
MICHIGAN STATE UNIVERSITY
Children's Hospital LOS ANGELES
NHS Great Ormond Street Hospital for Children
ABAIM
American Board of Artificial Intelligence in Medicine
MIS
Intelligent Health | 2023 International Summit

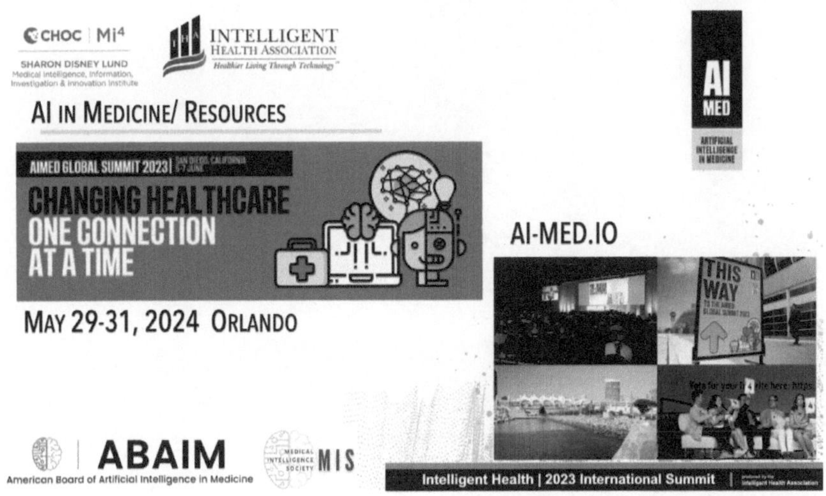
CHOC Mi4
SHARON DISNEY LUND
INTELLIGENT HEALTH ASSOCIATION
AI IN MEDICINE/ RESOURCES
AI MED
AIMED GLOBAL SUMMIT 2023
CHANGING HEALTHCARE ONE CONNECTION AT A TIME
AI-MED.IO
MAY 29-31, 2024 ORLANDO
ABAIM
American Board of Artificial Intelligence in Medicine
MIS
Intelligent Health | 2023 International Summit

# Chapter 15:

## ABC Roundtable

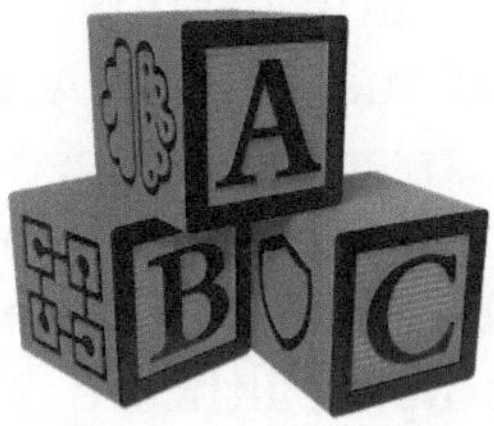


**David Metcalf, PhD**

**Dexter Hadley, MD, PhD**

**Max Hooper, PhD**

**Harry Pappas**

**Vikram Dhillon, MD**

### *Editor's Note*

The unique perspective of the authors and editors provides opportunity for multiple perspectives to be shared and appreciated in the chapters and the overall context of this first edition and early conversation. We hope you will engage with us in upcoming events to add your voice to the conversation and to continue the advancement of these game-changing technologies for health. Potential chapters that might be inserted between the others.

## Dr. David Metcalf

It's so good to look at a summary of the great work that has happened in the process of writing this book as a community and I'm so pleased that we can come together and really have this summation and think about some of the things that we've learned in the process of the connect points between ABC, AI, Blockchain, and Cybersecurity in the post-quantum era and what that looks like. The great voices that we've had, the case studies, the examples that we've had and what that's meant. It's been so great to work with all of you and to see the unique perspectives that each of you represent too in the medical field, the research field, in the associations and standards making, and in investing and pull all of those unique perspectives together to curate a fine collection of some of the best thinking and best early examples of where ABC is coming together. I was really struck by Colonel Wilson Ariza and his perspective on this from what the military and government needed and started to see the same thing with the perspective of what so many other places within pharmaceutical, within hospitals, within the Allied Healthcare Systems, insurance, all of the community that makes up healthcare, the research community and that really seeing it resonate with ABC across the board. It's been great to work with all of you on other book projects, too. I'd like to pull from that experience, too, and first call on Vikram Dhillon, Dr. Vikram Dhillon, to talk a little bit about his experience within the writing of this book and the connective tissue between our other books and the work of the other authors in this book. Vikram, over to you.

## Dr. Vikram Dhillon

Thank you so much, Dr. Metcalf. A couple of major learning points for me during the writing process and more importantly, as things have unfolded outside in the largely in the AI community. More recently, we saw in OpenAI, one of the one of the major leaders in the AI industry with ChatGPT. They had a bit of back and forth between leadership and there was a concern at that point about decentralization, the fabric of the blockchain, the foundation, technological foundation of blockchain and the promise of decentralization to create equitable members and more importantly, to create a landscape where power is not concentrated within single points of failure. Those really shined and coming out of that OpenAI even mentioned that they have been thinking about decentralization as a means to propel AI forward and more importantly, to propel AI research forward. In the next few years, particularly with layer two and layer three scaling solutions, I imagine that blockchain will make a comeback, not in the traditional sense that it had the past few years. But I suspect that blockchain will have a much deeper role in terms of the technology, in terms of the glue that ties together seemingly unrelated processes and makes the job of an immutable record much smoother, more efficient and more financially sort of viable. In addition to that, integrating AI into the blockchain has been a goal for many, many years. It seems that the AI world right now is going through this, what would be the equivalent to a Cambrian explosion where more applications, more papers are coming out week by week. And it seems in the next few years, we'll get to see a native blockchain and artificial intelligence set up where not only does the blockchain itself become suitable for artificial intelligence applications, but more importantly, all the derivatives. So smart contracts, being able to look at transactions, being able to trace the transactions, zero-knowledge proofs, just even smart wallets, all of these are going to have a layer of AI integrated in them to be able to carry out a lot of the simple tasks in the blockchain, to be able to diagnose simple issues with user to user interaction, and more importantly, to help developers build and deploy applications, next generation of applications onto the blockchains. I'm very excited to see where the blockchain goes, particularly in terms of decentralized management. That's a very, very true, like a bonafide way to showcase how incredibly advantageous the blockchain can be in providing solutions to a problem that not only exists now but will continue to compound as more and more larger AI companies build products that affect our lives.

## Dr. David Metcalf

Great perspective, we get the development perspective as well as the MD perspective on that too. And Dr. Hadley, Dexter, I'd love to hear from you on some of your thoughts as a medical professional and a researcher.

## Dr. Dexter Hadley

I think the most interesting thing, I thought that point was well taken. I think the idea of developers seems to be going away. You just talk to the computers today and they tell you, you know, they build your apps for you. The need for a really hardcore developer seems to be going away. What is most concerning to me, I think, is, you know, OpenAI just released custom GPT agents or, you know, you can fine tune OpenAI's GPT now on anything. So literally anybody and their mother can build a chatbot today. The problem is the data. I see the blockchain as necessary, at least in healthcare. It's what's going to happen with UnitedHealth, with a couple of the other healthcare companies. That's total nonsense until the data is diverse, is valid, it's not over 50, anyone's population. And that's a huge problem. You know, I don't think you can overcome it. I read an article yesterday, Zuckerberg and Threads, Threads.app is going to compete with Mastodon. Mastodon is a fully decentralized network on the blockchain. Threads wants to be, I guess, because people stop using Facebook. And it's more of the same, where you're going to get, Facebook is garbage for medical community driven AI, like my chapter sort of alludes to stuff. So, I think it's about the data, dummy, not really so much about as far as the blockchain and sort of the community aspect of this. I think the key for this to work in medicine equitably is really about building communities, from my perspective as a physician, I guess.

## Dr. David Metcalf

Great, it's good to have that perspective, too, and some current events there, too but yes, we want to make sure that we're looking at this from that perspective, too, and thinking about equitable, ethical and fair use.

## Dr. Dexter Hadley

Well, let me finish in a sense, right, because the data is now, well, let me add to what I said, just because it just popped into my head. If we're training AI to read mammograms, the mammograms better be not generated by a GAN Generated Adversarial Network). I think that's where the cyber can fit into this very well. You know, you can have bad players just become almost a national, what country, I think Sweden, or one of them, is about to implement AI mandated mammograms, right? So, AI as the standard of care, reading of the mammogram plus a physician. So, I feel like that is coming to health care, where there's money to be made. I read an interesting article yesterday about Threads and Zuckerberg and these guys want to take over the decentralization, like they did for social media. Anybody can build a Facebook, but there's only one Facebook. So, I feel like that's just an interesting perspective. It recently occurred to me that, you know, that it's less about the development and more about the data and the integrity of the data. And all this ABC should really or could really maintain the integrity of the data.

## Dr. David Metcalf

Yeah, good perspective, good perspective. Thank you. Harry, let's go to you. You've been such an organizer and convener of the community that's growing around all of these emerging technologies in health care. Give us a little bit of perspective on what you've been seeing and some of the thoughts that you have.

## Dr. Harry Pappas

Thank you, David. But I want to just want to make a couple of comments with Dr. Dexter Hadley's comments. Bad data. You know, this is going to be a recurring nightmare. And the industry should be concerned about false data, bad data going into the repository. And then skewing the net data the wrong way. Dexter, you know what I'm talking about. You know, if you've got a character out there somewhere in some country or some political group who wants to skew the curve one way or the other, they can do that by feeding the system bad data. Am I right or not on that?

## Dr. Dexter Hadley

And then it becomes a political weapon, right? It's going to be the same as Facebook and all the sensationalism.

## Dr. Harry Pappas

Yeah, I had this discussion with a few AI leaders just before the holidays. And, you know, we went over this checklist because one of the things that we're working on, David, and I'm glad you're going to be at CES. Dexter, I'm glad you're not going to be at CES. But, you know, we had this discussion with a number of AI thought leaders who are using AI in the OR. They're using AI in the EU and so forth. Well, we haven't seen the beginning or the end of any of this. And then when you combine it with cybersecurity and you combine it with blockchain, now you're really compounding the issues. But let me tell you why we're all at CES. Because in 2025, what I've suggested to a number of clinicians is that we take our traditional intelligent hospital model that we've been producing around the world but add a layer of AI. Add a layer of cybersecurity. So, if we build out an operating room with the standard technology, standard medical devices, medical equipment, consumables, RFID, RTLS, all those technologies, and then you layer AI on top of that. What's the impact? What's the impact on the patient? What's the impact on the surgeon, the clinician? And what about a medical device that's AI equipped, like an infusion pump? I was talking to an infusion pump manufacturer in Germany a couple of weeks ago, and I said, what was the impact going to be? Where's the data coming from? Where's the data going? Well, we're still trying to figure this out. And so, I'm a surgeon in the OR, and I'm looking at the data up on the data monitor on the dashboard. How do I know it's real? How do I know what AI, ChatGPT is telling me? I don't know. David, am I making myself clear?

## Dr. David Metcalf

You are, Harry. Those are some of the big questions that as we go through the process of writing this book, there's as many questions as there are answers, because we are so early in this process of seeing these trends connect.

## Dr. Harry Pappas

And this is why I agree with you that we should have a version two of the book, maybe six, seven, eight months. No, because...

## Dr. David Metcalf

Yeah, it's moving so fast. You're right. You're right. It looks like Vikram would like to add in a quick comment too, but let's call on him for a second. Vikram?

## Dr. Vikram Dhillon

Sorry, I know I had already passed my turn, but the discussion was very interesting. So, I wanted to add a quick comment here. Two things. One, I completely agree with the statements made. The quality of data, especially the quality of training data that we use moving forward is going to be incredibly important. And I think blockchain and more importantly, security has a big role in this because generating false data and having the equivalent of guardrails to stop that data from polluting your training datasets is going to become crucial. And not only using cryptographic hashes, but more advanced cryptographic and statistical techniques to limit the quality of bad data, to be able to remove it, to be able to detect it are crucial moving forward. And blockchain as well as security, particularly more advanced ciphers may play a very, very important role in this, in being able to tell us that the quality of data we're using is not only off standard, but also not harmful in the way that it can destroy the models that we're training.

## Dr. Harry Pappas

That's where it resonates. Go ahead.

## Dr. David Metcalf

Yeah, Harry, that's what I was going to say too. That some of the problems that we identify and that others identify with AI, the provenance and the verification and trust associated with blockchain technology and the ability to have a cyber infrastructure that can withstand even the most current generation and future generations of cyber compromises to privacy, as well as to the verification and validity of that data is really at the core of ABC across many different aspects of the healthcare industry and other industry segments too that we're going to be exploring in other volumes within the series. So, I'm really glad that you brought that up and that that's resonated with all three of you so far. I'd like to give Dr. Hooper a chance to talk, not only having the financial and investor background, but also the expertise of having gone through some of the first cohorts at MIT, London School of Economics in blockchain and some of the other advanced technologies, looking at how AI influencing that and give his perspective. And then we'll circle back around to everybody. Max, over to you.

## Dr. Max Hooper

Yes, David, thank you. And really, the way I see this is the convergence, ABC being the convergence, really, of the digitization of the capital markets. And there's so many different ways to perceive this. But, you know, like we were talking earlier that as we work through this process, we learn about more and more new things and new innovations. And, you know, one of the big surprises, I think, by a lot of people was that the tokenization platforms started really, really working in 2023. But it was what they were doing is putting together treasury bills. And U.S. treasury bills were like a major thing that happened, you know, as well as different types of bond financings. And so, we just start talking about the financing and the liquidity needs around the world. And then you start seeing what, you know, ABC can do. I mean, it's just, you know, blockchain smart contracts, you know, decentralized autonomous organizations, you know, all those things coming together helps make the transactions more complete, faster, reduce intermediaries and those type of things. So, then you get into AI being able to analyze all the financial data in real time, detect fraudulent activities. And then you have cybersecurity playing their part, which comes in to make it invalidated. So, it truly is a unique thing that is happening with ABC. And the capital markets finally have come together in a way and are poised for trillions of dollars of activity around the world when this is more mainstream.

## Dr. David Metcalf

I think that that's because when we look at financial transactions and health transactions and where they mix in reimbursement, in insurance, in some of the other areas, the two are inextricably linked to each other. And I think we're going to continue to see that the value and validity of those records, you mentioned smart contracts and the ability to track, verify and validate as being something really important to this whole process. I appreciate that you added that, Max. I think that's really a great point for us all to consider and is so prevalent as a theme throughout the whole of the book. And also, all of the lead up conferences, sessions, interviews, and writings that we saw that make up the collective thought of a whole community during this time. So, what I'd like to do is to get from each of you maybe one aha moment or something that came out during the time of the writing of the book that really resonated with you and that picks up on the theme that you each mentioned, too, for what we have and what we learned during this time as a community. I'll start with something that happened back at last year's HIMSS at the AIML conference. I heard a few people say this, so I won't attribute it to one particular person, but there was a couple of sessions where they said, don't worry, everyone, AI is not going to replace your doctor. But doctors who use AI will replace your doctor. And I'd love to get any comments from those with an MD on the roundtable today, but also to think through some of the implications of that for trusting that in a Human and System Integration, HSI, and what that might mean for how you have the best of human intelligence. The best of artificial intelligence and using those in unique ways with the validation and security and privacy that blockchain and post-quantum cybersecurity can provide for us. Those are some of the things that have been most telling to me during this timeframe. Let's go around the table again.

## Dr. Dexter Hadley

So, I'm a pathologist. We do something called cytology, or a failed pathologist, I don't practice, but the reason I don't practice is because to get one positive, you have to go through 2000 negatives. No human wants to actually do that. Same for Melanoma. Melanocytic reasons on the skin. It's a phenomenon in medicine that there's many more false positives than true positives. Breast cancer is one in 2000. False positive mammograms for everybody. So, what doctor wants to go write notes of every little incident that happened on the admission? Like my mom got admitted for four days to the hospital. So, I'm pushing back on this idea that doctors don't want AI in their profession. We do. I think we do. I think it takes the bull out of the profession and it lets us use our brain for what is supposedly the art of medicine. I try to allude to this in my chapter where I say basically AI is going to make the art of medicine more scientific. AI is going to make the art of medicine more scientific. It will allow our human brains to do what computers, at least currently, cannot do. Maybe it might change one day. But nobody wants to sit and write a shit ton of notes after working 12 hours. No surgeon wants to go resect margins and send when a computer can do it easier. So, I agree. Doctors with AI are going to replace doctors without AI.

## Dr. Harry Pappas

Yeah Dexter, let me respond to that. I think the key, there's a number of factors here. Number one, I go back to education and why we started the Intelligent Health Association. Somebody's got to be out there in a vendor neutral manner and educate today's physicians. But also, what are we doing about educating the next generation of physicians based on AI and generative AI and conversational AI? What are we doing about showing the physician, hey, you need to get trained to how to use all this. How do you incorporate it into your practice? I had a talk with my family physician just before the holidays. And he says, I don't want to even talk about AI. I said, you don't plan to use it? No, it's not perfected yet. It won't be perfected for another 10 years. So how do you overcome these issues using education, whether it's face to face or online? Somebody's got to provide this vendor neutral educational platform. And we're talking about doctors. And Dexter, what about this? What about physical therapists? What about nurses? Who's going to educate all these people to start to utilize and trust AI?

## Dr. Dexter Hadley

So, here's my pushback on it. So, the average surgeon reads textbooks cover to cover. I'm not lying. Don't you want your surgeon reading textbooks cover to cover? I mean, isn't it a better idea to fine tune AI on four or five Grey's Anatomy or whatever, textbooks, than ask the questions? I mean, it's a better way. That's how I'm teaching my medical students. We're having a whole class along those lines. Who can go read 100,000 clinical trials for oncology? No one person can. Only the pharma companies and so on and so forth. So, to make unmanageable mountains and corpora of information, text, numbers, images, pixels, waves, whatever you want, accessible by our little human brain, you have to have AI. I don't accept the argument. I accept people who have no idea, really, might think so. But Microsoft just made $100 million. I mean, probably just off of that ChatGPT thing. This is coming and it's here. I think at least to answer your question, Harry, I'm teaching my med students and I'm figuring that out. Can AI diagnose cases? OpenAI says it can. I'm going to test it come April or whenever this course starts, that I'm working on. So, I think a lot of it is just noise and politics from relatively ignorant people. So, I would like to change that and really see how doctors use this thing in my classroom. Because I could do that. I'm in a position to do that. So maybe I should add it to the chapter, David. I think that might be a nice conclusion. So, I'm going to add that in. That's the future of medical education.

## Dr. David Metcalf

That's a good point. And that's what having an independent non-profit association like the Intelligent Health Association and the standard, like what we heard through from Oida and John on the Linux foundations, open voice network and the Trustmark brand to be able to know that you can trust the information. These are all important things and important ways that I think all of us on this particular roundtable are going to continue to help educate on all of these areas. AI, blockchain, cybersecurity, the interconnection of those and many other emerging technologies, too, that we've only begun to start to integrate or think about. And I think that that's a really important point that you bring up, Harry. I do want to come back and make sure we have a chance to hear from Vikram and then also Max, too. Max, over to you.

## Dr. Max Hooper

Yeah. I mean, I think there's a lot of fear of change, and that's what's going on in an awful lot of this as far as people wanting to accept or not accept or when they accept or how they align with different groups to do this. But, I mean, to me, what Dexter said is right there. I mean, this is the educational tool that makes things more efficient and more effective. So not being a medical person, but just from a business and efficiency standpoint, it makes total sense to me.

## Dr. David Metcalf

Great point. Great point. So, with that, we kind of round the corner on thinking about some of the aha moments, and we've really come to how do we make sure that all of us are as smart as we can be in this area and that the whole of the team can benefit from this new technology from our unique perspectives. And then make sure that we are educating those that we serve, whether it's medical, whether it's the financial side, whether it's the association standard side, the developer community, the standards side, the research community. And Dr. Dillon, would you like to comment on that as well, too?

## Dr. Vikram Dhillon

So actually, I wanted to come back to something that was mentioned early in the discussion. One of the big learning points for me, or I suppose realization as I was writing the book, so many of the ideas from when blockchain was sort of at its peak of the hype cycle, so many of those ideas are still applicable. They're still very, very much applicable to this new world of artificial intelligence. So, data integrity, just base security of your training data, and more importantly, the implementation lessons that we learned. It seems to me that implementation in the AI world is happening in two phases. The first phase is just underlying architecture. So, do we have enough capacity to be able to run AI models on local devices, like the phones? And now there's some open source models that can even run on a simple iPhone. Once the baseline implementation is done, then the next level is deploying the more advanced applications. Blockchain went through the very much the same phase. Early on, it was a concern of do we have enough nodes? Is the network going to scale? And once that problem was solved, we were able to then do a lot of very interesting and sophisticated tech work on it. Similarly, I feel that an AI will have a next layer of applications that are built on the blockchain once both the AI and the blockchain-based infrastructures are available at MOS.

## Dr. David Metcalf

Great point.

## Dr. Harry Pappas

David, I know we're running out of time, but one of the things I've been looking at, because as you know, I talk to a lot of people in a given day, and I talk to people from Melbourne, Australia to Kuala Lumpur and everywhere in between. Nobody's educating the consumer. The consumer has to understand how AI can improve their health and well-being. And what questions should the consumer be asking his healthcare professional? I was at the dentist the other day, and we started talking about 3D printing in dentistry. He says, that stuff doesn't work. I said, well, what about AI in dentistry? He said, I'm not interested. And so, I'm a consumer. I'm asking healthcare professionals, you know, and the consumers have got to be educated, that when you go to your family physician, here are some of the questions to ask him when he gives you your lab reports. I went through this recently, and I said, how accurate are these lab reports? He said, what do you mean? He says, they're all computer automated, they're this, they're that. I said, yeah, okay, I get that. But how accurate are they? Well, you know, we're starting to use AI in comparing your lab reports with 10 million other people. But what does that do to the consumer? Okay, how does it alter the care cycle? You know, so there's a lot of questions that are coming up. And this is why one of the things, David, we want to talk about at CES is, you know, how will AI affect or blockchain and cybersecurity affect the consumer who cares about their health, their well-being? Forget about them being 90 years old. Health and wellness is for everybody. So how is all these technologies, cybersecurity, blockchain, AI, how's that all going to impact the average consumer? So that's a question that I'm asking a lot of people, whether it's Columbia University or Penn Medicine, as I did this morning. So, I just wanted to throw that out that we really, at the same time we're trying to educate the clinicians, somebody should be out there trying to educate the consumer so they're aware of the implications and the impact. Thanks, David.

## Dr. David Metcalf

Yeah, no, that's a great point. And when we look at not just AI, which has had a lot of executive orders and actions recently and guidance, but also quantum computing and how we keep all these records safe when there is an opportunity for there to be a skeleton key, in essence, that can be a one or a zero at any given time and break through the current levels of encryption that we have and the ciphers. How do we inform the rest of the people that make decisions about our systems in the government that maybe aren't as technical, how they can protect themselves, their work, and like you said, in this case, talking about health, the health consumer, the patient, if they're a patient already, and make sure that we are able to protect that, protect their privacy, and then verify that, so things like blockchain and smart contracts, and leverage the intelligence of this collective AI and human intelligence. I think that that's really a lot of the big question for the future, too. And I'd love to hear from each one of you about any vision that you have for the future of ABC and where these different technologies will either collide or be cooperative and synergistic, and what your thoughts are. Vikram, you want to go first?

## Dr. Vikram Dhillon

Yeah, I think one of the most exciting things that we're going to see, and it's only a matter of time before we actually see this, is being able to provide sort of guardrails. So, NVIDIA had recently a product launch where they created this open source guardrails project, which essentially monitors the outputs from a large language model, and be able to do that at scale to different product offerings, and then tie in microtransactions from a blockchain. So, you can offer this idea of guardrails and security, so to speak, for AI models, implement microtransactions, and do something on the blockchain that it actually does very well, which is transactions. So, I'm very excited to see this cybersecurity as a service type model, or rather cybersecurity as a microservice type model being offered to AI products using underlying blockchain. I think that intersection may be a very, very interesting idea that will take shape in some form in the next two, three years or so.

## Dr. Dexter Hadley

It's an advertising model for security, right? So, ChatGPT wants to sell ads on your custom fine-tuned model. Threads wants to sell, Facebook wants to be the ad server. So, it seems like this is already happening, and cybersecurity is another layer, right? So, to me, if Facebook takes control of Mastodon, which is what it seems like it wants to do, it's going to have Facebook cybersecurity built in. I feel like that's coming for health as well. Every other day, some hospital is getting hacked for some nonsense with crappy security. So, I think the writing is on the wall. We can use all kinds of analogies like that is coming to health. Yes, it's a little bit different, the privacy and whatnot.

## Dr. David Metcalf

Thank you so much, Dexter. I'm glad to have your comments on the future and thoughts on *ABC*. So, thank you. Harry, how about you? What do you think that the future holds in this area?

## Dr. Harry Pappas

David, I'm looking at my Greek crystal ball. You know, I thought the WWW upended the world. I thought the iPhone upended the world. But I think AI, blockchain and cybersecurity are going to beat everything. I see it as I talk to payers, providers, technology companies, building AI into wearables, building AI into diagnostic equipment. I think we're not even scratching the surface. My biggest fear, David, and this is why I'm working with the Linux Foundation and the Trustmark Initiative. And it's not OK just for the US to set up guardrails. I think this is an international problem. Because the players, good players, bad players are all over the world. And if bad data, if we allow bad data or bad guidelines to prop up, it'll destroy the system. And I often wonder, David, whether in Space Odyssey, the HAL computer was infected with bad data. OK, think about that.

## Dr. David Metcalf

Good point.

## Dr. Harry Pappas

So, I'm looking at this and I see the positives. But I'm also starting to think about the negatives, because we really got to understand the negatives. The positives, I think, are self-evident. I can see it. Like Dexter said, no doctor is going to sit there and read a thousand pages and look at these test results. You know, when I went to my doctor recently and he gave me my A1C, I said, well, what's that compared to? Oh, I don't know. I said, well, what's it based on? Is it based on a million samples or 10 million samples? He said, I don't know. I can't answer that. So, you're creating standards and you're creating these indexes based on what? OK, so I think we have a long way to go. I think it's exciting. The guardrails have got to be there, but across the board for everybody around the world. OK, and the consumer has got to understand why the guardrails are needed. So, I think the industry has got to self-regulate and self-guardrails, set up self-guardrails. Those are my thoughts, David.

## Dr. David Metcalf

I think you're right. It's been so refreshing to at least see that some of the organizations like IEEE, Linux Foundation, some of our friends who are promoting Trustmark are represented in the book. But also, just the good work that they're doing for advocacy, for education, for standards making. And that all those organizations we mentioned are international organizations. They are not just looking at this from one geography's perspective. They're trying to take into account things like TECFA and the GDPR regulations and some of the other regulations and some of the standards that we're seeing. And now we need to think about the standards that are coming out for blockchain, the standards that are coming out for AI and some of the executive orders, and some of those around next generation cybersecurity. This post-quantum timeframe that we're looking at and the examples of the executive orders that have come out too. Those are all examples of some of the need that we have and ways that we can inject that trust, re-inject that trust back into society and into the structures we have for society. Whether that's government, whether that's trusting your doctors, trusting your hospitals. Those are the things that we can help re-establish if we're careful. And if we're not, then I'm concerned like you are, Harry. Dr. Hooper, you have a thought on this?

## Dr. Max Hooper

Yes, it's a little bit different, I think, than totally the medical view of this. But I'm going to respond a little bit to Harry's comment about how the consumer is affected. I noticed that the supply chain management, when I was reading all this, really kind of jumped out at me that when you take the blockchain and make an immutable record, and then you can track movement of goods and ensure transparency and accountability, all of a sudden things start working a lot better. And we've all seen the big supply chain issues that have affected the consumer. But additionally, then AI comes in and helps optimize logistics, predicts the demand for the goods so the pricing can be stabilized, the effect of delivery is done correctly. And then, you know, when cybersecurity comes in and identity management and all the things to that, to me, all these are outcomes that do affect the consumer or can affect them in a good way once they're all implemented and coordinated. So that, to me, of course, I'm always thinking like the capital structure and how business is done and how the money flows around and where the things that block it and the supply chain has been a big, certainly a big issue in the last few years.

## Dr. David Metcalf

Great point. Great point. So, any final words or comments from anybody as we wrap up and think about not only what we've learned as this book, but really this book forming community around this idea and looking ahead at so much work still to be done. And this might only be, if the series of time were a book, this would only be chapter one. And we have multiple chapters yet to be written. And we're excited about the idea of next editions of this that will advance this idea and also take some of these ideas into other vertical industry segments like you've talked about, Max. The idea that the connective tissue between healthcare records and the connective tissue with transactions, financial, fintech records, and Harry, as you mentioned, education, government records, government standards, all of these things benefiting from this connection between AI, blockchain, and cyber in the next generation and post-quantum. So, I'm so thrilled that we've gotten a chance to work on this together as a team and that while this has come together fairly quickly, we've got a good, broad, and diverse representation of the ideas and how this technology can be helpful to society. And some of the guardrails that we need to look at that we need to be mindful of as we think about this powerful technology and making sure that it's used appropriately for the good of society, for freedom, for diversity. And for the ideals that we look at a tech-positive, forward-looking, innovative society that benefits all members of society. That's what I think the promise of this ABC, AI, blockchain, and cyber for healthcare can be.

## Dr. Harry Pappas

David, thank you for bringing this all together and thank you for making this book possible.

## Dr. David Metcalf

Thank all of you. And we'll continue on to the finish line and look forward to seeing many of you at HIMMS and other conferences around the globe as we continue to educate, advocate, and explore the next generation of technologies for healthcare.